Specialist Training in
ONCOLOGY

Dedication

This book is dedicated to our mothers (Thankamma and Margaret) who gave us life and the encouragement to write, and to our families for keeping us sane during the preparation of this book.

Commissioning Editor: *Louise Crowe*
Development Editor: *Fiona Conn*
Project Manager: *Beula Christopher*
Designer: *Kirsteen Wright*
Illustration Manager: *Gillian Richards*
Illustrator: *Jennifer Rose*

Specialist Training in
ONCOLOGY

TV Ajithkumar MD FRCP (Edin) FRCR

Consultant in Clinical Oncology
Norwich and Norfolk University Hospital
Norwich, UK

Helen M Hatcher PhD MRCP

Consultant in Medical and Teenage and Young Adult Oncology
Cambridge University Hospital
Cambridge, UK

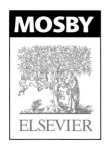

MOSBY

ELSEVIER

Edinburgh London New York Oxford Philadelphia St Louis Sydney Toronto 2011

MOSBY
ELSEVIER

© 2011 Elsevier Ltd. All rights reserved.

ISBN 978 0 7234 3458 0

British Library Cataloguing in Publication Data
A catalogue record for this book is available from the British Library

Library of Congress Cataloging in Publication Data
A catalog record for this book is available from the Library of Congress

Notices

Knowledge and best practice in this field are constantly changing. As new research and experience broaden our understanding, changes in research methods, professional practices, or medical treatment may become necessary.

Practitioners and researchers must always rely on their own experience and knowledge in evaluating and using any information, methods, compounds, or experiments described herein. In using such information or methods they should be mindful of their own safety and the safety of others, including parties for whom they have a professional responsibility.

With respect to any drug or pharmaceutical products identified, readers are advised to check the most current information provided (i) on procedures featured or (ii) by the manufacturer of each product to be administered, to verify the recommended dose or formula, the method and duration of administration, and contraindications. It is the responsibility of practitioners, relying on their own experience and knowledge of their patients, to make diagnoses, to determine dosages and the best treatment for each individual patient, and to take all appropriate safety precautions.

To the fullest extent of the law, neither the Publisher nor the authors, contributors, or editors, assume any liability for any injury and/or damage to persons or property as a matter of products liability, negligence or otherwise, or from any use or operation of any methods, products, instructions, or ideas contained in the material herein.

ELSEVIER your source for books, journals and multimedia in the health sciences

www.elsevierhealth.com

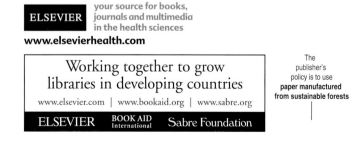

Working together to grow libraries in developing countries

www.elsevier.com | www.bookaid.org | www.sabre.org

ELSEVIER   BOOK AID International   Sabre Foundation

The publisher's policy is to use paper manufactured from sustainable forests

Printed in China

Contents

Contributors

TV Ajithkumar MD FRCP (Edin) FRCR
Consultant in Clinical Oncology
Norwich and Norfolk University Hospital
Norwich, UK

Mark Beresford MA, MRCP, FRCR, DM
Consultant Clinical Oncologist
Bristol Oncology Centre and
Honorary Senior Lecturer
University of Bristol
Bristol, UK

Ellen Copson BSc, MB BS, MRCP, PhD
Consultant Medical Oncologist
Southampton University Hospitals Trust and Salisbury
Foundation Trust
Southampton, UK

Emma de Winton BSc, MRCP, FRCP
Consultant Clinical Oncologist
Royal United Hospital
Bath, UK

Albert A Edwards BSc MBBS MRCP
Specialist Registrar in Clinical Oncology
St Bartholomew's Hospital
London, UK

Helen M Hatcher PhD MRCP
Consultant in Medical and Teenage and Young Adult
Oncology
Cambridge University Hospital
Cambridge, UK

Ruheena Mendes MRCP, FRCR
Consultant Clinical Oncologist
University College London Hospitals NHS Trust
London, UK

Christine Parkinson PhD, MRCP
Associate Clinical Lecturer
Department of Oncology
Cambridge University Hospitals NHS Foundation
Trust
Cambridge, UK

Christopher Williams FRCP, DM
Consultant Medical Oncologist
Bristol Haematology and Oncology Centre
Bristol, UK

Jessica Wrigley MB BChir (Cantb), MRCP
Academic Clinical Fellow
Department of Medical Oncology
Cambridge University Hospitals NHS Foundation
Trust
Cambridge, UK

Preface

It is a startling fact that one in three people will develop cancer in their lifetime and one in four people will die of cancer. It is therefore important to most people in the health sector to have a basic understanding of cancer and its treatments.

When we started our training in oncology and were faced with new patients every day, what we felt was needed was a book which summarized the most common cancers and their treatments. There are many books which discuss the scientific basis of cancer, but we wanted to know what to tell the patient about what treatments they may have and what their outcome might be. This is true for many health professionals, both those in training (including students) and those whose main speciality is not cancer management, but which brings them into contact with cancer patients regularly, e.g. general practitioners, specialist nurses and pharmacists.

We wanted to provide an overview of clinical presentation, required investigations and treatment options according to stage and fitness. We have tried to explain the practical elements of treating cancer patients from radiotherapy planning to chemotherapy prescription, the rationale behind them and what the patients are likely to ask about these treatments.

Oncology is one of the most rapidly changing areas of medicine with the developments of new therapies constantly evolving. With the modern computer-literate patient, we are repeatedly challenged to be up to date, which is difficult in such a dynamic specialty. In some instances, we have included website addresses, which are useful either for your patients or yourselves.

In essence, this is a handbook of practical guidance and knowledge for all those who come into contact with patients going through their cancer journey. It is the culmination of years of teaching and our own knowledge journey, which we hope provides the reader with rapid access to essential information.

TV Ajithkumar and
HM Hatcher

Acknowledgements

We are indebted to those who took time in their busy lives to provide their expert comments on the manuscript:

- Professor Ann Barrett
- Professor Ian Judson
- Dr Mike Shere
- Dr Sharon Straus

We owe thanks to several of our colleagues for the provision of figures and illustrations:

- Dr Matt Beasley, Dr Priyanka Mehta, Neil Ogborne, Henry Lawrence, Alison Stapleton and Helen Appleby at Bristol Oncology Centre.
- Dr Andrew Medford at Glenfield Hospital.
- Mr Rob Grimer at Royal Orthopaedic Hospital, Birmingham.
- Dr Evis Sala, Cambridge University Hospital, Cambridge.
- Varian Medical Systems.

We thank Sue Shadbolt for her excellent organizational and computer skills in assisting with the preparation of figures.

We are grateful to Timothy Horne, Janice Urquhart and Fiona Conn at Elsevier for commissioning this book and supporting us throughout its development and production.

Finally, we thank all those who helped us through our training and the knowledge from senior colleagues to students whose questions led us to search deeper.

Part I

Basic principles of cancer management

Clinical approach to cancer patients

TV Ajithkumar and HM Hatcher

Introduction

Cancer is a global healthcare problem. In the year 2000, cancer accounted for 12% of approximately 56 million deaths worldwide from all causes. It is estimated by 2050 more than 27 million cancer cases per year will be diagnosed and result in 17.5 million deaths. In the UK, 1 in 3 adults will develop some form of cancer during their lifetime and 1 in 4 die from cancer.

A suspicion of cancer or diagnosis of cancer is the beginning of a difficult journey. In many ways it is like climbing a mountain for the first time; a journey filled with uncertainty and challenges which carries no guarantees (Figure 1.1). Patients often carry additional anxieties if there have been perceived delays so that a knowledge of warning signs of cancer and an understanding of referral and treatment is essential for any healthcare professional.

Patients presenting to their primary care physician with warning signs of cancer (Box 1.1) should be referred to a specialist centre for an urgent evaluation. In the UK and many parts of the World, cancer treatment is organized around a multidisciplinary team which consists of physicians, surgeons, cancer specialists, radiologists, pathologists and clinical nurse specialists. Many investigations for suspected cancer are done either in 'one-stop' (e.g. for breast cancer) or 'two-stop' clinics (e.g. lung cancer) to expedite diagnosis and treatment.

Investigations for a suspected cancer

Initial investigations are to establish a histological diagnosis of cancer, to assess the extent of local disease, and to look for metastatic disease. Further investigations are done to evaluate suitability for standard or trial treatment and to assess the severity of any co-morbid medical conditions.

Diagnostic investigations

Diagnostic investigations are undertaken in a logical order, with blood tests including relevant tumour markers and simple imaging, and proceed to the diagnostic imaging of choice for particular tumour types. Imaging helps to determine local and distant metastatic staging. Confirmation of the diagnosis can be obtained by cytology or biopsy. Many tumours require biopsy for

> **Box 1.1: Warning signs of cancer**
> - Rapid weight loss
> - Haemoptysis/persistent cough/hoarseness of voice for >3 weeks
> - Rectal bleeding/melaena/altered bowel habit
> - Haematuria
> - Breast lump
> - Progressive dysphagia
> - Persistent headache
> - Persistent non-specific symptoms

© 2011, Elsevier Ltd
DOI: 10.1016/B978-0-7234-3458-0.00006-3

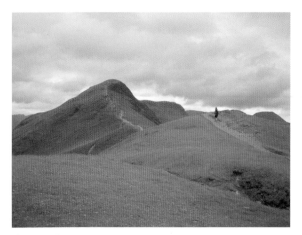

Figure 1.1
The diagnosis of cancer can be a lonely and challenging experience.

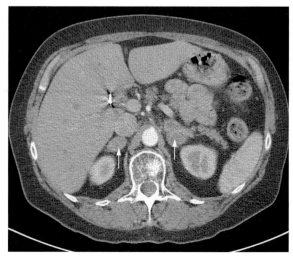

Figure 1.3
CT scan abdomen shows bilateral adrenal metastasis in small cell lung cancer.

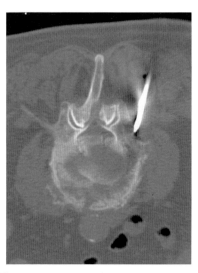

Figure 1.2
CT guided biopsy from vertebral body.

further characterization and immunohistochemical assessment. Biopsies can be obtained by core biopsies, and guided biopsies using imaging or endoscopic visualization (Figure 1.2). All patients need a definite histological diagnosis if specific cancer treatment is contemplated. Rarely, treatment can be undertaken when the radiological appearance and tumour markers are typical (e.g. choriocarcinoma, germ cell tumours).

Staging investigations

Once the histological diagnosis is established, further investigations are undertaken to stage the

cancer. The choice of investigation depends on the primary and pattern of metastasis. For example, the common sites of metastasis in lung cancer are regional lymph nodes, adrenals and liver; hence all patients with a lung cancer have CT scan of chest and abdomen (Figure 1.3). All patients who are planned to undergo curative treatment, particularly an extensive surgical resection, need additional investigations to assess their suitability for radical treatment. Functional imaging is more sensitive than anatomical imaging in detecting distant metastasis (e.g. PET scan staging alters conventional staging in up to 25% of patients). Endoscopic ultrasound and thoracoscopy and laparoscopy are also used in staging in appropriate situations (Chapters 9, 11).

Staging

The purpose of staging is to assess the extent of disease, choose the appropriate treatment and to assess likely outcome of the disease. Staging is also important in the comparison of results between treatment centres. The TNM system has been developed for many cancers. TNM staging denotes tumour, node and metastatic status. T staging is generally based on the size of the tumour (usually according to defined size criteria, e.g. in breast cancer) or depth of

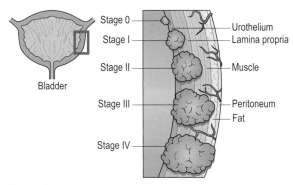

Figure 1.4
Staging of cancer.

Box 1.2: TNM staging descriptors

Prefix
- c – clinical staging: based on physical examination, imaging and endoscopy.
- p – pathological staging: after surgery and histopathological examination. Some tumours have different c and p staging (e.g. breast cancer) whereas others have only p staging (e.g. colon cancer).
- y – denotes staging after neoadjuvant therapy (p. 163).
- r – recurrent tumour: restaging following a disease free interval.
- a – autopsy staging.

Grading (G)
- Gx – cannot be assessed.
- G1 – well differentiated.
- G2 – moderately differentiated.
- G3 – poorly differentiated.
- G4 – undifferentiated.

L – lymphatic invasion
- Lx – cannot be assessed.
- L0 – no lymphatic invasion.
- L1 – lymphatic invasion.

V – venous invasion
- Vx – cannot be assessed.
- V1 – microscopic invasion.
- V2 – macroscopic invasion.

R – residual tumour after surgery
- R – no residual tumour.
- R1 – microscopic residual tumour.
- R2 – macroscopic residual tumour.

Multiple tumours
- Multiple tumours in one organ – the tumour with highest T category should be identified and the multiplicity of the number of tumours is indicated in parentheses, e.g. T1 (m) or T1 (3).
- In simultaneous bilateral cancers of paired organs, each tumour is classified independently.

invasion in hollow organs (e.g. oesophageal cancer, bladder cancer) or local spread to neighbouring organs or subsites (e.g. supraglottic cancer) (Figure 1.4). N staging is based on pattern of spread along the lymphatic chain, or number of nodes involved or size of nodes involved. It may be clinical or pathological. M1 denotes distant metastasis. Composite staging involves grouping various T, N and M combinations into 4 stages and each site has different stage grouping (e.g. see p. 80). Other descriptors of TNM staging are shown in Box 1.2. Other cancers are staged by slightly different systems such as FIGO for many gynaecological cancers (Chapters 13, p. 197).

Prognostic factors

Many factors influence the prognosis of cancer apart from staging. Two generally important prognostic factors are performance status (see below) and significant weight loss (≥10% weight loss in last 3 months). A poor performance status (WHO 3–4) and significant weight loss suggest poor prognosis.

Multidisciplinary management

In the UK, all patients with suspected cancer are managed within the multidisciplinary team. This journey starts from the referral with suspected cancer to the end of the treatment and into follow-up or death.

Consultation with patients and breaking the news

When patients attend oncology clinics many of them may have some idea about the details of their cancer and a rough outline of their further management. However, most patients are in shock and may take a long time to come to terms with a diagnosis of cancer. This gets particularly difficult for an inquisitive patient, who will search for more information on the internet and some

Box 1.3: Tips on consultation

Dos

- Introduce yourself to the patient and family – mention your role in the care.
- Get a precise and focused history to understand the current symptoms, performance status and weight loss.
- Get a clear idea of their support at home, which will be required to physically and mentally help them through treatment.
- Take a good family history as this may affect the chances of further malignancies or screening for other family members.
- Do a relevant clinical examination.
- Ask patient and family what they know so far (the usual answer is 'not much' – they are not trying to trick you, but haven't taken in everything they have been told – be patient and sympathetic).
- Reiterate the situation – discuss the details of investigations. Offer them an opportunity to look at their scan pictures, if they wish to.
- Discuss the treatment options and their relative advantages and disadvantages.
- Be clear and realistic about the aim of treatment (e.g. cure, improving chances of cure, prolonging life, improving symptoms).
- Many patients would like you to give them some suggestions regarding what do you think is the best option and why (though it is the era of informed consent, you may need to help them to make a decision regarding their treatment!).
- Formulate a simple plan of treatment and explain this to the patient.
- Always encourage patients and their relatives to ask questions and be candid in giving an answer.
- If you need any extra tests or investigations, explain how it is going to affect the treatment plan (make sure you chase the results of the tests you requested and let the patient know the result in time).
- Discuss details and logistics about treatment and get their consent.
- Give them contact details if they need further clarification and emergency numbers if things go wrong.
- Introduce them to your team, particularly clinical nurse specialists.
- Keep a positive, caring, sympathetic and professional attitude.

Don'ts

- Don't give life expectancy in fixed terms. Though many patients on palliative treatment ask about their life expectancy, it is better to refrain from giving some answers like 4–5 weeks or less than 6 months. It is always a good idea to ask patient whether they would like to get some figure or just a rough idea. It is better is put in terms like 'weeks to months' or 'months to years'. If you are forced to give a figure, give a broad range and explain that the figure is an average. For example, for some with lung cancer with disseminated liver metastasis the estimated life expectancy will be around 3–6 months, but explain that in the best case scenario it might be more than 6 months and in the worst case less than 3 months.
- Don't be too authoritative.
- Don't try to answer a question if you don't know the right answer.
- Don't give equivocal results or bad news over phone – you don't know what is going on the other end of the phone or what support the patient has. If you have good news, just let the patient know as soon as possible. Anxiety for the patient is often greatest when awaiting a scan result. Some centres have a policy of telephoning with good results, but beware that an intelligent patient will know when there is bad news if a result is not given (patients talk to each other as well as to professionals).

of the information overload can add to the anxiety. A clinician role is to help the patient to cope with the situation, and give them clear directions on further management and aim (Box 1.3).

Assessing fitness for treatment

Assessing fitness for treatment is an important part of decision making. It is mainly based on the performance status of patient, active co-

morbidities at the diagnosis, likely responsiveness of the particular tumour type and calculating the tolerance to any planned treatment.

Performance status (PS): Performance status helps to quantify the physical well-being of patients and helps to determine optimal treatment, make treatment modifications (including dose modification of chemotherapy) and to measure the intensity of supportive care required. It should be clearly documented at the beginning

Table 1.1: Karnofsky performance status (KPS) and WHO score

KPS		WHO (KPS)	
Score (%)	Description	Score	Description
100	Normal, no signs of disease	0 (90–100)	Asymptomatic, fully active and able to carry out all predisease activities without restriction
90	Capable of normal activity, a few symptoms or signs of disease	1 (70–90)	Symptomatic, restricted in physically strenuous activity but ambulatory and able to carry out light or sedentary work
80	Normal activity with some difficulty. Some symptoms or signs		
70	Self-caring, not capable of normal activity or work	2 (50–70)	Capable of all self-care but unable to carry out any work activities ; <50% in bed during day
60	Needs some help with care, can take care of most personal requirements		
50	Help required often, frequent medical care needed	3 (30–50)	Capable of only limited self-care; >50% in bed during the day
40	Disabled, requires special care and help		
30	Severely disabled, hospital admission needed but no risk of death	4 (10–30)	Completely disabled and cannot do any self-care. Totally confined to bed or chair
20	Very ill, needs urgent admission and required supportive care		
10	Moribund, rapidly progressive fatal disease		
0	Death	5	Death

and throughout treatment. There are a number of scoring systems and the two most commonly used are Karnofsky performance status (KPS) and WHO score (Table 1.1). Patients are generally eligible for curative treatment only if PS is 0–1, palliative anticancer treatment when PS is 0–2 and generally no anticancer treatment is given if PS 3–4. However, in certain situations, when the disease is very responsive to treatment and rapid deterioration is due to the current disease process, modified curative treatment is considered (e.g. germ cell tumours). If performance status deteriorates rapidly during anti-cancer treatment, treatment is either stopped or modified.

A proper assessment of active co-morbidities is important in predicting side effects to proposed cancer treatment. For example, patients with severe COPD with poor pulmonary function tests (FEV1 <1) are not considered for surgery or radical radiotherapy even if the tumour is very

small and potentially curable. Similarly, many chemotherapy drugs have systemic organ effects which need to be taken into account when planning anticancer treatment.

Implementing planned treatment

For many early stage cancers, delay in treatment is proven to compromise the chances of cure (e.g. germ cell tumours), and in tumours with rapid proliferation (e.g. Burkitt's lymphoma which has a doubling time of <24 hours) even a few day of delay in initiating treatment can be detrimental. Hence it is important to start curative treatment as soon as possible.

Follow-up during treatment

Follow-up during treatment is to assess response to treatment, monitor toxicity and modify further treatment. Toxicity should be monitored alongside treatment so that patients on a 3 weekly cycle of chemotherapy will be seen every 3 weeks prior to each treatment to modify the dose or adjust supportive treatments. For patients who have had significant toxicities on a previous cycle, they may be seen in between the cycle dates. Patients undergoing radiotherapy will often be seen at least once throughout their treatment to assess acute toxicities and prescribe supportive measures as necessary.

The optimal timing to assess tumour response to treatment varies depending upon the type of cancer treatment. For example, radiotherapy and hormonal agents generally take a 3–4 months to show any response to treatment, whereas chemotherapy response is faster (6–9 weeks). Hence, investigations to assess response to treatment should be planned according to the appropriate time scale. However if there is any clinical suspicion of progression while on treatment, prompt investigations are required prior to planned investigations.

Support during treatment

From the moment of diagnosis of cancer, a person's life is changed forever. It affects not only their physical health, but their mental health is also challenged. Different individuals deal with this process in different ways but each should be offered appropriate support for their needs. This may involve psychological support or something more practical such as directing them to possible sources of financial support. Many people are working at the time of diagnosis and their future employment may be affected depending on their job and employer. Laws exist to protect individuals, but those who are self-employed will only be protected if they had pre-existing insurance. Relationships are frequently challenged by the diagnosis of cancer and the journey through its treatment, and it is not uncommon for couples to split up at this time. Financial worries may continue after treatment has completed as it affects the ability to gain new life insurance or a mortgage. Those living in countries which require health insurance will notice an increase in premiums or difficulty obtaining further health insurance. Local health providers such as general practitioners will have a key role in coordinating some of this care and providing additional necessary services such as physiotherapy and occupational therapy.

At the time of diagnosis, an individual should therefore be provided with sources of information to help them through all these areas to facilitate their treatment and return to health. The key areas are:

- Psychosocial support.
- Income support.
- Macmillan team.
- Cancer care in the community.

The potential sources of this support can be in the form of documents from helpful websites or organizations, local cancer support groups, and named key workers such as specialist nurses or Macmillan nurses. It should be emphasized at the start of diagnosis and treatment that it is natural to require the help of others at some point in the journey and that it will only help their overall outcome. The special needs of children diagnosed with cancer and their family is discussed on p. 320.

Cancer screening

Several cancers now have proven screening programmes which have been seen to improve either the incidence or outcome of invasive cancers, e.g. breast and cervix. For other cancers screening programmes are in development to try to minimize the mortality from this disease.

Genetic screening

Patients with a suspected genetic component to their cancer need referral to a clinical genetics department. Chapter 5 (p. 45) deals with the recommendations for referral to clinical genetics and further management for the patient and their family.

Follow-up after treatment and management of recurrence

Almost all patients who have been treated with curative intent need some regular follow-up to detect an early potentially curable recurrence and a second cancer. The frequency and mode of

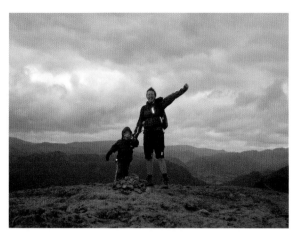

Figure 1.5
Successful treatment of cancer is often a cause for celebration, but people will also need help getting down from the mountain at the other side.

follow-up depend on the pattern of recurrence of individual cancers, which are dealt with individually. It is still debatable whether early detection of a metastatic recurrence improves overall survival in most cancers.

Beyond cure and survivorship

For many patients treatment will be possible and they will succeed in climbing the mountain of diagnosis, treatment and its complications (Figure 1.5). However the long-term impact of this on their lives must not be underestimated and many patients feel at their most lost at the end of treatment or when follow-up is discontinued (see also p. 58, late effects). An understanding of this process will help facilitate any further care that is necessary to return them to a functional life.

Further reading

Referral guide for suspected cancer, NICE. Available from
http://guidance.nice.org.uk/CG27/Guidance/pdf/English

Principles of surgical oncology

2

TV Ajithkumar

Introduction

Surgery remains the major mode of cure for many cancers. The majority of solid tumours are treated initially with a curative resection if possible. The proportion of patients who can undergo a curative resection depends on the stage at presentation and tumour site. Curative surgery may result in disruption of cosmesis and function. Hence surgery also has an important role in reconstructive surgery to maintain body image and ability to return to normal functioning life.

The potential role of surgery in the management of cancer includes:

- Diagnosis and staging.
- Curative.
- Palliative.
- Reconstructive (oncoplastic) surgery.
- Risk reduction surgery.
- Minimal access and robotic.

Diagnosis and staging

Diagnosis

Histological diagnosis is obtained from tumour tissue by fine needle aspiration cytology, core biopsy, incisional biopsy and excisional biopsy. Choosing the right technique is based on the location of tumour, anticipated type of the tumour and reliability of the method to make a definite diagnosis.

Fine needle aspiration (FNA) yields quick result and shows cellular characteristics but not architecture. FNA serves as good screening tool prior to more definitive diagnostic methods. FNA is useful for diagnosis of enlarged lymph nodes, aspiration of cysts, diagnosis of thyroid nodule and confirmation of recurrent or metastatic disease.

Core biopsy helps to visualize architecture as well as to perform immunohistochemical studies. It is useful in the diagnosis of solid masses such as breast lumps or liver metastases. However, core biopsy should not be used in lymphoma (which requires extensive immunohistochemical stains) or for soft tissue or bone sarcoma.

Incisional biopsy is used when core biopsy is non-diagnostic and excision biopsy is not appropriate. The common indication is a suspected sarcoma needing neoadjuvant treatment or definite resection. Care should be taken when planning incision biopsy to ensure that the site of biopsy is within the area definite surgery and should only be undertaken by surgeons who will undertake the final surgery. A poorly planned incision biopsy can lead to unnecessary morbid surgery.

Excision biopsy involves removal of the entire mass or skin lesion. It is important to make sure that this procedure does not compromise a later wider excision if necessary. The specimen needs to be oriented in three dimensions for the pathologist to determine surgical margins.

Frozen section is occasionally used preoperatively to confirm diagnosis when previous histologic diagnosis is not available (e.g. solitary lung lesions), to decide need for further surgery (e.g. lymph node dissection) and ensure adequate surgical margins.

Staging

Various surgical procedures such as endoscopy and staging laparotomy aid in defining the extent

© 2011, Elsevier Ltd
DOI: 10.1016/B978-0-7234-3458-0.00007-5

of disease as well as obtaining histological confirmation of metastatic disease. These are covered in detail for specific malignancies. One example is the use of laparoscopy as an adjunct to detect small peritoneal and liver metastases reduces the number of 'open and close' laparotomies by less than 5% in stomach cancer.

Curative surgery

Surgery plays a significant role in curative treatment of cancer. For many cancers surgery is the primary modality of treatment. A decision regarding curative surgery is made after careful consideration of various patient and tumour related characteristics at a multidisciplinary meeting with surgeons, oncologists, radiologists and pathologists. At this meeting staging and diagnosis will be reviewed along with information concerning the patient. Patient-related factors which influence the choice of curative surgery include age, performance status and co-morbidities. Tumour-related factors include chances of long-term benefit and potential surgical risks and complications.

Surgery of the primary tumour

Curative surgery is aimed at removal of the malignant tumour with a clear margin of normal tissue ('R0' resection) with reconstruction of the surgical defect if appropriate. Based on the extent of removal of cancer, resections are classified as follows which is part of the TNM staging:

- R0 – all margins are histologically free of tumour.
- R1 – microscopic residual disease after resection.
- R2 – gross residual disease after resection.

The tumour should be orientated and marked at the time of surgery such that any positive margins can be identified anatomically should the need for re-excision arise.

Depending on the type of cancer and anatomical site, curative surgery can be:

- Wide local excision (e.g. breast cancer).
- Removal of part of the organ and surrounding tissue at risk of spread (e.g. partial gastrectomy).
- Removal of an entire organ with or without important adjacent structures (e.g. total abdominal hysterectomy with bilateral salpingo-oophorectomy).

At the time of surgery exposure and shedding viable tumour cells should be avoided if possible. Certain tumours have a propensity to recur along surgical incision lines or drainage sites e.g. mesothelioma and sarcoma. A curative resection is aimed at a gross visible margin as imaging modalities will not identify microscopic disease. This gross margin depends on the type of malignancy and pattern of local spread. An adequate gross margin helps to ensure adequate microscopic margin of resection. Table 2.1 shows examples of the gross resection margin and microscopic resection margin for some common tumours.

Multimodality treatment has affected the surgical approach to many cancers. The use of radiotherapy, chemotherapy or both has led to the use of less radical procedures with an improvement of quality of life.

Surgery of regional lymph nodes

Some tumours spread to regional lymph nodes in a predictive fashion. In these cancers, local lymph nodes in continuity with lymphatics are removed along with the primary tumour. This provides important staging information as well as a therapeutic advantage to minimize the risk of a regional recurrence, preventing more extensive surgery in the future. Various methods are used to screen pathological involvement of lymph nodes before extensive lymph nodes dissection is undertaken. These include:

- FNA of enlarged regional lymph nodes.
- Node sampling – involves cherry picking of 4–5 regional lymph nodes (e.g. breast cancer).
- Sentinel node biopsy – is based on the principle that tumour spread to a single node (sentinel) prior to spreading to other nodes in an 'ordered' fashion and lymph nodes can be identified by using blue dye or radioisotopes (Figure 2.1).
- Lymph node dissection

However, in many situations the role of lymph node dissection in overall survival remains controversial. In practice, patients with involved

Table 2.1: Gross resection margin and minimal microscopic resection margin for curative resection

Tumour type	Local spread pattern	Gross margin	Microscopic margin
Breast cancer	Circumferential	1 cm	1–5 mm
Lung cancer	Within the same lobe	Lobectomy	
Oesophageal cancer	Longitudinal submucosal	5 cm	1 mm
Stomach cancer	Submucosal and towards serosa	1 cm	1 mm
Colon cancer	Submucosal and towards serosa	3 cm	1 mm
Rectal cancer	Towards serosa	3 cm	1 mm
Squamous cell carcinoma skin	Peripheral	1 cm	1 mm
Malignant melanoma	Deep	1–2 cm	1 mm
Head and neck cancer	Within the anatomic compartment	Anatomic compartment	1 mm

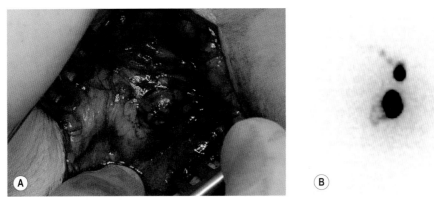

Figure 2.1
Sentinel node biopsy. Sentinel node is identified by either use of blue dye (A) or radioisotope (Tc-99m albumin nanocolloid). Picture B shows an intense uptake above the injection site with smaller less distinct nodes.

lymph nodes undergo node dissection whereas the role of elective lymph node dissection is dependent on the site of cancer, type of cancer and other prognostic factors. Benefits of nodal dissections in different cancers are discussed in the corresponding chapters.

Metastatectomy as part of curative surgery

Resection of isolated metastatic lesions is useful for a selected group of patients in certain cancers (Box 2.1). In general this is undertaken for patients with surgically resectable metastatic disease at presentation or in a very select group of patients with good performance status with a long disease-free survival after treatment of the primary tumour. In the absence of proper randomized studies it is not known whether the observed therapeutic benefit is actual or due to the strict selection process (selection bias). The common situations are resection of isolated or limited liver metastases in colorectal cancer which results in 20–40% 5-year survival (p. 164). Pulmonary metastatectomy in sarcomas leads to a 5-year survival of 20–25% (p. 259). An alternative is the evolving use of radiofrequency ablation.

- Liver – selected patients with colorectal cancer.
- Lung – selected patients with colorectal, kidney and testicular cancers and sarcoma.
- Adrenal – selected patients with resectable lung cancer and isolated adrenal disease.
- Brain – solitary metastasis with controlled/ potentially curable systemic disease.

Box 2.2: Potential indications for risk reducing surgery

Surgery	Indication
Bilateral mastectomy	BRCA1/2 mutations
	Familial breast cancer
	Unilateral breast cancer in <40 years
Bilateral oophorectomy	BRCA1/2 mutations
	Familial ovarian cancer
Total proctocolectomy	Familial adenomatous polyposis or APC mutations
	Hereditary non-polyposis colon cancer – germline mutations
Thyroidectomy	RET oncogene mutation MEN 2

Salvage surgery

Surgery is useful as a salvage measure after primary treatment failure or recurrence after definitive treatment. It is only appropriate for fit patients with a good chance of prolonged survival. Examples include abdomino-perineal resection after chemoradiotherapy for anal cancer, and exenteration in cervical cancer after chemoradiotherapy. In patients with prior limited surgery or chemoradiotherapy, a second chance of cure is aimed with surgery. Examples include mastectomy for local recurrence after conservative surgery for breast cancer and neck node dissection for isolated nodal recurrence after chemoradiotherapy for head and neck cancer.

Palliative surgery

The aim of palliative surgery is to improve or prevent significant symptoms (e.g. pain, bleeding and obstruction) which are likely to occur without intervention. It can also enhance the effect of chemotherapy (e.g. in ovarian cancer where it improves survival). Debulking surgery of the primary tumour can produce good symptom control and improve quality of life by preventing complications due to uncontrolled disease (e.g. loco-regional surgery in breast cancer prevents fungation and symptomatic axillary disease).

Reconstructive (oncoplastic) surgery

Extensive resection often results in disruption of normal anatomy and subsequent cosmesis and function. Plastic surgical techniques are useful in correcting the anatomical defects and improving cosmesis (e.g. reconstructive breast surgery) and function (e.g. in head and neck surgery).

Risk reduction surgery

Less than 5% patients have a genetic component to their cancer (p. 45). Increasing understanding of the development of genetically associated cancers has led to prophylactic surgery for some patients. Box 2.2 shows the indications for common prophylactic surgeries. Appropriate genetic testing and counselling is, however, an absolute pre-requisite prior to any prophylactic surgery. Women with BRCA1 and BRCA2 mutations have a high risk of breast cancer which is reduced by 90–95% with bilateral mastectomy. However, the decision to undergo prophylactic mastectomy should be done after careful discussion on explaining the future quality of life, potential surgical risks and wishes of the patient. Alternative risk reduction methods such as use of tamoxifen and prophylactic oophorectomy after completion of family should also be considered. Another example is FAP and prophylactic colectomy (p. 50).

Minimal access and robotic surgery

The role of minimal access surgery is being increasingly studied in the management of solid tumours. It is being more often used in abdominal malignancies and studies show that laparoscopic surgery results in the same long term survival as that of open surgery, with no increased risk of abdominal wall recurrence, less surgical morbidity and quick return to normal function. Laparoscopic surgery is an accepted modality of surgical treatment in gastric, kidney, adrenal and colorectal cancers. Video-assisted thoracic surgery for stage I lung cancer is a particularly attractive option for elderly patients.

Robotic assisted surgery is being studied in prostate and renal cell cancers. This technique may result in minimal surgical trauma with better toxicity profile.

Further reading

Sabel M, Sandak V and Sussman J. Essentials of surgical Oncology. 2006, Elsevier.

Principles of radiotherapy

3

TV Ajithkumar

Introduction

After surgery, radiotherapy is the most effective curative treatment for cancer, contributing up to 25–30% of cure. At least half of the patients with cancer require radiotherapy at some time in their illness of which about 60% are treated with curative intent, often in combination with surgery and chemotherapy. Radiotherapy involves use of various types of ionizing radiation, and X-ray is the commonest type of radiation used. Other forms of radiation include electrons, protons, neutrons and gamma radiations from radioactive isotopes. This chapter intends to review the principles of practical radiotherapy (Box 3.1) and a detailed discussion on radiobiology and mathematical modelling are beyond the scope of this chapter.

Indications for radiotherapy

Radiotherapy is indicated if it cures or improves the chances of cure, improves local tumour control, achieves symptom control or improves the quality of life. There are already adequate data on these various indications for radiotherapy for different neoplasms. With current understanding of radiation biology and improved techniques, more indications are evolving, particularly for tumours previously thought to be radioresistant (e.g. liver and pancreatic cancer).

Intent of radiotherapy

Radiotherapy treatment is given with either curative or palliative intent. Curative treatment involves either radical radiotherapy (radiotherapy given either alone or in combination with chemotherapy or biological agents) or adjuvant radiotherapy (given after definitive treatment of tumour, usually surgery). Palliative radiotherapy is intended to improve symptoms (e.g. bone pain) or prevent tumour related complications (e.g. ulceration in breast cancer).

Methods of delivery of radiotherapy

Radiotherapy is either delivered by a radiation source placed away from the body (teletherapy or external beam radiotherapy), by placing a radiation source into the tumour (interstitial brachytherapy, e.g. small tongue cancer) or in a body cavity containing the tumour (intracavitary brachytherapy, e.g. cervical cancer) or by intravenous or oral administration of nonsealed radionuclides. Depending on the site and type of cancer, radiotherapy is delivered by either one of these techniques or a combination. Sometimes radiotherapy is delivered concurrently with chemotherapy or biological agents to improve the chances of cure (see below).

External beam radiotherapy (EBRT)

EBRT commonly utilizes X-rays and electrons. Before the 1950s, radiotherapy units were kilovoltage machines which produced X-rays with limited penetrability. These machines, which are still used in some centres, can be one of the following:

- Superficial X-rays – operate at a potential of 50–150 kVp and tube current of 5–10 mA and useful to treat superficial skin cancers.

© 2011, Elsevier Ltd
DOI: 10.1016/B978-0-7234-3458-0.00008-7

1. Indication for radiotherapy
2. Intent of radiotherapy
3. Which is the best way to deliver radiotherapy?
   - External beam radiotherapy alone (e.g. head and neck cancer)
   - Brachytherapy alone (e.g. early stage cervical cancer)
   - External beam radiotherapy and brachytherapy (e.g. advanced stage cervical cancer)
   - External beam radiotherapy with concurrent chemotherapy (e.g. squamous oesophageal cancer)
   - External beam radiotherapy with target agents (e.g. advanced head and neck cancer)
   - Radioisotopes (e.g. well-differentiated thyroid cancer)
4. Obtaining informed consent
   - Benefit of radiotherapy
   - Explaining the process
   - Expected side effects – short-term and long-term
5. Radiotherapy planning and delivery
   - Position of patient and immobilization
   - Localization of tumour (CT or MRI)
   - Target volume definition
     - Tumour volumes (GTV, CTV, PTV)
     - Normal organs
   - Planning technique
     - Conventional (2D)
     - Conformal planning (3D)
     - Intensity-modulated radiotherapy (IMRT)
     - Image guided radiotherapy (IGRT)
   - Treatment planning
     - Beam arrangement
     - Beam size and shape
     - Energy of beam
     - Wedges, shields, bolus
   - Evaluation of treatment plans – homogenous dose to PTV and dose to critical organs
   - Prescription of radiotherapy treatment
   - Treatment verification and corrections
6. Supportive care during radiotherapy
7. Treatment modifications during treatment (e.g. bank holidays, toxicities and interruptions)
8. Care after radiotherapy and survivorship issues

- Deep (ortho – 'orthodox') X-rays – operate at a potential of 150–500 kVp and tube current of 10–20 mA. These are useful to treat thick skin cancers and rib lesions. In many centres, these machines are being replaced by electron beam treatment.

Electrons from gun are accelerated before they hit the target. The X-rays produced from the target are collimated by primary collimators in the direction of patient. This beam is further modified by flattening filter, secondary collimation and multileaf collimators before reaching patient's surface.

Modern radiotherapy is based on megavoltage X-rays (photons) and electrons. Megavoltage X-rays are produced by artificial acceleration of electrons through a vacuum to impact on a target in machines called linear accelerators (LINACs) (Box 3.2). The energy of the X-rays is proportional to the speed of electrons. Electrons are produced when the target in a linear accelerator is removed from the path of the electron beam (Box 3.2). Modern LINACs have facilities to produce both photons and electrons. Electrons have a predictable penetrability and hence are useful when it is important to limit the radiation dose to a deeper organ. Characteristics of photons that are useful in their clinical use are:

- Greater penetration compared to lower energy X-rays, which helps in delivering a higher proportion of dose to the deep tumour compared to the surface dose.
- Skin sparing effect – the maximum absorbed dose is deposited a few millimetres beneath the skin. This helps to deliver higher dose to depth without causing significant damage to skin and subcutaneous tissue (Box 3.3).

Brachytherapy

Brachytherapy involves placing radioactive sources at a very short distance from or in contact with, the tumour. Rapid fall off of radiation dose at increasing distance from the source permits delivery of a high dose of radiotherapy to the tumour with sparing of surrounding normal tissue. Short half life and high specific activity of isotopes allow delivery of the dose over a short period of time. The spatial distribution of sources is based on a complex set of rules.

The previous problems of radiation safety for patients and staff, and prolonged treatment time, have become history with modern brachytherapy machines (Figure 3.3). Clinical applications of brachytherapy are as follows:

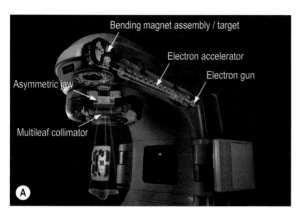
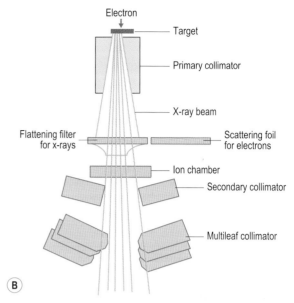

Figure 3.1
A & B, Linear accelerator. (Courtesy of Varian Medical Systems.)

Box 3.3: Choosing the energy *(Figure 3.2)*

Electrons have a definite range (range in centimeters is approximately half of beam energy in MeV) and selection of electron is based on the depth needed to treat (effective treatment depth in centimeters, as defined by 90% isodose in centre, is approximately one-third of the beam energy in MeV). With increasing energy, the surface dose decreases and hence if higher dose is needed at the surface, a bolus is used (p. 23). Bolus is also used to bring up high dose region to surface to avoid radiation to underlying critical structure. Higher energy electron beams exhibit a lateral constriction of 90% isodose line *(Figure 3.2B)* which need to be taken into consideration while deciding the field size at surface.

Photons have a skin sparing effect and maximum dose is deposited at a depth from surface. Dose at a depth increases with energy of photos. 6–10 MV is generally used, however in large patients with very deep seated tumours >10 MV yields a better dose distribution.

- Curative treatment as a single modality – e.g. prostate cancer, cervical cancer.
- Adjuvant after surgery – e.g. breast cancer.
- Curative treatment with external beam radiotherapy – e.g. cervical cancer, prostate cancer, anal cancer.

- Palliative treatment – e.g. intracavitary treatment for bronchial cancer and oesophageal cancer.

Radionuclide treatment

Systemic administration of radionuclides, which emit gamma-radiation, is a useful treatment for cancer. In well differentiated thyroid cancer, ^{131}I is given to patients after thyroidectomy (p. 282). Strontium-89 and samarium-153 are used for palliation of bone metastases, particularly from prostate cancer.

Informed consent

Once a decision is made to treat with radiotherapy, this decision should be communicated to the patient. The patient should be informed of the intention of treatment, potential benefits and side effects, both short term and long term. It is also an obligation to explain to the patient the potentially serious short and long term consequences of treatment in order to obtain truly informed consent. Often patients would like to know details of how radiation works (Box 3.4), dose and length of treatment, rationale for a number of treatments (fractionation – the process of giving the total dose of radiation as small doses

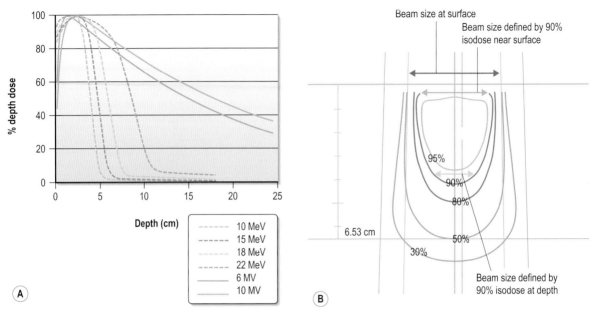

Figure 3.2
A, The percentage of depth dose of electrons (MeV) and photons (MV). B, Electron beam isodose curves – Note the constriction of 90% isodose at depth which necessitates addition of wider margins to beam width for adequate coverage of tumour at depth.

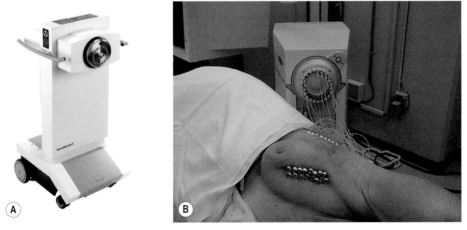

Figure 3.3
Brachytherapy machine and its application. A, High dose rate (HDR) afterloading brachytherapy machine which is fully computer controlled and completes treatment in a few minutes. B, Interstitial brachytherapy in breast cancer (Courtesy of Varian Medical Systems).

over a period of time) (Box 3.5) and side effects (p. 348). Side effects of radiotherapy depend on the area of treatment, total dose and dose per fraction. These can be acute (occurring during radiotherapy and within 3 months of completion of radiotherapy) or chronic (occurring 3 months after completion of radiotherapy).

Radiotherapy planning and delivery

Position and immobilization

Radiotherapy aims to deliver a uniform (homogenous) therapeutic dose of radiation to the tumour

Box 3.4: How does radiation work?

Therapeutic use of radiotherapy is born out of empiricism. Science caught up with empirical clinical use later to provide explanations for various patterns of response to treatment. The cancer cell has an unlimited capacity to multiply and radiotherapy is aimed to prevent this unlimited multiplication. The conventional explanation of radiation effect is based on radiation damage to DNA caused directly by photons and indirectly by free radicals which are produced when photons interact with water molecules in the tissue (see Figure 3.4). There are three different types of radiation damage to DNA:

- Lethal – irreversible, irreparable leading to cell death.
- Sublethal – under normal circumstances cells can be repaired in a few hours unless additional sublethal damage (another dose of radiation) occurs which makes the damage lethal.
- Potentially lethal – the component of radiation damage can be modified by the post radiation environment.

However, DNA damage is not the only mechanism of radiotherapy action. Radiotherapy can also influence genes controlling the cell cycle (e.g. RB gene, p53) and alter the expression of various genes resulting in expression of cytokines, growth factors, structural proteins or enzymes. Radiation damage to cell membrane sends signals to the nucleus and these signals affect cell behaviour.

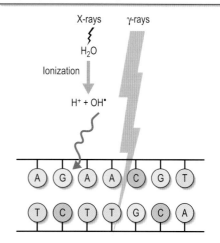

and areas of microscopic spread with minimal possible dose to the adjacent organs. This necessitates accurate reproduction of treatment position on a daily basis. Patients are positioned and immobilized to ensure optimal beam delivery while maintaining a comfortable position. The common positions are either supine or prone.

Immobilization depends on the site of treatment and intent. Radical treatment needs better immobilization techniques as the dose delivered is often very high. Examples of site specific immobilization devices used are as follows:

- Brain tumours – for radical treatment: Perspex shell or stereotactic frame and for palliative treatment: thermoplastic shell.
- Head and neck cancers – Perspex shell.
- Breast cancer – chest board with cross bar to fix the arms above the head.
- Chest – head support and knee support or stereotactic body frame.
- Abdomen and pelvis – knee support or stereotactic frame or vacuum bags.
- Limbs – vacuum bags.

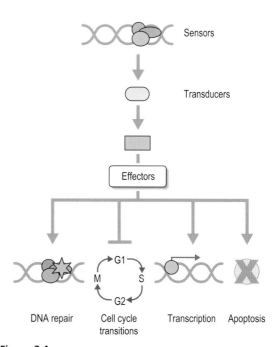

Figure 3.4
Mechanism of radiation induced cell damage.

Box 3.5: Rationale for fractionation

Radiotherapy usually results in equal damage to both normal cells and cancer arising from them. However, normal cells and cancer cells differ in their ability to recover from radiation damage. This differential capacity of normal cells to repair and re-grow is exploited in eradication of tumour cells. Radiation sensitivity of cells is dependent on the phase of cell cycle they are in: G2 and M are radiosensitive whereas S phase is radioresistant. At the time of radiotherapy, the cancer cells are in various phases of cell cycles; some of them will be in the sensitive phase when there is a good chance of cell kill and some will be in the resistant phase.

Rationale of fractionation is explained by 5 Rs. Some of the Rs lead to more cancer cell kill, whereas others lead to better repair of normal cells.

- Redistribution of cells – delivering radiotherapy as multiple treatments allows tumour cells to reassort into more radiosensitive phase leading to more cancer cell damage.
- Reoxygenation – many cancers have hypoxic areas within the tumour and normal cells do not have any hypoxic areas. Hypoxic areas are relatively resistant to radiotherapy. With each fraction, radiotherapy reduces the number of cancer cells and allows some of the hypoxic areas to become more oxygenated leading to better cancer cell radiation damage.
- The inherent radiosensitivity of the tumour is important in achieving a cure or control of tumour. Some tumours are very radiosensitive (e.g. lymphoma and seminoma) whereas others are relatively radioresistant (e.g. melanoma, sarcoma). Most tumours are moderately radiosensitive. Cure can be achieved with a smaller dose of radiotherapy in very radiosensitive tumours (e.g. germinoma, p. 275)
- Repair of sublethal damage – reducing the dose per fraction helps to repair damage of normal tissues more effectively than tumours. Normal tissue may be able to repair sublethal damage if the interval between two fractions of radiotherapy is at least 6 hours. However, some types of cancers also have quick ability to repair radiation damage leading to radioresistance (e.g. melanoma).
- Repopulation – fractionation helps rapidly populating normal tissues such as skin and gut to repopulate and hence recover from radiotherapy damage. Again, cancer cells also have the capacity to repopulate especially when radiation treatment is very prolonged or interrupted (gap correction, see later).

Localization of tumour

Localization of tumour is to define various treatment volumes (Box 3.6). Conventional localization (2-dimensional, 2D) is with orthogonal X-rays using special treatment planning machines

Box 3.6: Volumes in radiotherapy *(Figure 3.5)*

The following are the volumes in radiotherapy:

- GTV – Gross tumour volume – is the gross disease or radiologically visible tumour – this area has 10^9 cancer cells. In the figure, the T2W MRI shows hyperintense low grade brain tumour.
- CTV – Clinical target volume – is the volume which contains GTV and/or subclinical microscopic disease (10^6 cells) which need to be treated to an adequate dose to achieve the aim of treatment. The CTV depends on the pattern of local spread of specific tumours. In the figure, note the outer border of CTV merges with that of PTV as there is no possibility of microscopic spread beyond the inner layer of the skull.
- PTV – Planning target volume – is a geographical concept which denotes the CTV and margins for geographic variations and inaccuracies during treatment. The margin added to CTV to derive PTV depends mainly on the immobilization device (e.g. 2–3 mm with stereotactic frame). PTV has two components:
  - IM (internal margin) – is a margin added to CTV to compensate for normal anatomical movements and variations in size, shape and position of CTV during treatment. In the figure, there is very little anatomic movement of CTV and hence IM is almost zero, whereas in a lung tumour, it may be around 1–4 cm depending on the location of the tumour and depth of breathing.
  - SM (set up margin) – a number of factors can cause uncertainties such as daily variation in position of the patient, mechanical uncertainties of the equipment, transfer set up errors etc. In brain tumour treatment, if a Perspex shell is used a 5 mm margin is added.
- TV – treated volume – is the volume enclosed by an isodose surface, selected and specified by the oncologist as being appropriate to achieve the purpose of treatment.
- IrV – irradiated volume – is that tissue volume which receives a dose that is considered significant in relation to normal tissue tolerance.
- PRV – planning organ at risk volume – refers to the definition of margins around organs at risk for injury by radiation.

Please note, even if the actual tumour (GTV) is small, after adding various margins as above the irradiated volume is much bigger. This is one of the limiting factors in delivering a high dose to tumour without having significant irradiation to normal tissue. Studies show that a 4–5% increase in dose increases the tumour control probability by 10% and hence newer developments are aiming at better localization of tumour and reduction of various margins to increase the dose to the actual tumour.

called simulators. These are diagnostic X-ray machines, which can mimic all the positions and movements of a treatment machine (Figure 3.6A) and some of these machines have a CT scan facility. 2D localization is appropriate for palliative treatment. Radical radiotherapy utilizes a planning CT scan or advanced techniques to define the various tumour volumes in 3-dimensions. Modern computer software allows co-registration of the planning CT scan with an MRI or PET scan (Figure 3.6B), which improves the

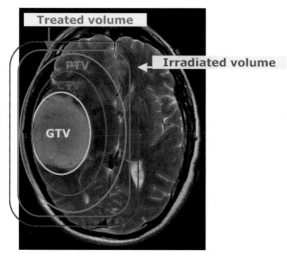

Figure 3.5
Volumes in radiotherapy.

accuracy of GTV delineation. Planning CT scan is usually taken at a slice interval of 1.5–5 mm. A slice thickness of <3 mm helps to get better resolution of digitally reconstructed images (DRRs) which are used to check accuracy of treatment delivery (see later in Box 3.12).

Planning technique

Conventional (2D) simulator planning uses simple beam arrangements such as single field radiotherapy or parallel opposed beams. In conformal (3D) planning various volumes and organs at risk (OAR) are delineated individually on every slice of cross-sectional imaging and a treatment plan produced by a planning computer. Intensity modulated planning (IMRT) is a further improvement of 3D planning, which is aimed at ensuring homogeneous dose to the tumour with less dose to organs at risk. This technique has particular advantage with concave-shaped target volumes with OAR located in the concavity. The technique is also useful in sparing critical organs from radiotherapy toxicity (e.g. parotid gland sparing in head and neck cancer).

Image guided radiotherapy (IGRT) is a further advance in radiotherapy planning and delivery where the real time position of the tumour is taken into consideration (Figure 3.7). 3D, IMRT and IGRT use multiple beams to obtain the optimal treatment plan.

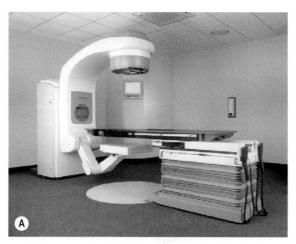

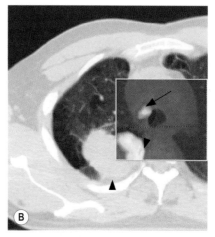

Figure 3.6
Localization of tumour. A, Simulator used for conventional localization as well as for plan verification (courtesy Varian Medical Systems). B, Co-registered planning CT with PET scan showing primary tumour (arrow head) and PET positive right paratracheal node (arrow).

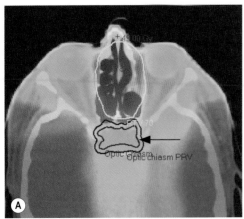
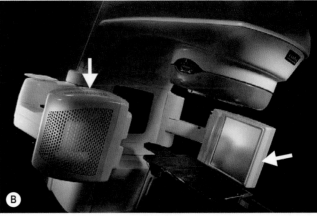

Figure 3.7
A&B, IMRT and IGRT. A, IMRT is a conformal technique which helps to selectively avoid/limit radiotherapy dose to critical structures. This IMRT plan aims to give 70 Gy to ethmoid cancer (yellow line represents 70 Gy) while keeping the dose to the optic chiasma (arrow) to less than 50 Gy. B, IGRT – specialized radiotherapy machine with on-board imaging system (arrows) allows real time imaging and correction of error. (Courtesy Varian Medical Systems.)

Box 3.7: Radiotherapy planning (see Figure 3.8)

Three fields are used and the dose is prescribed at the intersection point as 100% of prescribed dose

Note the beam arrangement –

- Only one beam passes directly through the spinal cord so as to keep cord dose within tolerance
- Beams enter only through the side of disease. No beams are entering through the normal lung side
- Beams are sized according to the beam's eye view and are of different dimension

Box 3.8: Beam shaping (Figure 3.9)

In the early 1950s radiotherapy beams used to be either square or rectangular. There was an option to shield part of the field with lead or equivalent material. When conformal radiotherapy started evolving, individual blocks were made based on the BEV of individual beams to shape the radiotherapy fields using cerrobend (an alloy of bismuth, lead, tin and cadmium with a melting point of 70°C and hence easy to make different shapes). Currently beam shaping is achieving with MLCs (see Figure 3.9).

Treatment planning (Box 3.7)

Direction of beam

The direction of beam depends on the location of PTV and OARs. Generally beams are placed so that they are equi-angled, entering the body through the side of disease and avoiding passing directly through the OARs if possible.

Beam size and shape

Conventional radiotherapy uses either rectangular or square fields with appropriate blocking of beams over critical organs (by shields, see below). Conformal radiotherapy shapes every beam according to the 'beam's eye view' (BEV). The exact shaping of the beam used to be attained by shaped blocks. With the advent of multileaf

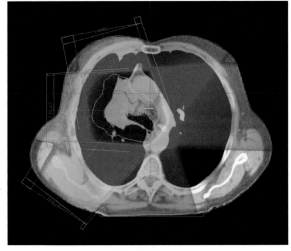

Figure 3.8
Radiotherapy planning.

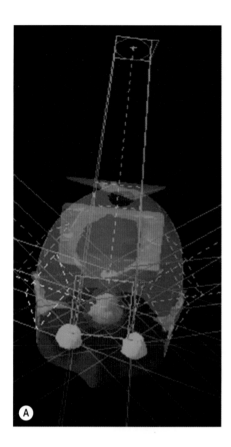

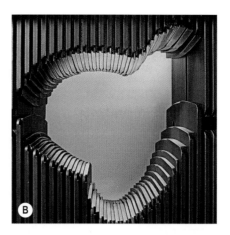

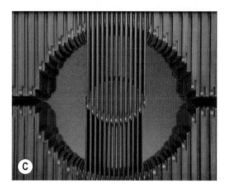

Figure 3.9
Beam shaping using BEV (A) and MLCs (B&C).

collimators (MLC), shaping of beams becomes increasingly easy (Box 3.8).

Energy of the beam

For superficial lesions and lesions lying within a limited depth, electrons are used and energy of the electron beam depends on the depth which needs to be treated (Box 3.3). For deep seated tumours, megavoltage energy is used, usually 6 MV photons; in some patients a higher energy with high penetration is necessary to improve the dose homogeneity.

Wedges, shields and bolus

In multifield radiotherapy, wedges are necessary to alter the beam profile, thereby ensuring a homogeneous dose to the target volume (Box 3.6). Wedges also act as a tissue compensator for sloping external surface.

Shields are used to avoid irradiation of part of the radiotherapy field. In the modern machines it is achieved by individual leaves of multileaf collimators.

Bolus (a tissue-equivalent material placed directly on the patient's skin surface) is used to bring up the radiation dose to the surface. The commonly used tissue equivalent materials are slabs of paraffin wax, gauze coated with petrolatum or synthetic-based substances. Megavoltage radiotherapy has a skin sparing effect (i.e. delivering maximum dose at a point deep to the skin) which may be a disadvantage when treating a superficial PTV (e.g. chest wall after mastectomy). Hence in order to bring up the maximum dose to the surface bolus is placed on the surface of the treatment volume. Bolus is also used to bring up the high dose radiation towards the surface to avoid higher doses to the deeply situated OARs.

Evaluation of treatment plan

Once treatment is planned, it is necessary to evaluate the treatment plan before it is accepted for treatment. In difficult situations, such as when an OAR is lying near the PTV, the planning physicists come up with more than one plan for the oncologist to evaluate and choose one for treatment. Evaluation of the plan takes the following steps (Box 3.9):

- Homogenous dose to the PTV – ideally, the whole of the PTV should be covered by 95% isodose and the recommendation is that PTV dose should be within –5% and +7% of the

Box 3.9: Evaluation of a treatment plan
(Figure 3.10)

Treatment plan evaluation is to ensure that the PTV receives a homogenous dose and the doses to the OAR are within tolerance. Spatial distribution displays ensure that 95% isodose encloses the PTV (Figure 3.10A & B). Dose volume histogram (Figure 3.10C) is helpful to indicate underdosage to PTV as well as excessive dose to OAR.

prescribed dose. This is confirmed by looking at the dose distribution at every slice of plan or looking at the dose volume histogram (DVH). DVH plots the total dose against the percentage of target volume or OAR irradiated (Box 3.9). Hotspots are areas outside the PTV which receive a dose >100% of the specified PTV dose. Hotspots are considered significant only if they exceed >15 mm in diameter, except in small organs (e.g. eye, optic nerve) where <15 mm diameter has to be considered significant.

- Dose to OAR – dose to the OAR should not exceed their tolerance dose. Tolerance dose (TD) is the dose beyond which there is a risk of dose limiting toxicity. TD is stated as TD5/5 (dose at which there is 5% risk of occurring dose limiting toxicity at 5 years) and TD5/50

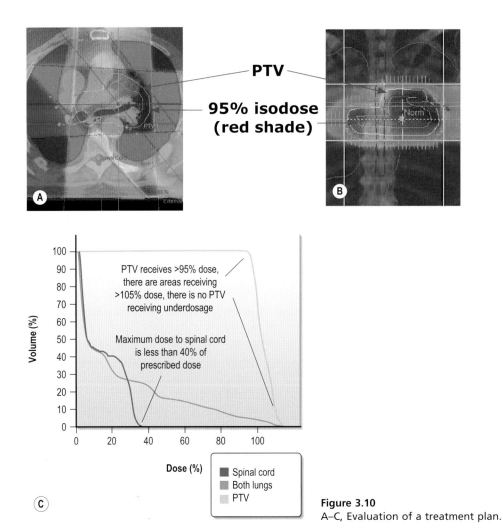

Figure 3.10
A–C, Evaluation of a treatment plan.

Table 3.1: Normal tissue radiation tolerance dose (treated with 2 Gy per fraction)

Organ	TD5/5 (Gy) Whole	2/3rd	1/3rd	Dose limiting toxicity
Brain	45	50	60	Necrosis
Brain stem	50	53	60	Necrosis
Colon	45	–	55	Obstruction, perforation and ulceration
Heart	40	45	60	Pericarditis
Kidney	23	30	50	Renal failure
Lens	10	–	–	Cataract
Liver	30	35	50	Hepatitis
Lung	17.5	30	45	Pulmonary fibrosis
Oesophagus	55	58	60	Stricture
Optic apparatus	50	–	–	Blindness
Parotid	32	32	–	Xerostomia
Rectum	60	–	–	Necrosis, fistula, stenosis
Retina	45	–	–	Blindness
Spinal cord	47	50	50	Myelitis
Small intestine	40	–	50	Obstruction, perforation
Stomach	50	55	60	Ulceration, perforation

(dose at which there is 50% risk of occurring dose limiting toxicity at 5 years. The aim of treatment plan evaluation is to limit the dose to OAR below TD5/5. Table 3.1 gives the approximate TD of various organs.

- Dose to other normal tissue – it is important to check that there is no increased dose to the entry and exit of the beam and there are no sensitive structures in the path of the radiation beams.

Dose prescription for radiation treatment

The prescription point of radiotherapy depends on the type of plan. For a single beam, the prescription point either lies in the point of maximum dose (d_{max}) or at a depth. For parallel opposed beams the prescription point is mid-plane whereas for all 3D and 4D planning the prescription point is often at the isocentre or at the intersection of points.

For electrons, dose is prescribed at 100%; however, it is necessary that 90% isodose covers the PTV.

The prescription should indicate the total dose, number of fractions, dose per fraction, and duration of treatment (e.g. 50 Gy in 20 fractions over 4 weeks). Conventional fractionation is to deliver one radiotherapy fraction per day for 5 days a week. There are a number of alternate fractionation regimes (Box 3.10). The total dose of radiotherapy depends on the type of cancer, site and bulk of disease (Box 3.11). Gray (Gy) is the usual measure of radiotherapy which is defined as 1 joule of energy per 1 kg of material. The subunit is centigray (cGy) which is 1/100 of a Gray. Radiotherapy alone for cure needs a dose of >60–65 Gy as 1.8–2 Gy per day whereas adjuvant radiotherapy uses 50–60 Gy. Most studies indicate a direct relation between the dose and chances of control and cure.

Treatment verification and corrections

Accurate position and immobilization during planning and treatment are important in accurate delivery of radiotherapy. In spite of this, treatment delivered can be different from the planned

Box 3.10: Fractionation schedules

- Conventional fractionation – delivers 1.8–2 Gy single fraction per day, 5 times weekly.
- Accelerated fractionation – aims to shorten the treatment time by delivering larger than standard size fractions five times weekly or more than five fractions per week of 2 Gy. Multiple fractions may also be given daily. The acute toxicity is greater with this and late toxicity is either the same as (if complete repair of sublethal damage occurs) or greater than conventional fractionation. It is useful for tumours with a rapid growth rate.
- Hyperfractionation – aims to improve tumour control probability with the same late effects as conventional fractionation. It delivers a larger number of smaller than conventional dose fractions per day and the total dose is 10–20% higher than standard fractionation while total treatment time remains the same. It is useful for tumours with slow growth.
- Accelerated hyperfractionation – combines the principles of hyperfractionation and accelerated fractionation.
- Continuous accelerated hyperfractionation (CHART) – treatment is given as 1.5 Gy per fraction, three times daily 6 hours apart for 12 continuous days. Proved to improve local control in lung cancer.
- Hypofractionation – delivers more than 2 Gy per fractions and less than five fractions per week.

Box 3.11: Tumour control probability (TCP), normal tissue complication probability (NTCP) and therapeutic ratio (Figure 3.11)

For many types of cancer, a higher dose of radiotherapy produces better tumour control. After fractionated radiotherapy, the total number of cancer cells surviving depends on the initial number of cells and the proportion of cancer cells killed with each treatment. Studies show that visible disease needs more dose than microscopic disease (to pathologically detect microscopic disease, cell aggregates of $\geq 10^6/cm^3$ are needed) and subclinical disease (cannot be detected microscopically). For example a dose of >65 Gy is needed to control visible epithelial tumours, whereas the dose needed to control microscopic disease is 60–65 Gy and 50–60 Gy for subclinical disease.

The aim of radiotherapy is to deliver a dose of radiation to destroy the tumour without leading to serious normal tissue complications. Therapeutic ratio is used to represent this concept where it is the ratio of the tumour control probability (TCP) and normal tissue complication probability (NTCP) at a specified level of response (usually <5% or 0.05) for normal tissue.

The probability of tumour control without normal tissue complications is highest in the therapeutic window. The further the NTCP curve to the right of the TCP (see Figure 3.11) cure it is easier to achieve a tumour control with minimal toxicity (A) and a larger therapeutic ratio. When NTCP and TCP (C) get closer the therapeutic ratio gets smaller.

In practical radiotherapy a better therapeutic ratio can be achieved by:

- Advanced treatment planning (3D, IMRT or IGRT)
- Accurate target localization which helps to reduce safety margins
- Sophisticated dose delivery

treatment. Hence it is important to ensure that treatment delivery is within the tolerance limit of accepted variation from the planning. The accepted tolerance generally depends on the immobilization method; e.g. a variation of <5 mm is acceptable with Perspex. The accuracy of planned treatment can be verified by:

- Verification of treatment position before treatment using simulator – the simulator X-rays are compared with DRRs for accuracy in terms of isocentre and comparison of bony landmarks if feasible and comparison of individual fields (Box 3.12).
- Verification of treatment during treatment with portal imaging – a comparison is made with DRR to assess the position of isocentre in at least two views (anterior and posterior), position of beam in relation to bony or other visible landmarks (Box 3.12) and shape of individual fields.
- Real time verification of treatment with correction for variation is the back bone of image guided radiotherapy.

Box 3.12: Verification of treatment (Figure 3.12)

DRR (Figure 3.12A) is used to verify treatment accuracy. This is commonly done by comparison of DRR with the treatment verification film (Figure 3.12B). The treatment set-up is checked by comparing the position of isocentre, bony landmarks and the positions of MLCs or beam shaping block for the same beams. If a systemic error is found during verification, it needs to be corrected before proceeding with further treatment and the corrected treatment plan should be verified for accuracy of treatment set-up.

During the process of verification two types of errors in treatment set up can occur:

- Systemic Σ – error between planning and treatment. This needs correction before proceeding with further treatment.

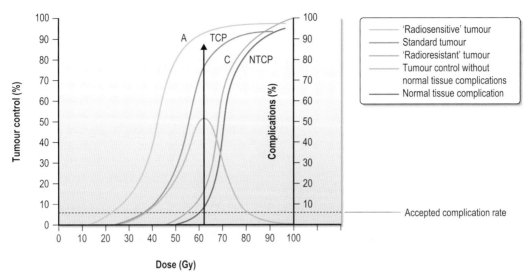

Figure 3.11
TCP and NTCP (see Box 3.11).

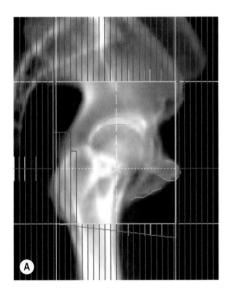

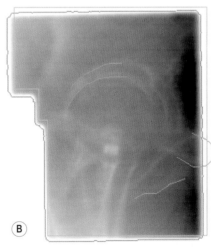

Figure 3.12
A&B, Verification of treatment.

- Random ∂ – variations and uncertainties that arise between each fraction of treatment. It is difficult to correct this error as this does not occur consistently.

During determination of PTV, these errors are taken into consideration to add a margin to PTV. The suggested margin is $2.5\ \Sigma + 0.7\partial$.

Supportive care during radiotherapy

It is important to follow up patients regularly during radiotherapy to assess and manage radio-therapy toxicities, to monitor nutritional status and check blood counts. Studies have shown that during radical radiotherapy of head and neck, lung, oesophageal and cervical cancer, it is important to maintain a haemoglobin level of >12 gm/dl (a level lower than this may result in 10–12% less chance of disease control). The importance of level of haemoglobin is less clear in other cancers. However, symptomatic anaemia needs to be corrected. It is also important to make sure that the blood counts remains safe (i.e. platelet count of $>100 \times 10^9/dL$ and neutrophil count of $>1.5 \times 10^9/dL$) during radiotherapy especially when it is given concurrently with chemotherapy or when a significant amount of bone marrow bearing area is being irradiated. Blood counts below the safe threshold necessitate either withholding chemotherapy or suspending chemotherapy until the blood count recovers.

Treatment modifications during treatment

Gap correction

One of the common situations is an interruption during radiotherapy due to holidays, non-attendance or intolerable toxicity. This might need modification of treatment. Studies have shown that tumours exhibit accelerated repopulation during radiotherapy. Accelerated repopulation implies an increase in multiplication of cancer cells which often starts with partial shrinkage of tumour after radiotherapy or chemotherapy. Prolonged interruption of radiotherapy results in decreasing efficacy of radiotherapy due to accelerated repopulation. Using modelling analysis, an increase of total treatment duration by 1 day may reduce local control by 1.4%. Hence attempts should be made to avoid prolongation of overall treatment. Still, occasionally treatment gets prolonged, when adjustment should be made to complete the treatment in the planned overall time by:

- delivering twice daily fractions, at a minimum of a 6-hour interval
- treating over the weekend
- use of biologically equivalent dose in fewer fractions to achieve planned overall time.

If treatment still cannot be completed within the planned overall time additional fractions may be considered. A rough estimate is an additional dose of 0.6 Gy per every day of increase in overall treatment time.

Care after radiotherapy and survivorship

Some patients have persistent acute radiotherapy side effects up to 3 months after completion of radiotherapy. Management of these side effects is multidisciplinary, involving a number of healthcare professionals including an oncologist, nurse specialists, therapeutic radiographers, dietician and speech and language therapists (SALT).

In the long term, there are a number of side effects needing special attention. Patients receiving radiotherapy to whole or part of the brain are at risk of cognitive impairment, cerebrovascular accidents, hormonal deficiency and second cancer (p. 58, late effects). Radiotherapy to the chest is associated with increased risk of second cancer and radiation damage to heart, particularly in patients receiving radiotherapy for left breast cancer. Pelvic radiotherapy often results in menopause and infertility in women and sexual dysfunction and infertility in men. Radiotherapy induced or promoted second cancer is an important survivorship issue. After cancer treatment, people often face an array of challenges including psycho-social functioning and economic well-being. As physicians, our triumph is not just in curing or controlling cancer, but also in helping cancer survivors to lead a high quality life in the society. For a detailed discussion on cancer survivorship, see p. 58.

Advances in radiotherapy

Based on experimental studies, there is a direct correlation between the radiation dose and chances of control of cancer, though not linear. However, various uncertainties in the radiotherapy planning process often lead to a large treatment volume (see Box 3.6). Advances in radiotherapy are aimed at understanding and controlling these uncertainties in radiotherapy planning. By doing so, we will be able to give a much higher dose to the tumour and areas of possible spread with minimal dose to the surrounding normal organs. The areas under research include advanced immobilization, improved radiotherapy with image guidance and incorporation of molecular imaging for tumour volume delineation.

Measures to improve efficacy of radiotherapy

Various measures are being studied to improve the efficacy of radiotherapy. These include alternative fractionations (Box 3.10), use of radiotherapy with concurrent chemotherapy, radiation sensitizers and recently, biological agents. The examples of alternative fractionation proven to improve tumour control include CHART for non-small cell lung cancer, 6 fractions per week in head and neck cancer and radiosurgery.

Concurrent chemotherapy is proven to have a role in the primary management of oesophageal, cervical and anal cancers (see corresponding chapters). Chemotherapy improves local control by tumour kill as well as acting as a radiation sensitizer.

Biological agents

Based on the current evidence, radiotherapy (as well as chemotherapy) causes logarithmic kill of cancer cells and as we know a logarithmic kill does not end in zero cells, but in at least one cell. To achieve permanent tumour control, this last tumour cell which is capable of producing a recurrence (so called tumour rescuing unit or clonogenic tumour cell) must be killed. Clinical use of radiotherapy is based on inactivation of clonogenic cells. Addition of biological agents is thought to improve the radiation effect as well as cause a direct tumour kill. The following biological agents are being studied as radiation modulators:

- Inhibitors of epidermal growth factor receptor (EGFR) – EGFR is expressed in solid tumours such as head and neck squamous cell cancer, glioblastoma and non-small cell lung cancer. Overexpression of EGFR is associated with poor prognosis and radioresistance. Hence EGFR inhibition is thought to improve radiosensitivity and these agents also have a direct cell kill effect. An example of success of such a combination is a recently reported randomized study of radiotherapy with or without cetuximab (an EGFR inhibitor) in locally advanced head and neck cancer which has shown that addition of cetuximab improves local control (median duration of 24.4 months vs. 14.9 months $p = 0.005$) and median survival (49 months vs. 29.3 months $p = 0.03$). Cetuximab is also being studied in lung cancer.
- Anti-angiogenesis inhibitors – anti-angiogenesis molecules have an indirect cell kill effect. They are also thought to modify radiation effect by various mechanisms such as improved

tumour oxygenation, decreased vessel density, increased tumour cell loss and radiosensitization of endothelial cells. Examples of anti-angiogenesis inhibitors under study include bevacizumab and thalidomide.

Re-irradiation

With more effective systemic treatment, the overall life expectancy of cancer patients is increasing. This often results in recurrence of disease with symptoms (such as bone pain, cough etc.) at a previously irradiated site. The conventional thinking has been that a heavily irradiated tissue will not tolerate further treatment. However, recent data suggest that re-irradiation is often possible. Modern techniques help in re-irradiation with optimal sparing of critical structures. Examples are re-irradiation for head and neck tumours with spinal cord sparing and re-irradiation with radiosurgery or partial brain radiotherapy after whole brain radiotherapy for recurrent brain metastasis.

Future directions

Progress in radiotherapy is driven by advances in computer technology. In contrast to the advances in chemotherapy, based on a structured evaluation of efficacy and side effects of new drugs, advances in radiotherapy are often based on technological safety for clinical use rather than its proven clinical benefit compared with the existing method of radiotherapy delivery. A better physical dose distribution of radiotherapy delivery is often a surrogate measure of clinical benefit of a new technology. However, just a good radiotherapy plan itself is not capable of delivering a better clinical result. Hence it is important in future to critically evaluate the true clinical benefits of very costly technological advances compared with the existing less costly alternatives.

Further reading

Barrett A, Dobbs J, Morris SL, Roques T. Practical Radiotherapy Planning, 4th Edition. London: Hodder Arnold, 2009.

Principles of systemic therapy

4

HM Hatcher

Introduction

Systemic therapies form the basis for medical oncology and a significant amount of clinical oncology in the UK. The description is broad and can be thought to include any treatment which is given to a patient which will be absorbed systemically and could potentially affect the whole body. Traditionally this would be thought to be chemotherapy but the definition also includes hormonal treatments, chemical adjuncts, immunotherapy, biological agents and systemic radiotherapy treatments. Each will be discussed and examples given with reference to the appropriate chapters for more detail.

This chapter gives an overview of the practical aspects of various systemic therapies (Box 4.1). A detailed pharmacological discussion is beyond the scope of this book but further reading is suggested for those interested.

Aim of systemic treatment

Before recommending or prescribing a systemic treatment the aim of the treatment has to be understood (Box 4.2). This, in addition to a knowledge of the specific disease and treatments that are effective for that tumour, will dictate the type of treatment offered and its likely intensity (Box 4.3). Treatment intensity should be greatest in those conditions where the intention is cure, and there is some evidence in certain tumours (e.g. bone tumours) that increased toxicity during chemotherapy is related to improved survival. When the treatment is not curative significant toxicity is unacceptable.

In acute leukaemias the curative chemotherapy is given in various phases (Box 4.4).

Chemotherapy

Chemotherapy involves the treatment with cytotoxic chemicals to kill cancer cells. Its benefit depends upon the high proliferation rate of cancer cells compared with the non cancer cells in the body. The discovery of nitrogen mustard and its effects on proliferating cells was discovered in both World Wars, but only put into practice to treat leukaemias and lymphomas in the 1940s (Figure 4.1). Later that decade aminopterin was shown to induce remissions in leukaemia, although the majority of patients relapsed and died. In the following 10 years different classes of chemotherapeutic agents were discovered. Most of these were directed against DNA synthesis or cell division. In the 1970s cytotoxic agents were seen to impact significantly on the cure of specific cancers such as testicular cancer and leukaemia (Box 4.5). This improvement in survival was due not only to the development of new drugs but also to the understanding of how to combine them.

Classes of chemotherapy drugs

Chemotherapy agents are divided into different categories according to their mechanism of action. The rationale behind chemotherapy is to inhibit or kill rapidly dividing cancer cells. This may be due to the drug acting at a particular point in the cell cycle (cell cycle-specific) or is independent of the cell cycle (cell cycle-non specific) (Figure 4.2). Boxes 4.6 and 4.7 give examples of different classes of drugs in each of these categories with some specific examples.

© 2011, Elsevier Ltd
DOI: 10.1016/B978-0-7234-3458-0.00009-9

Box 4.1: Types of systemic treatments

- Chemotherapy (single agent or in combination)
- Targeted treatments:
  - hormonal treatments e.g. tamoxifen, arimidex, goserelin
  - antibodies e.g. rituximab, cetuximab
  - small molecules e.g. imatinib, erlotinib
- Other agents:
  - bisphosphonates, e.g. pamidronate, zoledronic acid
  - immunological agents, e.g. interleukin-2, interferon

Box 4.2: Aim of systemic treatment

Curative
Chemotherapy is given as the definitive treatment for cure, e.g. acute leukaemia, choriocarcinoma.

Adjuvant
Treatment is given after a definitive treatment such as surgery or radiotherapy with the aim of destroying micrometastatic residual disease, and thereby increasing the chances of cure, e.g. chemotherapy after surgery for breast cancer.

Neoadjuvant
A treatment is given before a definitive treatment such as surgery to facilitate the procedure and/or improve chances of cure, e.g. chemotherapy is given to patients with osteosarcoma prior to resection and replacement with prosthesis. This has the benefit of assessing pathological response to chemotherapy such that adjuvant chemotherapy can be modified if necessary.

Palliative
A treatment is given to improve the quality of life and symptoms of a patient without the intention of cure. It may prolong the life of the individual but this is not necessarily the case. Quality of life is the prime assessment.

Box 4.3: Dose intensity and dose density

Dose intensity refers to the total amount of drug delivered to the patient over a week. This may be given as a single bolus or in a number of treatments over a few weeks but intensity reflects the actual average dose per week. Maintaining the intended dose intensity (as prescribed on the chart) has been shown to be important in the survival of certain types of cancers (e.g. breast cancer). In those patients whose treatment was delayed or dose reduced (resulting in reduced intensity) relapses occurred more frequently.

Dose density refers to the method of giving a drug in small repeated amounts frequently rather than as a single high dose less often.

Box 4.4: Phases of chemotherapy treatment in haematologic malignancies (p. 310)

Induction
Initial intense chemotherapy designed to rapidly reduce tumour burden and aim for remission.

Consolidation
Continued treatment to reduce the tumour burden further to the point of remission where no tumour cells are detectable.

Maintenance
Ongoing lower dose treatment to maintain remission. Evidence from ALL studies show improved survival with prolonged low-dose chemotherapy and intrathecal methotrexate (p. 310).

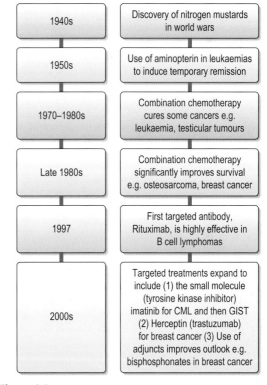

Figure 4.1
Milestones in the development of systemic therapy for cancer.

How does chemotherapy work?

Tumour cells are detectable by conventional means at 10^9 cells (equivalent to 1 g tumour or 1 cm tumour) and continue to grow without treatment. Patients usually die if they remain untreated or after unsuccessful treatment when the tumour load reaches 10^{12} cells. When a

Box 4.5: Examples of tumours in which chemotherapy has a significant impact

Cured with chemotherapy
- Childhood acute leukaemia
- Testicular cancer
- Ovarian germ cell tumours
- Choriocarcinoma
- Wilms' tumour

Associated with improved survival
- Breast cancer
- Osteosarcoma
- Ewing's sarcoma
- Ovarian cancer
- And several others

Box 4.6: Cell cycle specific chemotherapy drugs

Antimetabolites	S phase	e.g. methotraxate, capecitabine
Vinca alkaloids	M phase	e.g. vincristine, vinorelbine
Taxanes	M phase	e.g. paclitaxel, docetaxel
Epipodophyllotoxins	G2, S, premitotic, topo II	e.g. etoposide
Camptothecans	S phase, topo I	e.g. irinotecan, topotecan

Box 4.7: Cell cycle non-specific chemotherapy drugs

Antitumour antibiotics	e.g. doxorubicin, mitomycin-C
Alkylating agents	e.g. ifosfamide, chlorambucil
Nitrosoureas	e.g. lomustine, carmustine

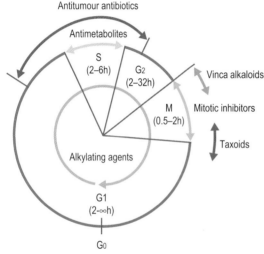

Figure 4.2
Cell cycle showing phases of cell replication and division. Cancer cells progress rapidly through this but may be inhibited at various points.

tumours receive additional courses of chemotherapy to bring down the number of tumour cells to an absolute minimum. However this does not necessarily result in complete removal of tumour cells at the end of chemotherapy and it is believed that the normal body immunosurveillance will help to achieve a cure in some instances. In some patients, cancer can grow back at any point of time (relapse) during the conventionally undetectable phase (see Box 4.8). In some other patients, the tumours do not respond to chemotherapy (resistance to treatment) which requires change of treatment (Figure 4.3).

Rationale for combining chemotherapy agents

In clinical practice cancer cells tend to develop resistance to a single drug by further gene mutations, or development of cellular pumps which reduce the dose of drug received by the tumour cells. Consequently the tumour will have a period of sensitivity followed by a rebound tumour regrowth. This may be partly due to the fact that not all tumour cells are passing through the same point of the cell cycle at the same time. Combining drugs allows the oncologist to direct agents with different activities or against different parts

chemotherapy regime is given to a sensitive tumour it causes cell death in a proportion of the cancer cells (log kill). In a chemo-sensitive tumour, each course of chemotherapy (see Box 4.9) results in a proportional cell kill and with a few courses of chemotherapy, tumour may not be detectable by conventional means (called complete response to treatment). At this point there is a possibility of $<10^9$ cells remaining and stopping treatment at this point may lead to an early progression/relapse of disease. Hence patients with chemo-sensitive

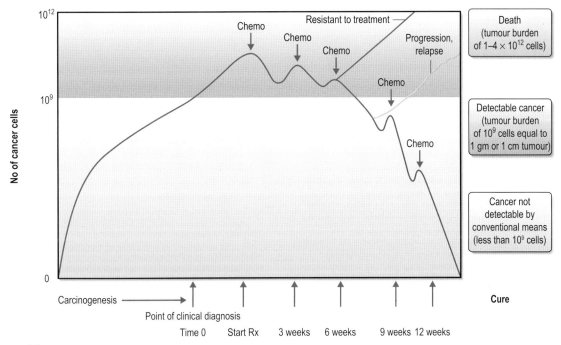

Figure 4.3
Cancer growth and response to treatment.

Box 4.8: Why not give treatment more often to prevent tumour regrowth?

Unfortunately giving treatment at an increased frequency (or intensity) also increases the toxicity of the treatment. Although some regimens have been able to achieve increased dose frequency with additional drugs to support the patient (e.g. use of granulocyte-colony stimulating factor [G-CSF] to avoid life-threatening neutropenic sepsis).

Figure 4.4 shows response of the bone marrow to chemotherapy after chemotherapy given on day 1. Neutrophils fall to their minimum between days 10 and 14 in a standard 21-day cycle. If G-CSF is given the neutrophils may not drop to such a low number.

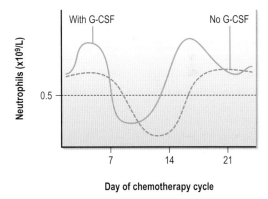

Figure 4.4
Neutrophil response during a cycle of chemotherapy.

of the cell cycle simultaneously. The idea is that this increases cell kill at the time of each treatment but also reduces the development of drug resistance.

Planning a combination chemotherapy regimen requires some knowledge of the mechanisms of action of the individual drugs, their dosing for particular cancers and their toxicities (see Box 4.10).

Actions of specific drug classes (Figure 4.6)

Cell cycle phase specific drugs act on cells within a particular phase of the cell cycle.

Antimetabolites

These drugs are developed to mimic naturally produced metabolites, purines, pyrimidines or

Box 4.9: Cycles of chemotherapy

What is a cycle?
A cycle is a complete treatment from the first day of one cycle to the first day of the second cycle. For many regimens this means a 3 or 4 week period of time (depending on the dose determining toxicity and its recovery period). Over that time drugs may all be given on day 1 only or can be given at several time points in those few weeks.

How many cycles of chemotherapy?
For curative treatment, further cycles of chemotherapy are needed after a conventional clinical response, to tackle the clinically undetectable tumour burden (Figure 4.3). Hence the amount of chemotherapy may vary from a few cycles to months to years depending on the specific cancer (e.g. acute lymphatic leukaemia needs more than a year of chemotherapy, whereas in choriocarcinoma two more courses of chemotherapy is given after a complete tumour marker response).

For many adjuvant treatments, traditionally 6 cycles of chemotherapy are given. (e.g. breast cancer usually 6–8 courses of chemotherapy depending on the regime).

In palliative treatments it is important to assess response (usually after 2–3 courses of chemotherapy) before continuing with treatment but if responding patients may continue for up to 6 (to 8) cycles depending on toxicity and the drugs involved.

The concept of a cycle does not fit with certain therapies such as hormonal treatments or with tyrosine kinase inhibitors as these drugs are continued for a finite number of years or until progression.

Box 4.10: How do you decide which drugs to combine for a given cancer?

- Activity and scheduling: Each drug must have shown activity for that type of cancer when given as a single agent and be given in a similar scheduling and dosing (synergistic activity).
- Mechanism of action: Ideally the drugs should have different, complementary mechanisms of action (a measure to prevent resistance).
- Toxicities: The toxicities of the drugs should also be different to minimize overall toxicity.

e.g. Combination of gemcitabine and carboplatin in lung cancer:

Activities and scheduling
- Carboplatin and gemticabine – each has a single agent response of $\leq 20\%$ in lung cancer and is given 3-weekly.

Mechanism of action (Figure 4.5)
- Carboplatin (cell cycle non-specific) act by forming DNA adducts which prevents DNA synthesis
- Gemcitabine (cell cycle specific) – pyramidine antimetabolite

Toxicity
- Carboplatin: dose limiting toxicity is thrombocypenia
- Gemcitabine: dose limiting toxicity is neutropenia

Combination of carboplatin and gemcitabine results in 30–50% response rate and the dose limiting toxicity is thrombocytopenia.

folates essential to the synthesis of nucleic acids and DNA (S phase) preventing the correct incorporation of purines or pyrimidines in the DNA structure. They therefore prevent DNA replication and lead to cell death. They are most effective against tumours with a high growth fraction and similarly have predominant toxicities on normal tissues with high cell turn over (e.g. mucosal epithelium and gastrointestinal tract). Examples are methotrexate, cytosine arabinoside, capecitabine, gemcitabine and 5-fluorouracil (5-FU).

Vinca alkaloids and taxanes

Either derived from plant alkaloids or synthetic derivatives of them, they interfere with mitotic spindle assembly in M phase causing metaphase arrest. Vinca alkaloids are extracts of the periwinkle plant. They bind to microtubular proteins which are essential to the formation of the mitotic

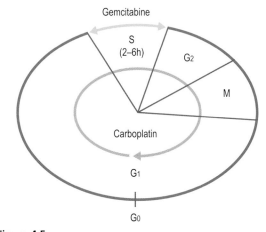

Figure 4.5
Rationale for the combination of gemcitabine and carboplatin.

spindle of dividing cells. Taxanes cause mitotic arrest by forming abnormal spindle fibres. One of the common toxicities of these agents is peripheral neutropathy. Examples are vincristine and paclitaxel.

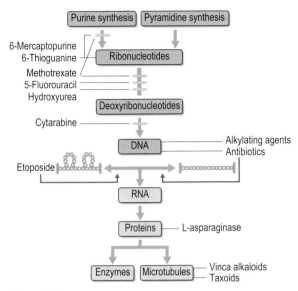

Figure 4.6
Sites of action of various chemotherapeutic agents.

Box 4.11: Sanctuary sites

Systemic treatments by definition are thought to act at all areas of the body via the bloodstream. However there are areas which have been referred to as sanctuary sites as traditionally chemotherapy is not thought to access them via the bloodstream. These are the central nervous system and the testes. The central nervous system is separated by tight junctions from the cerebral vasculature such that most drugs do not cross the blood–brain barrier. For this reason disease in this area often has to be treated directly by the intrathecal route or using radiotherapy. Some fat soluble drugs e.g. nitrosoureas are thought to be able to cross this barrier. It is also possible that in advanced disease where the vasculature is abnormal and friable that many drugs will be able to enter the brain even if not lipid soluble.

The testes are also a sanctuary site such that testicular biopsies may be performed to assess involvement in acute leukaemia and in testicular tumours, the cancerous testicle needs to be removed even after intensive chemotherapy.

Epipodophyllotoxins

A plant derived compound (from the mandrake plant) which acts at several parts of the cell cycle. They prevent entry into G1/2 and the S phase but also have activity on topoisomerase II. Topoisomerases are the enzymes responsible for maintaining the topology of DNA. Common toxicity is myelosuppression. An example is etoposide (VP-16).

Camptothecans

This group inhibit topoisomerase I, a nuclear enzyme responsible for maintaining nuclear structure, which interferes with both transcription and replication of DNA by preventing DNA supercoiling. They act in S phase. Their name is derived from the tree *Camptotheca acuminata*. Examples are irinotecan and topotecan.

Cell cycle phase non-specific drugs act at any point in the cell cycle.

Antitumour antibiotics

This group of drugs interfere with DNA-directed RNA synthesis by intercalating between the base pairs of DNA and generating toxic oxygen-free radicals, causing single or double stranded breaks. Most of these drugs are isolated from a number of *Streptomyces* bacteria. Common tox-icities include mucositis and myelosuppression. Examples are epirubicin and bleomycin.

Alkylating agents

These bind to DNA adding alkyl groups to the cancer cells which results in cross-linking and strand breakage of the DNA with destruction of the DNA template. Destruction of the DNA template stops replication and leads to cell lysis. Examples are chlorambucil and platinums such as cisplatin and carboplatin.

Nitrosoureas

Nitrosoureas are lipid soluble alkylating agents which also destroy DNA preventing any further DNA synthesis. Due to their lipid solubility they can cross the blood–brain barrier into the CNS (see Box 4.11) and are used in several CNS protocols. Examples are lomustine and carmustine.

Delivery of chemotherapy

Consent

Prior to the prescribing and administration of chemotherapy, a definite histological diagnosis (exceptions include germ cell tumours and choriocarcinoma where elevated tumour markers in the appropriate clinical setting is sufficient) and informed consent is necessary. Informed consent

Box 4.12: What do your patients want to know about their systemic treatment?

- The intended benefits (improvement in survival or symptoms)
- Names of the drugs
- Major and frequent side effects
- What to do and who to call with problems and when
- How the drugs will be given (oral, IV bolus, IV infusion)
- How long it will take to give the drugs
- How often will they have treatment and for how many cycles
- When they need to come back to hospital for treatment and for an appointment

is obtained after detailed discussion of benefits and side effects of the treatment (Box 4.12).

Prescribing chemotherapy

Prescribing and reviewing chemotherapy charts is an important role of an oncologist. Many hospitals now have charts which have preprinted chemotherapeutic and supportive drugs on the charts (Figure 4.7) which require only a dose calculation, patient details and test results to be added. Others have electronic systems with that information included. Some of these charts are very simple with all supportive drugs included. In some hospitals however the entire chart has to be written by hand and safety checks are

Oncology Centre: Chemotherapy Prescription Chart							Carboplatin

DATE:

Hb		Neuts		Wt		**Dose Modifications/Other Instructions:**	**Addressograph or** Name:
WBC		Serum Creat		SA			Date of Birth:
Platelets		Cr/Cl or EDTA		Height			Hosp Number:

Cockcroft formula - please complete to show workings:

Male: [1.25 x (140-age) x weight (kg)] =   Female: [1.05 x (140-age) x weight (kg)] =
     Serum creatinine (μmol/l)   Serum creatinine (μmol/l)

Calvert formula:
Dose (mg) for AUC5 =
(EDTA GFR (ml/min) + 25) x 5 =

Performance status 0 1 2 3 4

Consultant:

Cycle 1 of 6		ALLERGIES:					Ward/Dept:

Date	PREMEDICATION	Dose	Route	Rate	Special Instructions	Drs sig	Time	Check	Admin
	Ondansetron	8mg	po	Stat	≥ 30 mins pre chemo				
	Dexamethasone	8mg	po	Stat	≥ 30 mins pre chemo				

Date	CYTOTOXIC DRUGS	Dose	Route	Rate	Volume	Special Instructions	OP Pharm Cyto Pharm	Batch Number Date	Start Time Stop Time	Admin Check
Day 1										
	Carboplatin AUC 5/6/7 5% Dextrose	mg	IV	30 mins	500ml					

Date	TTO's	Dose	Route	Freq	Instructions	Instructions continued
	Domperidone	20mg	po	QDS	PRN for 5 days post chemotherapy	
	Ondansetron	8mg	po	OM	For 5 days post chemotherapy	

NB: Next cycle due in 21 days

Figure 4.7
A sample chemotherapy prescription chart.

- Is the allergy box filled in and does it contain anything which causes concern for the chemotherapy or supportive drugs?
- Is this the correct chart for that treatment?
- Is the performance status appropriate for the type and intent of treatment?
- Are the height and weight accurate and up to date?
- Is the body surface area correct? (Have your own calculator or check on a computer).
- Has the baseline imaging been performed and the mid treatment imaging booked to allow assessment of response?
- Has a GFR been performed (for drugs such as carboplatin, ifosfamide)?
- Has a MUGA been performed (for anthracyclines and herceptin)? Does the next MUGA need to be booked?
- Has the patient previously received a similar drug which limits the dose and (e.g. anthracyclines) has the cumulative dose been recorded?
- Are the appropriate blood results available and are they in the correct range for the drugs being given? Has there been a significant deterioration in a blood result which could be attributable to one of the chemotherapy drugs?
- Does the dose need modifying on the next cycle due to toxicity? (you may only know this after reviewing the patient).
- Does the patient have significant co-morbidities which due to the toxicities of the chemotherapy may require dose reduction?

Box 4.14: Prescribing carboplatin: AUC and the Calvert formula

The required dose is calculated by the following formula:

$$Dose = AUC \times (GFR + 25)$$

where AUC is the area under the curve. It refers to increasing dosages which have an increasing effect until the effect plateaus and any increase in dose results only in increased toxicity. In general AUC values are in the range 5–7 in adults but up to 9 in children.

especially important in that case. Before the chart is written, given that chemotherapy is toxic, a number of calculations and checks have to be made. These are summarized in Box 4.13.

Chemotherapy is generally calculated based on the surface area of an individual. This is an historic phenomenon based on the extrapolation of doses administered to animals (given as dose per surface area) in preclinical models. However the initial human surface area calculations were based on hemi-body moulds created from wrapping brown paper around a small number of cadavers some of whom were children. In addition many other drugs are given to adults in a flat (or standard) dosing such as paracetamol. Some studies suggest that giving everyone the dose calculated for the average surface area of 1.7 m^2 was as effective as calculating the specific

dose for an individual, but for most drugs the use of surface area calculations continue.

Some drugs are not metabolized in the same way. Carboplatin is the classical example of this type of drug. During the original phase I studies the dose limiting toxicity of carboplatin was thrombocytopenia. However, unlike other drugs, there appeared to be no relationship between the dose administered according to mg/m^2 and the degree of thrombocytopenia. It was known that carboplatin is excreted almost entirely by the kidney and Calvert and colleagues then realized that the drug's toxicity was related to the glomerular filtration rate (GFR). This gave rise to the Calvert formula which is used to prescribe carboplatin (Box 4.14). It requires knowledge of the GFR, ideally calculated by nuclear medicine scan.

Some recent drugs, especially the small molecules such as the tyrosine kinase inhibitor, imatinib, are given as a standard dose which is the same for all patients. For imatinib the standard dose is 400 mg per day.

Routes of chemotherapy administration

Systemic treatments can be given by a number of routes. Chemotherapy is usually given intravenously (IV) but some drugs can be given orally and some as both IV and orally. For some intravenous drugs there are several ways to administer it. For example, 5-fluorouracil (5-FU) can be given as a daily bolus for 5 days every 3 weeks (Mayo regimen) or as a 48 hour continuous infusion every 2 weeks (modified de Gramont) (p. 165). This drug needs prolonged or repeated exposure as it acts in S phase but these two methods produce different toxicity profiles with the Mayo regimen producing more significant stomatitis and myelosuppression whereas modified de Gramont produces significant palmoplanter erythema. Although many clinicians believe the two methods to be equally effective, randomized trials have not been performed for all cancer types so that some oncologists will only prescribe the method used in the original trials.

Some drugs can also given either intrathecally (Box 4.15 and Figure 4.8) or via the intraperitoneal route (Box 4.16 and Figure 4.9).

More recent drugs again have a range of administration routes from intravenous, e.g. monoclonal antibodies, to subcutaneous, e.g. vaccines, to oral, e.g. tyrosine kinase inhibitors. Patients often prefer an oral route of administration or a short intravenous infusion to minimize their time in the hospital but they need to understand that toxicities from oral drugs (e.g. capecitabine) can be as great as those from intravenous drugs and that oral chemotherapy is not a 'gentle option'.

Toxicity recording

In order to minimize side effects and to evaluate how changes in treatment have affected these side effects or the patient's symptoms due to the cancer, accurate recordings of drug toxicity (Box 4.17) must be made. Ideally this should be recorded on a flow chart so that progress can be monitored. It also allows the clinician to record dates of future scans which can be reviewed prior to further treatment. Toxicity should be scored according to an internationally accepted system such as the National Cancer Institute Common Toxicity Criteria and Adverse Events version 3 (NCI CTCAE v3) which can be found at: http://www.fda.gov/cder/cancer/toxicityframe.htm.

Dose adjustment

Although supportive drugs to minimize side effects are usually given prophylactically significant toxicity can occur. Initially the aim would be to change or add to the supportive drugs to reduce toxicity, e.g. different or additional anti-emetics for nausea control, or use of G-CSF to prevent neutropenic sepsis. If the toxicity has

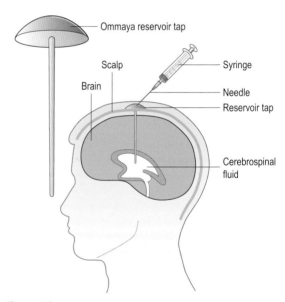

Figure 4.8
Ommaya reservoir.

Box 4.15: Intrathecal (IT) chemotherapy. WARNING – this route can be hazardous!

Drugs delivered directly into the CSF via the intrathecal route can be used to prevent or treat meningeal disease. Prophylactic treatment is given commonly in ALL and in high grade lymphomas likely to involve CNS.

It can be given via lumbar puncture or a central reservoir (Ommaya reservoir) placed by a neurosurgeon in the ventricles.

Extreme care must be taken to prevent administration of a drug not licensed for intrathecal administration as this can be, and has been, fatal. Strict policies should therefore be adhered to and IT chemotherapy should not be given on the same day as intravenous chemotherapy.

Drugs safe to give intrathecally:

- Methotrexate
- Cytosine arabinoside
- Thiotepa

Box 4.16: Intraperitoneal chemotherapy

Surgical placement of a catheter directly into the peritoneum to administer chemotherapy via the peritoneal fluid has been used in several malignancies, notably ovarian cancer and mesothelioma. It allows for large concentrations of drugs to be placed in close contact with peritoneal metastases. Much lower concentrations will also enter the bloodstream. It has shown to be effective in ovarian cancer but is associated with increased toxicity (both systemic and local) and abdominal pain.

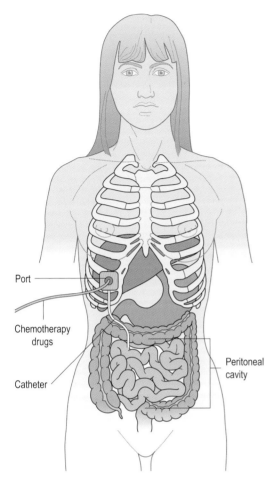

Port

Chemotherapy
drugs

Catheter

Peritoneal
cavity

Figure 4.9
Diagram to show intraperitoneal port and catheter.

been significant, such that it has not resolved with adjustment of supportive drugs, a dose reduction should be made. For example recurrent neutropaenic sepsis which occurs even after prophylactic G-CSF requires dose reduction. For clinical trials there will also be specific instances when this should occur and the protocol must be followed in this case. In general, a reduction of 20–25% is made but this depends on the drugs being given, whether all or only one of them is likely to be the cause. It also depends on the intended outcome of the treatment and the likely effect that dose reduction will have on the outcome. For example it is known that the survival benefit from adjuvant chemotherapy can be reduced by a reduction in dose intensity.

Box 4.17: Chemotherapy toxicities

Acute toxicities are those which occur within a treatment cycle in contrast to late effects which can occur many years later and are covered in (p. 58). Each drug will have its own specific acute toxicities but the following are common to many classes of drugs:

- Nausea and vomiting: tend to occur within hours or days of the chemotherapy but should be controlled with appropriate anti-emetics.

- Diarrhoea and constipation: can occur due to chemotherapy, e.g. diarrhoea after ifosfamide or due to anti-emetics, e.g. constipation with 5HT3 antagonists such as ondansetron.

- Mucositis: inflammation of the gastrointestinal tract is common with some antimetabolites and anthracyclines. It tends to peak the week after day 1 of treatment.

- Myelosuppression causing anaemia or neutropaenia is common to many classes of chemotherapy. It usually occurs 7–10 days after treatment but in some drugs such as nitrosoureas it occurs later (3–4 weeks) which accounts for the longer treatment cycle.

- Infection: is a common source of morbidity for chemotherapy patients but the risks should be minimized by avoiding treating with neutrophil counts which are too low. Dental assessment should also be made before treatment to reduce the risk of oral sepsis and invasive dental procedures should be avoided during chemotherapy. Infection risk is greatest 7–15 days after treatment but can occur at any time which is why fever in a patient on chemotherapy should always be taken seriously.

- Fatigue: a common side effect of many treatments which tends to become more significant over the course of a treatment. It can occur at any time in the cycle but tends to be worse within the first few days of treatment. Patients given steroids as part of their antiemetics can experience increased fatigue the day after the steroids stop.

- Hair loss: is common with many (but not all) drugs. It starts within two weeks of the first treatment so wig referrals should be made before treatment to best match hair colour and style. Alternative is use of scalp cooling which only works for selected chemotherapy regimes.

- Taste change: is very common and can add to problems with appetite.

When consenting patients, do not forget the late effects (p. 58) as these can be significant. Figure 4.10 gives an example of a toxicity chart.

However if the patient has suffered a life-threatening infection associated with the treatment, the risk of death as a complication of continuing the same dose of treatment may be greater than that of recurrence of the cancer.

Toxicity chart												
Trial name:												
Treatment protocol:						**Date:**		**Cycle:**				
Toxicity:	0	1	2	3	4		0	1	2	3	4	
Performance status						Neuropathy						
Fatigue						Stomatitis (oral)						
Nausea/vomiting						Alopecia						
Diarrhoea						Cardiac						
Constipation						Bilirubin						
Haematological (max)						ALT						
Transfusions since last	Plts					Blood pressure						
cycle (units)	Red cells					Height (if myeloma)						
Days in hospital						Weight						
Days on IV antibiotics						Days on antifungals						

Figure 4.10
Example of a toxicity chart.

Complementary therapy interactions

Many patients, especially with advanced cancer, take additional treatments or complementary therapies. Each hospital has a different policy about whether patients are allowed to take complementary medicines alongside their chemotherapy. However it is important to take a full history of these and ensure that certain complementary treatments which can interact with chemotherapy or other drugs. A specific example is St John's wort which many patients take for mild depression. It is metabolized by the cytochrome p450 isoenzymes, especially CYP 3A4 and can significantly interfere with the doses of several systemic treatments including etoposide and the tyrosine kinase inhibitor, imatinib.

Other classes of systemic therapy

Although chemotherapy has been the mainstay of systemic therapy, the development of alternative methods of treatment has occurred in the last 20 years, many of which have made significant improvements in survival. Some of these have been developed against a particular target spe-

cific to the cancer, whereas others have broader actions.

Hormone treatments (Table 4.1)

The observation that breast cancer can regress after oophorectomy and that prostate cancer can be controlled by orchidectomy suggested that some cancers may be hormone sensitive. Since the observation that surgical measures to reduce hormone levels were effective, drugs were developed which would achieve a similar effect. In the 1990s dramatic improvements in breast cancer survival were seen with the introduction of the anti-oestrogen, tamoxifen, to women with oestrogen receptor positive breast cancer. This led to the developments of other drugs which target the production of oestrogen (such as the aromatase inhibitors) as well as examining the role of hormone treatments in other hormone sensitive cancers such as prostate cancer. These are discussed in more detail in the breast and prostate chapters (Chapters 10 and 12). In general these treatments are taken for many years to prevent recurrence or control the disease and can be effective without chemotherapy. In fact there is evidence to suggest that they should not

Table 4.1: Medical hormone treatments

	Example	Mechanism of action
Breast cancer		
Anti-oestrogen	Tamoxifen	Binds with oestrogen receptor
Aromatase inhibitors	Arimidex, exemestane	Inhibits peripheral conversion of androgens to oestrogens by the enzyme aromatase
Prostate cancer		
LHRH antagonists	Goserelin	Negative feedback inhibition of LH from pituitary which decreases testosterone from testis
Corticosteroid	Hydrocortisone	Suppression of adrenal androgen production

be given alongside chemotherapy, particularly for anti-oestrogen therapies in breast cancer as it is thought that these cytostatic agents (e.g. tamoxifen) causes cell cycle arrest preventing the action of chemotherapy which is dependent on rapidly dividing cells for its action.

Bisphosphonates

Bisphosphonates represent a good example of an adjunct in the treatment of cancer. These agents were originally developed to treat osteoporosis but have been shown to be active in stabilizing bony metastases in a number of malignancies and have also been shown to reduce visceral metastases in breast cancer. The exact mechanism for this latter activity is unknown. They can be given intravenously or orally. Examples include pamidronate and zoledronic acid.

Antibodies

Antibodies are immunoglobulins produced by plasma B cells in response to antigens. Several tumour cells express specific antigens which are not produced by normal cells and these have been the target for the development of monoclonal antibodies to these specific antigens. To date the most successful drugs in this class are rituximab and transtuzumab. Rituximab is directed against CD20 found on B cells and the addition of rituximab to standard chemotherapy for B cell lymphomas has significantly improved survival. Transtuzumab has been developed to target the HER-2 receptor which is found in 25% of breast cancers. Initially used in metastatic disease but then in the adjuvant setting for women with HER-2 receptor positive breast cancer, this has also seen a significant improvement in survival.

Other antibodies have been developed with a wider range of action such as bevacizumab which targets the vascular endothelial growth factor receptor. This has shown some improvement in survival in several cancers, which are covered in appropriate chapters. The toxicities of these drugs are different to cytotoxics with allergic reaction being one of the most significant.

Immune therapy

In addition to antibodies, which may be considered an immune treatment, there are also a group of drugs which act by modifying the immune response of the host (patient) in general, rather than targeting a specific molecule or receptor. Examples in this group include interferons and interleukins. High dose interferon has been used in melanoma (p. 235) and interleukin-2 has some efficacy in renal cell carcinoma (p. 176). Interferon and interleukin both produce systemic side effects of an immune response which resemble a viral infection, e.g. fever, fatigue, myalgia and headache.

Small molecules

Small molecules are drugs developed with a specific target, usually to a cellular pathway or molecule within that pathway. Examples include tyrosine kinase inhibitors (TKIs) and mTOR inhibitors. TKIs can be specific to a particular tyrosine kinase, e.g. imatinib, or may have activity across a number of kinases, e.g. sunitinib. Figure 4.11 shows an example of a tyrosine kinase signalling pathway using c-KIT. Once the receptor is bound it sets off a cascade leading to further cell proliferation. Some of the cascade steps are common to pathways involved in many cancers such that effective inhibitors to one protein could be useful drugs in a range of cancers.

Systemic radiotherapy

In general radiotherapy is directed against a specific site in the body. Generally a radioisotope scan is done to assess the uptake by the specific tumour prior to giving definitive radioablative dose (for example, see p. 282). Doses can be repeated several times but there is a risk of late myelodysplastic syndromes.

Assessment of response to treatment

Systemic treatments are often given to treat metastatic disease or neoadjuvantly prior to surgery. In these cases an assessment needs to be made to ensure that the treatment is effective (Figure 4.12) so that an alternative treatment may be considered and to avoid inappropriate toxicity. Most often this assessment is made radiologically (e.g. by CT or MRI) by Response Evaluation Criteria in Solid Tumours (RECIST) criteria (Boxes 4.18 and 4.19, Table 4.2). An understanding of these terms is necessary in the management of all cancers, even if alternative means of assessment may also be used (e.g. see section on gastrointestinal stromal tumours, p. 261).

However for some tumours or in the adjuvant setting RECIST terms may not adequately describe response. In adjuvant treatment where the aim is to cure, the overall survival and sometimes the progression free survival are the key indicators of success. For clinical trials this may take many years to assess so sometimes other indicators are used. These include pathological response for tumours such as bone tumours or breast cancer in whom the patients have been given neoadjuvant treatment. The degree of cell necrosis or pathological response reflects prognosis in these groups. For gastrointestinal stromal tumours which have been treated with a targeted treatment, imatinib, the response assessed by RECIST criteria may not reflect the true response. For these tumours, and other sarcomas there may not be an obvious reduction in the size of the tumour, and yet the patient feels better. Radiologically this is usually accompanied by a change in the density of the tumour becoming more cystic and less dense. For gastrointestinal stromal tumours new criteria (Choi criteria) have been applied to these tumours to take these changes into account (p. 263).

In addition, particularly in the context of clinical trials the term Clinical Benefit is used. This takes into account not only the obvious CR and PR RECIST responses but also those tumours

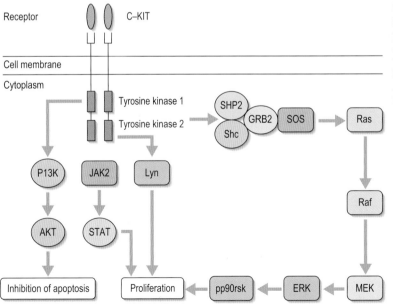

Figure 4.11
Simplified diagram to show signalling pathway of the tyrosine kinase c-KIT and the cascade that follows once the receptor is bound. Targets are being developed to several proteins along this pathway including raf, MEK, P13K and AKT.

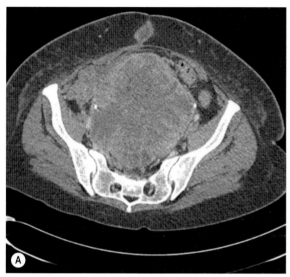
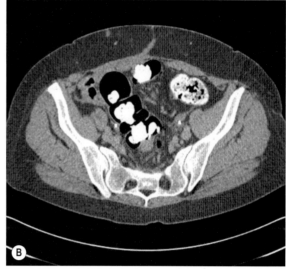

Figure 4.12

CT scan showing a large recurrent uterine sarcoma prior to chemotherapy (A) and after 6 cycles of treatment demonstrating a complete response (B). The patient went on to have radical radiotherapy and remains free of disease 6 years later.

Box 4.18: Definition of lesions for RECIST evaluation

- Measurable lesions – lesions that can be accurately measured in at least one dimension with longest diameter ≥20 mm using conventional techniques or ≥10 mm with spiral CT scan.
- Non-measurable lesions – all other lesions, including small lesions (longest diameter <20 mm with conventional techniques or <10 mm with spiral CT scan), e.g. bone lesions, leptomeningeal disease, ascites, pleural/pericardial effusion.

Box 4.19: Confirmation of response by RECIST criteria

- The main goal of confirmation of objective response is to avoid overestimating the response rate observed. In cases where confirmation of response is not feasible, it should be made clear when reporting the outcome of such studies that the responses are not confirmed.
- To be assigned a status of PR or CR, changes in tumour measurements must be confirmed by repeat assessments that should be performed no less than 4 weeks after the criteria for response are first met. Longer intervals as determined by the study protocol may also be appropriate.

which may be stable by RECIST, but treatment has also been associated with an improvement in symptoms. For palliative treatments this is clearly important.

The future of systemic treatments (Box 4.20)

This chapter has highlighted the growth and growing diversity of systemic treatments for cancer from early fortuitous discoveries of chemotherapeutic agents to the idea of targeted treatments. The future of systemic therapies lies in the development of more specific and less toxic drugs, and the methods to best assess them. It also remains to be discovered how is the best way to

Box 4.20: The future of systemic therapies

- Finding new targeted molecules especially for those cancers with few treatments.
- Finding the best way to assess response for new therapies.
- Learning the best way to combine new therapies either with other new agents or with chemotherapy.

combine drugs, e.g. cytotoxic with a small molecule or a number of targeted small molecules without chemotherapy. This, along with the changing arena of clinical trials, represents one of the great challenges for the future oncologist.

Table 4.2: RECIST response criteria

Evaluation of target lesions	
Complete response (CR):	Disappearance of all target lesions
Partial response (PR):	At least a 30% decrease in the sum of the longest diameter (LD) of target lesions, taking as reference the baseline sum LD
Progressive disease (PD):	At least a 20% increase in the sum of the LD of target lesions, taking as reference the smallest sum LD recorded since the treatment started or the appearance of one or more new lesions
Stable disease (SD):	Neither sufficient shrinkage to qualify for PR nor sufficient increase to qualify for PD, taking as reference the smallest sum LD since the treatment started
Evaluation of non-target lesions	
Complete response (CR):	Disappearance of all non-target lesions and normalization of tumour marker level
Incomplete response/ stable disease (SD):	Persistence of one or more non-target lesion(s) or/and maintenance of tumour marker level above the normal limits
Progressive disease (PD):	Appearance of one or more new lesions and/or unequivocal progression of existing non-target lesions

Further reading

Eisenhauer EA, Therasse P, Bogaerts J, et al. New response evaluation criteria in solid tumours: Revised RECIST guideline (version 1.1). Eur J Cancer 2009;45:228–247.

Brighton D, Wood M (eds). The Royal Marsden Hospital Book of Cancer Chemotherapy. Edinburgh: Elsevier, 2005.

Arkenau H, Carden C and De Bono S. Targeted agents in cancer therapy. Medicine 2007;36(1):33–37.

Cancer genetics

E Copson

Introduction

The last two decades have seen rapid expansion in our understanding of the genetic origins of cancers. Between 5–10% of cancers are due to inheritance of alterations in genes that confer a high life-time risk of certain malignancies, such as breast, colorectal cancer (see Table 5.1), and very rare tumours.

Most of these so-called 'hereditary cancer predisposition syndromes' are due to mutations within a single allele (copy) of a tumour suppressor gene inherited in an autosomal dominant fashion.

Mechanisms of inherited cancer

Tumorigenesis involves contributions from two classes of genes. Oncogenes control cell growth and proliferation under normal circumstances, but once inappropriately activated or overexpressed can promote rapid clonal expansion. Tumour suppressor genes normally inhibit abnormal cell proliferation; reduced expression of these genes can result in uncontrolled cell division. Almost all hereditary cancer predisposition syndromes are due to the inheritance of a germline mutation in a tumour suppressor gene. The inherited mutation inactivates one copy of the gene and the subsequent development of a mutation in the remaining 'normal' copy of the gene results in failure of a cell to produce the tumour suppressor protein (Knudson 'two-hit' hypothesis – see Figure 5.1).

The concept of heritable cancer predisposition was originally developed from observations of an earlier age of onset of retinoblastoma in patients with a positive family history.

Inheritance of two alleles each carrying a mutation within the same tumour suppression gene is extremely rare and can result in a different and more severe phenotype than monoallelic mutation inheritance. For example, inheritance of one BRCA2 mutation from a single parent is associated with breast/ovarian cancer whilst biallelic BRCA2 mutations are a cause of Fanconi's anaemia.

Diagnosis

A hereditary predisposition towards developing malignancy is characterized by young age at presentation, an increased incidence of bilateral tumours, more than one primary tumour site and a family history of specific cancers. The first step requires a detailed family history containing all maternal and paternal cases of malignant disease, with particular emphasis on age of onset and the site of the primary tumour. Wherever possible, verification of these diagnoses should be gained from pathology records.

Analysis of DNA for mutations in known cancer predisposition genes is performed in a limited number of specialist molecular genetics laboratories using DNA derived from a peripheral blood sample. The gold standard is direct sequencing of the whole gene but this is generally not commercially viable for very large genes such as BRCA1/2. Screening for pathogenic mutations is therefore often limited to analysis of coding regions only, or regions of the genes which carry the greatest density of reported mutations. Additional tests are required to detect gene deletions. A full screen for unknown mutations will take several weeks to process. 'Predictive testing', in

Table 5.1: The risk of common cancers associated with inherited cancer syndromes

Tumour site	Genes associated with relative risk of >5.0	Cancer syndrome
Breast	BRCA1/2	Hereditary breast/ovarian cancer syndrome
	TP53	Li–Fraumeni syndrome
	PTEN	Cowden syndrome
	CDH1	Hereditary diffuse gastric cancer syndrome
	STK11	Peutz–Jeghers syndrome
Colorectal	APC	Familial adenomatous polyposis
	MUTYH	
	MLH1	Lynch syndrome (hereditary non-polyposis colon cancer)
	MSH2	
	MSH6	
	PMS2	
Pancreatic	BRCA2	Hereditary breast/ovarian cancer syndrome
	BRCA1	
	MSH2	Lynch syndrome (hereditary non-polyposis colon cancer)
	MLH1	
	STK11	Peutz–Jeghers syndrome
	TP53	Li–Fraumeni syndrome
	PRSS1	Hereditary pancreatitis
	SPINK1	Familial atypical mole malignant melanoma syndrome (FAMMM)
	CDKN2A	
Prostate	BRCA2	Hereditary breast/ovarian cancer syndrome
Endometrial	MLH1	Hereditary non-polyposis colon cancer
	MSH2	
	MSH6	
	PMS2	
Ovarian	BRCA1/2	Hereditary breast/ovarian cancer syndrome
	MLH1	Lynch syndrome
	MSH2	

which genetic testing is directed at establishing whether or not an individual has a specific mutation carried by another family member, is faster.

Genetic counselling

It is essential that any individual considering undergoing genetic screening for an inherited cancer predisposition syndrome receives expert counselling prior to testing and on receiving their result. Patients must be advised that failure to detect a mutation does not always mean that no mutation is present and that further results may become available in the future when genetic testing may become more sophisticated. The roles of genetic counselling are summarized in Box 5.1.

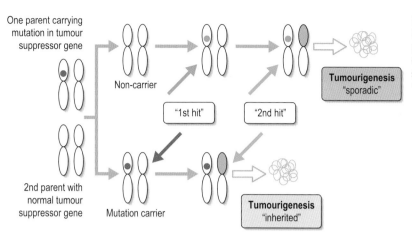

Figure 5.1
Comparison of tumourigenesis pathways in carriers and non-carriers of a mutation in a tumour suppressor gene – the Knudson 'two hit theory'.

Box 5.1: The roles of the genetic counsellor

- Explaining the difference between sporadic and inherited cancer risk.
- Facilitating the documentation of a detailed family history.
- Explaining alternative options to genetic testing, i.e. approximation of personal risk on basis of family history.
- Explaining the risk of passing on a mutation to offspring.
- Identifying the most appropriate family member to undergo genetic testing.
- Ensuring individuals understand the implications of a positive finding of a mutation in a cancer predisposition gene result, including current recommendations for screening and prophylactic interventions.
- Ensuring individuals understand the implications of a negative result, including population screening for common cancers.
- Ensuring individuals understand the implications of an ambiguous result.
- Helping to communicate test results to other members of the family.
- Ensuring individuals understand that genetic testing may result in discrimination by insurance companies.
- Focusing on family health.

Box 5.2: Women at increased risk of breast cancer

Women are generally considered to be at increased risk of breast cancer if they have:

- One close relative diagnosed with breast cancer under the age of 40, or
- Two close relatives (in same blood line) diagnosed under the age of 50, or
- Three or more close relatives diagnosed at any age

The remainder of this chapter will look in more detail at inherited breast and colorectal cancer, and the most common cancer predisposition syndromes.

Inherited breast cancer

Studies indicate that 20–30% of breast cancer patients report a positive family history of this condition (Box 5.2). Approximately 5% of all breast cancer cases are thought to be due to highly penetrant autosomal dominant cancer predisposition syndromes (Figure 5.2). The two most frequent highly penetrant breast cancer susceptibility genes are BRCA1 and BRCA2 where in some families lifetime penetrance for breast cancer can reach 80% but penetrance is clearly modified by other genetic and environmental factors. Much rarer syndromes including Li–Fraumeni, Cowden, Peutz–Jeghers and hereditary diffuse gastric cancer (HDGC) syndromes can be recognized either by other clinical manifestations or by the pattern of cancers in the family (Table 5.2). Lifetime breast cancer risk for carriers of these mutations is in the order of 20–100%. It is likely that most familial clusters of breast cancer are the consequence of multiple low penetrance cancer susceptibility genes acting in conjunction with environmental factors. Within the last few years a number of large case-control studies have identified variants in DNA repair genes (e.g. CHEK2, ATM, BRIP1 and

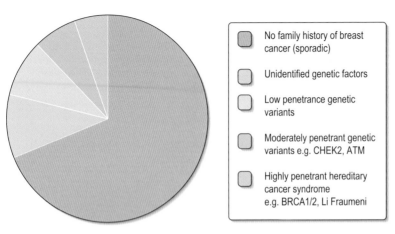

Figure 5.2
The importance of inherited factors in the aetiology of breast cancer.

- No family history of breast cancer (sporadic)
- Unidentified genetic factors
- Low penetrance genetic variants
- Moderately penetrant genetic variants e.g. CHEK2, ATM
- Highly penetrant hereditary cancer syndrome e.g. BRCA1/2, Li Fraumeni

Table 5.2: Cancer predisposition syndromes associated with an increased risk of breast cancer

Clinical syndrome	Gene	Population frequency	Breast cancer risk	Other component tumours
Hereditary breast cancer	BRCA1	1:1000	40–80% lifetime risk	Ovarian
Hereditary breast cancer	BRCA2	1:750	40–80% lifetime risk	Ovarian Prostate Pancreatic
Li–Fraumeni	TP53	<400 families worldwide	30–60% by age 45	Sarcoma Brain tumours Adrenocortical tumours Leukaemia
Cowden	PTEN	1: 300,000	25–50% lifetime risk	Thyroid Endometrial
Peutz–Jeghers	LKB1/ STK11	1:8900–1:280,000	30–55% lifetime risk	Colon Small bowel Pancreatic Ovarian
HDGC	CDH1	Unknown	20–40% lifetime risk	Gastric Colorectal
Ataxia Telangiectasia (homozygotes)	ATM	1:250	RR 2.3	Leukaemia Lymphoma

PALB2), which double the risk of breast cancer. The population prevalence of these variants seems to be in the order of 1–5%.

Hereditary breast/ovarian cancer syndrome

Clinical features
See Table 5.3.

Genetics and pathology

BRCA1 and BRCA2 act as classical tumour suppressor genes; inheritance of mutations occurs in an autosomal dominant fashion and loss of the unmutated allele is found in tumour specimens. The precise functions of the BRCA1 and BRCA2 gene products remain unclear but evidence indicates that these proteins are involved in DNA

Table 5.3: Clinical features of BRCA1 and BRCA2 hereditary breast/ovarian cancer syndrome

Feature	BRCA1	BRCA2
Gene locus	Chromosome 17	Chromosome 13
Population frequency	1 in 400 Increased to 1 in 50 in Ashkenazi Jews	1 in 400 Increased to 1 in 50 in Ashkenazi Jews
Inheritance	Autosomal dominant	Autosomal dominant
Lifetime risk of breast cancer (females)	40–80%	40–80%
Pathological features of breast tumours	Typically high grade with lymphocytic infiltrate and pushing tumour margins, ER, PR, HER-2 negative	No typical phenotype
Lifetime risk of ovarian cancer	40–60%	10–20%
Other associated tumours	Pancreatic	Male breast cancer Pancreatic Prostate

repair and transcription regulation, with additional roles in cell cycle checkpoint control and cytokinesis. Sporadic breast cancers do not contain BRCA1 mutations and very rarely demonstrate BRCA2.

Diagnosis

A number of scoring systems exist to estimate the likelihood of a family carrying BRCA1 or BRCA2 mutations, e.g. the Gail model. Most cancer genetic units recommend screening for BRCA 1/2 mutations if the chance of carrying a mutation is estimated at more than 20%. Oncologists should consider the possibility of an underlying BRCA1/2 mutation in breast cancer patients with the clinical features listed in Box 5.3.

Both BRCA1 and BRCA2 are extremely large genes but screening of all coding regions of the BRCA1 and BRCA2 genes for nonsense mutations can be done within 8 weeks, whilst predictive testing for known mutations can be accomplished within a week. Pre-natal and pre-implantation genetic diagnosis is now available. Over 20% of BRCA1 and BRCA2 screens identify missense mutations.

Primary prevention

For individuals with known BRCA1 or BRCA2 mutations, prophylactic double mastectomy is

> **Box 5.3: Clinical features indicative of a possible underlying BRCA1/2 mutation in breast cancer patients**
>
> - Young age at diagnosis (<35 years)
> - Strong family history of breast cancer, e.g.
>   - 2 first degree relatives with breast cancer, with average age at diagnosis <50 years
>   - ≥3 first or second degree relatives with breast cancer, diagnosed an average age of <60
> - Family history of breast and ovarian cancer
> - Family history of male breast cancer
> - Askenazi Jewish ethnicity
> - Bilateral breast cancer (if first diagnosed at <50 years)
> - (High grade ER/PR/HER2 negative tumour)*
>
> *BRCA1 only.

the most effective preventative measure, reducing the risk of breast cancer by up to 90%. More acceptable to many women is prophylactic oophorectomy which reduces breast cancer rates by 60% and ovarian cancer rates by 95%. The use of chemoprevention with tamoxifen remains controversial.

Secondary prevention

Regular breast screening by mammography, together with clinical breast examinations, has

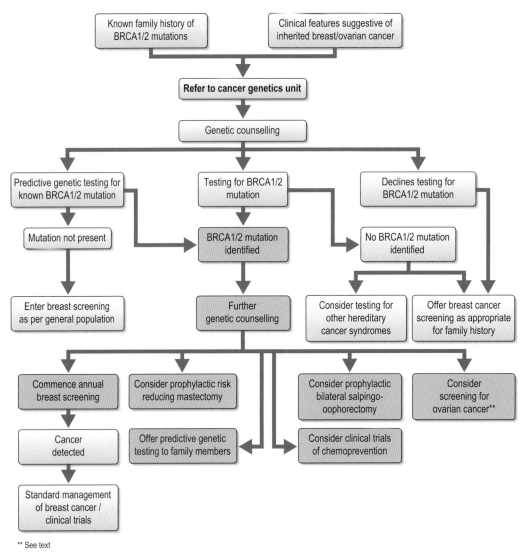

Figure 5.3
Algorithm for management of potential BRCA1/2 mutation carrier.

been recommended for all patients with known BRCA1 or BRCA2 mutations for some years. The 2006 National Institute for Health and Clinical Excellence (NICE) guidelines for the management of familial breast cancer include a recommendation for annual MRI surveillance of all BRCA1/2 mutation carriers aged 30–49 as this method of screening has proved more sensitive then mammography. Screening for ovarian cancer remains under investigation.

Treatment of BRCA associated breast cancer

The management of potential BRCA1/2 mutation carriers is summarised in Figure 5.3 and discussed in Chapter 10 on breast cancer.

Inherited colorectal cancer

Approximately 5% of cases of colorectal cancer are due to an underlying hereditary cancer syndrome, with an increased representation amongst

Box 5.4: Clinical features suggesting underlying inherited predisposition to colorectal cancer*

- Early age onset (<50 years) colorectal cancer or endometrial cancer
- Multiple colorectal carcinomas or >10 adenomatous polyps in same individual
- Individual with an HNPCC related tumour who has either:
  - ≥ One 1st degree relative with an HNPCC-related cancer at <50 years

  OR
  - ≥ Two 1st or 2nd degree relatives with an HNPCC-related cancer at any age
- History of multiple HNPCC related tumours in same individual
- Family with known cancer predisposition syndrome

* See Table 5.4 for HNPCC related cancers.

young colorectal cancer patients. Any features listed in Box 5.4 should raise the suspicion of a familial colorectal cancer syndrome.

Most familial cases are due to either hereditary non-polyposis colon cancer (HNPCC), also known as Lynch syndrome, which accounts for an estimated 2–3% of all colorectal cancers or familial adenomatous polyposis coli (FAP), which accounts for less than 1% of all colorectal cancers. The key features of these two syndromes are summarized in Table 5.4.

In addition, an increased risk of gastrointestinal cancer is also observed in Peutz–Jeghers syndrome, caused by the inheritance of mutations in STK11.

Familial adenomatous polyposis

Clinical features

FAP is characterized by the development of hundreds of colonic adenomatous polyps by the

Table 5.4: Clinical features of FAP and Lynch syndrome

Clinical syndrome	Familial adenomatous polyposis (FAP)	Lynch syndrome
Incidence	1 in 8000	1 in 1700
Clinical features	Extensive gastrointestinal adenomatous polyps from young age with extremely high rate of malignant transformation.	High risk of early onset colon cancer associated with elevated risk of distinct spectrum of extra-colonic tumours.
Risk of colon cancer	Almost 100% by age 40 80% by age 70 in 'attenuated FAP'	70–90%
Extra-colonic tumours	Desmoid tumours (12–17%) Upper gastrointestinal carcinomas (3–5%) Osteomas Thyroid carcinomas Hepato-pancreatic tumours	Endometrial carcinoma (30–60%) Ovarian carcinoma (9%) Stomach (19%) Duodenum Pancreas Urological (18%) Brain Sebaceous adenomas/carcinomas
Inheritance	Autosomal dominant	Autosomal dominant
Genes	APC	hMLH1 hMSH2 hMSH6
Pathogenesis	Activation of *Wnt* pathway and chromosomal instability (see text)	Defective DNA mismatch repair
Pathological features	Adenomatous polyposis	Microsatellite instability

age of 20, with a risk of malignant transformation of almost 100%. The average age of diagnosis of colon cancer is 39 years. Patients are also at increased risk of other tumours listed in Table 5.4.

Genetics and pathology

In more than 90% of FAP cases mutations are found within the APC gene on chromosome 5. Loss of the APC protein results in chromosomal instability due to loss of cytoskeleton control and activation of the *Wnt* pathway which promotes tumorigenesis.

Diagnosis

A clinical diagnosis of FAP can be made by flexible sigmoidoscopy at an early age. Genetic screening for APC mutations is recommended from the age of 10–12 years. Pre-natal diagnosis and pre-implantation genetic diagnosis is available for this condition.

Primary prevention

Carriers of APC mutations should undergo surveillance colonoscopy annually from the age of 10 to 15 years. Prophylactic colectomy by the age of 20 years is recommended for those found to have multiple adenomas on surveillance. The type of operation performed is dependent on the polyp load within the rectum and the age of the patient (see Table 5.5). The cyclo-oxygenase-2 inhibitor celecoxib and non-steroidal anti-inflammatory agent sulindac may both reduce duodenal adenoma formation but severe duodenal polyposis will require a Whipple's resection.

Secondary prevention

Long-term surveillance of the small intestine by upper endoscopy, starting from age 25–30 years, is also required as peri-ampullary carcinoma is the commonest cause of death in FAP patients who have undergone prophylactic colectomy. Regular abdominal examination and/ or imaging should also be considered it there is a family history of desmoids or hepatoblastoma.

Hereditary non-polyposis colorectal cancer

Clinical features

HNPCC is a hereditary cancer syndrome consisting of a high risk of early onset colorectal cancer with an increased frequency of endometrial, ovarian, gastric, duodenal, gastric and urological malignancies. Characteristically, the colonic tumours are predominantly right sided (70%) and there is an increased rate of synchronous and metachronous tumours.

Genetics and pathology

In up to 70% of patients with HNPCC, the underlying genetic defect is a germline mutation in one of three genes: hMLH1, hMSH2, hMSH6. These genes all encode DNA mismatch repair proteins. Defective mismatch repair promotes malignant transformation by permitting rapid accumulation of mutations in other genes, such as those that regulate the cell cycle.

Diagnosis

The National Comprehensive Cancer Network guidelines currently state that a clinical diagnosis

Table 5.5: Surgical options for patients with FAP

Age of patient and rectal polyp load	Recommended operative procedure	Advantages	Disadvantages
Teenagers with modest rectal polyp load Older patients with low rectal polyp load and attenuated polyposis	Total colectomy with ileorectal anastomosis	Can be performed laparoscopically Rapid recovery and lower complication rate Better bowel control	Surveillance of rectum required May require conversion to ileal pouch a few decades later
>20 years with classic FAP and high rectal polyp load	Procto colectomy with ileal pouch	Reduction of rectal carcinoma risk	Frequent defecation and risk of leakage Pelvic infection

At least three relatives must have a tumour associated with hereditary non-polyposis colorectal cancer (see Table 5.4) + all of the following criteria should be present:

- One must be a first-degree relative of the other two
- At least two successive generations must be affected
- At least one of the relatives should have the relevant cancer diagnosed before the age of 50 years
- FAP should be excluded

of HNPCC requires the following minimum criteria, based on the Amsterdam II criteria (Box 5.5).

Analysis of tumour tissue for high microsatellite instability (MSI), using a panel of five or six polymorphic markers, will be positive in more than 80% of patients fulfilling the Amsterdam criteria. Patients with evidence of MSI should be offered genetic screening for germ line mutations of hMLH1, hMSH2 and MSH6. Alternatively, immunohistochemical staining of colorectal tumours for the hMLH1, hSMH2 and hSMH6 proteins has been shown to be highly sensitive and specific in predicting an underlying MMR gene defect. The Bethesda guidelines can be used to identify patients with colorectal cancer where there is young onset or less striking familial clustering of cancers and in whom testing tumour samples for MSI can help direct genetic counselling and testing since less than 15% of sporadic tumours display MSI, but the vast majority of HNPCC related tumours show this phenomenon.

Primary prevention

The role of prophylactic colectomy in the management of patients with HNPCC remains controversial. Some specialists do recommend prophylactic hysterectomy and bilateral salpingo-oophorectomy on completion of child-bearing for female carriers of HNPCC associated gene mutations.

Secondary prevention

Annual colonoscopy screening from the age of 20–25 years is currently the most commonly advocated secondary prevention option for carriers of HNPCC associated gene mutations. Regular upper endoscopy screening should also be considered for HNPCC families with a history of gastric cancer and urine cytology for patients with a family history of urological tumours. All other surveillance recommendations are not evidence-based.

Female HNPCC mutation carriers should be screened for ovarian and endometrial tumours by pelvic ultrasonography with annual transvaginal measurements of endometrial thickness and/or endometrial aspirates.

Management of colonic carcinoma

Subtotal colectomy can be offered to HNPCC patients presenting with a colonic carcinoma, because of the high rate of synchronous tumours in these patients although this must be weighed against the functional consequences of extensive colonic resection.

Li–Fraumeni syndrome

First described in 1969, classic Li–Fraumeni syndrome (LFS), is a rare cancer susceptibility syndrome characterized by an autosomal dominant pattern of diverse neoplasms in children and young adults with a predominance of soft tissue sarcomas, osteosarcoma, and breast cancer and an excess of brain tumours, leukaemia, and adrenocortical carcinomas (see Box 5.6 for definition of classic LFS). Many additional tumours have also been reported in LFS families (see Table 5.6).

Genetics

Germline mutations of the TP53 gene (chromosome 17), are found in approximately 70% of families meeting the criteria for classic LFS criteria, but the detection rate drops as the criteria become less stringent. The protein product of TP53 is a regulator of the cell cycle and apoptosis. Loss of p53 results in cells with mutated DNA dividing in an uncontrolled fashion to form tumours.

Incidence

TP53 germline mutations have an estimated incidence of 1 in 5000. Penetrance is at least 50% by age 50.

Box 5.6: Clinical features of classic LFS

Definition of classic LFS according to Chompret criteria

Proband with sarcoma, brain tumour, breast cancer or adrenocortical carcinoma aged <36

+ ≥ one 1st- or 2nd-degree relative with cancer (other than breast cancer if the proband has breast cancer) < age of 46 years

OR

a relative with multiple primaries at any age

OR

a proband with multiple primary tumours, two of which are sarcoma, brain tumour, breast cancer, and/or adrenocortical carcinoma, with the initial cancer occurring <36 years, regardless of the family history

OR

a proband with adrenocortical carcinoma at any age of onset, regardless of the family history

Table 5.6: Component tumours of classic Li–Fraumeni syndrome and other tumours associated with LFS

Classic Li–Fraumeni component tumours	Other tumours associated with LFS
Breast carcinomas	Leukaemia
Soft tissue and bone sarcomas	Lung
Brain tumours	Gastrointestinal
Childhood adrenal cortical carcinoma	Ovary
(Choroid plexus tumours)	Lymphomas
	Paediatric tumours
	Melanoma
	Prostate
	Pancreatic
	(+ many others)

Diagnosis

TP53 mutations can be detected by sequencing of the TP53 gene.

Clinical management

Females with a proven TP53 mutation should be screened for breast cancer according to the NICE guidelines for high risk individuals, with annual breast MRI from age 30 (NICE recommend an individualized schedule for very high risk women and it may be appropriate to start MRI as young as 20 years in these rare cases).

There is no clinical evidence that tumours in LFS patients behave differently to sporadic tumours, although there has been concern that LFS patients are at a particular risk of second tumours following both chemo and radiotherapy.

Cowden syndrome

Cowden syndrome is an autosomally dominant inherited cancer predisposition syndrome characterized by multiple hamartomas and a high risk of thyroid and breast cancers, with other tumours also at increased frequency.

A clinical diagnosis of Cowden syndrome is currently made according to the International Cowden Consortium operational criteria (see Table 5.7).

Genetics

In 80% of Cowden syndrome families, the underlying mutation is in the PTEN (protein tyrosine phosphatase with homology to tensin) gene, located on chromosome 10. PTEN encodes a phosphatase which mediates cell growth,

Table 5.7: Criteria for clinical diagnosis of Cowden syndrome

Pathognomonic criteria	Major criteria	Minor criteria
Mucocutaneous lesions:	Include:	Include:
Facial trichilemmomas	Breast carcinoma	Genito-urinary tumours
Acral keratoses	Thyroid carcinoma	Lipomas
Papillomatous papules	Endometrial carcinoma	Fibromas
Mucosal lesions	Macrocephaly	Fibrocystic breast disease

proliferation, cell cycle arrest and/ or apoptosis, hence acting as a tumour suppressor.

Incidence

The incidence of Cowden syndrome is estimated to be 1 in 200,000. Inheritance of a germline PTEN mutation is associated with a 25–50% lifetime risk of breast cancer in females.

Clinical management

There is currently no consensus on screening. Individuals with known or suspected PTEN mutations should be referred to their local cancer genetics unit to seek up to date advice about surveillance.

Retinoblastoma

Retinoblastoma is a rare primary malignant tumour of the retina. Unilateral tumours usually present before the age of 4 years (median age 18 months) whilst bilateral tumours present even earlier (median age 13 months). Only 5–10% of patients have a positive family history. Second primary tumours are seen in a quarter of surviving patients with hereditary retinoblastoma, occurring up to 40 years after the initial event. These include sarcomas, melanoma, brain tumours, breast cancers and leukaemia.

Genetics

Germline mutations of the RB1 gene on chromosome 13 are found in over 80% of hereditary or bilateral cases of retinoblastoma and are inherited in an autosomal dominant fashion. The RB1 gene encodes a protein which acts as a transcription regulator, suppressing the expression of genes required for cells to progress through the cell cycle and into mitosis. Penetrance of RB1 mutations is variable and 'skipping' of generations may be observed.

Incidence

Retinoblastoma is very rare, with an incidence of 1 in 20,000 births worldwide. Approximately 45% of cases are hereditary.

Diagnosis

Identification of mutations within the retinoblastoma gene is complicated by the large size of this gene, with numerous different reported muta-tions. Pre-implantation genetic testing has been performed for this condition.

Management

Early identification of a RB1 mutation in the child of an affected parent can permit early diagnosis of retinoblastoma (with the aim of salvage of the eye), by regular fundoscopic examinations from birth. An increased frequency of second tumours has been associated with irradiation.

Von Hippel–Lindau syndrome

Von Hippel–Lindau (VHL) is a rare hereditary cancer syndrome consisting of haemangioblastomas of the retina and central nervous system (particularly cerebellar, medullary and spinal sites), associated with phaeochromocytomas and clear cell renal carcinomas. It is inherited in an autosomal dominant fashion. Hereditary phaeochromocytomas present earlier and are more frequently multiple than sporadic phaeochromocytomas but are less likely to undergo malignant transformation. Renal tumours occur in 25% of VHL families, presenting at a median age of 45 years. They are also more likely to be bilateral than sporadic renal carcinomas.

Genetics

The VHL gene is sited on chromosome 3. Mutations or deletions of the VHL gene are found in virtually all clinically diagnosed VHL families using modern genetic diagnostic methods.

Incidence

VHL syndrome is estimated to affect 1 in 35,000 individuals.

Clinical management

Screening for VHL tumours should be as set out in Table 5.8. Pre-natal and pre-implantation genetic diagnosis is now available for VHL when a mutation has been identified in a family.

Multiple neuroendocrine neoplasia syndromes

The multiple endocrine neoplasia (MEN) syndromes are autosomal dominant disorders characterized by the development of multiple benign and malignant tumours of endocrine glands. The

Table 5.8: Onset of clinical features of VHL and recommended surveillance

Age (years)	Clinical feature	Surveillance
1–10	Retinal angiomas	Retinal screening (from age 5)
11–20	Retinal angiomas Cerebellar haemangioblastoma Phaeochromocytomas	Retinal screening Consider CNS imaging Urinary/plasma catecholamines Start renal imaging by age 20
21–30	Cerebellar haemangioblastoma Phaeochromocytomas Renal cysts	Consider CNS imaging Urinary/plasma catecholamines Renal imaging
31–40	Renal cysts Renal carcinomas Endolymphatic sac tumours	Renal imaging Consider CNS imaging
41–50	Renal carcinomas	Renal imaging

Table 5.9: Clinical features of multiple neuroendocrine neoplasia syndromes

Syndrome	Component tumours	Comments	Genetic defect
MEN1	Parathyroid adenomas Pancreatic islet cell tumours Pituitary adenomas Carcinoid tumours Thyroid tumours	Present in up to 95% of cases Present in 50–75% of cases 25–65% of cases	Mutation in MEN1 gene, chromosome 11.
MEN2A	Medullary thyroid carcinoma Phaeochromocytoma Parathyroid hyperplasia	Up to 100% of cases Usually multifocal, bilateral 40% of cases 10–35% of cases	Mutation in extracellular cysteine codon of RET gene, chromosome 10

MEN2B	Medullary thyroid carcinoma
	Gangliomas
	Phaeochromocytoma
	Also
	  – skeletal abnormalities
	  – megacolon
		Up to 100% of cases
		Usually multifocal, bilateral
		Up to 100% of cases
		40–50% of cases
			Mutation in tyrosine kinase codon of RET gene, chromosome 10

key clinical features of MEN1, MEN2A and MEN2B are summarized in Table 5.9.

Genetics

MEN1 is caused by mutations in the menin gene located on chromosome 11. Menin is a tumour suppressor gene which interacts with a number of nuclear proteins including transcription factors.

Both MEN2A and MEN2B are associated with mutations of the chromosome 10 proto-oncogene RET which codes for a transmembrane receptor tyrosine kinase. The position of the mutation within the RET gene seems to determine whether the clinical features of MEN2A or MEN2 develop.

Incidence

The incidence of MEN is between 0.2–2 per 100,000.

Diagnosis

Direct mutation detection is now available for both the MEN and RET genes.

Clinical management

Regular screening of individuals from MEN1 families or known MEN mutation carriers should commence before the age of 10 and should consist of serum calcium and prolactin measurements. Consideration should also be given to measurements of pituitary, parathyroid and pancreatic hormones as well as imaging of the pituitary gland.

RET mutation carriers benefit from prophylactic thyroidectomy performed between the ages of 3 to 5 years. Screening for phaeochromocytomas should be performed from adulthood.

Summary

In any oncology clinic, a patient with an inherited cancer syndrome will be a rarity. However, identification of the correct underlying high risk genetic mutation can have significant consequences for both the patient and their family by ensuring that the appropriate clinical interventions are adopted to minimize their morbidity from malignant disease. It is therefore essential to document a full family history for all patients presenting with cancer and to refer all patients that do have clinical features suspicious of a hereditary cancer predisposition syndrome for expert assessment and advice.

Acknowledgement

With thanks to Professor Diana Eccles for her helpful comments.

Further reading

Eng C. Will the real Cowden syndrome please stand up: revised diagnostic criteria. J Med Genet 2000;37:828–830.

Callender GG, Rich TA, Perrier ND. Multiple endocrine neoplasia syndromes. Surg Clin North Am. 2008;88:863–895.

Foulkes WD. Inherited susceptibility to common cancers. N Eng J Med 2008;359:2143–2153.

Garber JE and Offit K. Hereditary cancer predisposition syndromes. J Clin Oncol 2005;23:276–292.

Gonzalez KD, Noltner KA, Buzin CH, Gu D, Wen-Fong CY et al. Beyond Li Fraumeni Syndrome: clinical characteristics of families with p53 germline mutations. J Clin Oncol. 2009;27:1250–1256.

Guillem JG, Wood WC, Moley JF, Berchuck A, Karlan BY, et al. ASCO/SSO review of current role of risk-reducing surgery in common hereditary cancer syndromes. J Clin Oncol 2006;24:4642–4660.

Kim WY and Kaelin WG. Role of VHL gene mutation in human cancer. J Clin Oncol 2004;22:4991–5004.

NCCN clinical practice guidelines in oncology: Colorectal cancer screening. www.nccn.org

NCCN clinical practice guidelines in oncology: Genetic/familial high-risk assessment: breast and ovarian. www.nccn.org

NICE clinical guideline 41: Familial breast cancer (issue date October 2006). www.nice.org

Late effects of cancer treatment and survivorship

6

HM Hatcher

Introduction

In the UK the estimated numbers of people living after a cancer diagnosis range from 1–1.5 million. With increasing cancer incidence and survival it is thought that this will rise to represent 1.5–2.5% of the adult population. The 5-year survival for children diagnosed with cancer is now 79% and for adult cancers is 64%. There are a number of medical, psychological, social and economic issues which can significantly contribute to a patient's morbidity and mortality after a diagnosis of cancer. This chapter aims to overview these issues.

Paediatric oncology and the history of survivorship

The median age of diagnosis of cancer in the general population is 70 years but the most significant increase in survival rates in the past 30 years has been in the area of paediatric oncology. Many children were treated in a clinical trial such that the initial survivorship data was gained from paediatric patients. The medical sequelae of cancer treatment as a child have profound consequences due to the current average life expectancy.

Given the dependence of children upon their parents and the developmental needs of a growing child some of their psychosocial survivorship issues are different to those of adults. In addition the families of children treated for cancer are significantly affected and many parents or siblings of childhood survivors suffer long-lasting psychological and social consequences even when the clinical outcome has been good.

Medical late effects

Late effects are dependent upon the original cancer, its treatment, the family genetics and the developmental stage of the individual when treated for cancer. Box 6.1 lists some of the major effects that can occur.

Second malignancy

Second malignancies are the second most common cause of death (after the primary cancer) in those diagnosed with cancer, and can either be a solid tumour or haematological (leukaemia or myelodysplastic syndromes). The risk of second malignancy is increased with combinations of chemotherapy and radiotherapy but is also dependent upon the underlying genetics of the individual and the sensitivity of the tissue irradiated (Table 6.1).

In general secondary solid tumours arise in sites of previous radiotherapy, especially if chemotherapy was also given. The total dose of radiotherapy delivered as well as the type and energy of the treatment and treated volume determine the risk. The tissues most likely to give rise to a secondary malignancy following radiotherapy are bone marrow, thyroid, breast and soft tissues (sarcomas) (Box 6.2).

Leukaemias and myelodysplastic syndromes have been found to relate to previous chemotherapy treatment, especially with etoposide, anthracyclines and alkylating agents. These leukaemias are characterized by a chromosomal abnormality at 11q23, tend to occur within 2 years of primary treatment and have a poor prognosis. Intensive regimens for Ewing's sarcoma or rhabdomyosarcoma have a risk of up to 20% at

© 2011, Elsevier Ltd
DOI: 10.1016/B978-0-7234-3458-0.00011-7

Box 6.1: Medical late effects of treatment

Second malignancy	e.g. leukaemia, sarcoma
Chronic health conditions	e.g. breathlessness, fatigue
Cardiological	e.g. arrhythmias
Neurological	e.g. peripheral neuropathy
Pulmonary	e.g. fibrosis
Endocrine	e.g. GH deficiency
Fertility	e.g. premature ovarian failure
Bone	e.g. osteoporosis
Renal	e.g. hypomagnesaemia

Box 6.2: Learning points

- Secondary tumours are often very aggressive and do not respond as well to treatment as primary tumours of the same histology.
- In Ewing's sarcoma, radiotherapy with greater than 54 Gy is associated with second malignancy but treatment with less than 45 Gy is associated with local recurrence.

Example box 6.1:

A 21-year-old woman was treated for Ewing's sarcoma of the right pelvis with neoadjuvant chemotherapy, debulking surgery, radiotherapy and further chemotherapy. She had a good response to treatment with only a small mass remaining which remained stable on CT scans for 5 years. With increasing symptoms of pelvic and groin pain at 8 years an X-ray then MRI was performed which showed a mass in the left acetabulum (Figure 6.1). The appearance of the mass was not typical for a Ewing's sarcoma and a biopsy was performed. The pathology showed an osteosarcoma. Despite staging showing no distant disease and treatment with chemotherapy, the tumour progressed rapidly, lung metastases developed and the patient died within a year.

Table 6.1: The most common second malignancy after treatment for cancer and some of the identified or proposed causative agents

Type of secondary malignancy	Identified or potential risk factors
Leukaemia	Chemotherapy, e.g. etoposide, anthracyclines
Sarcoma	Radiotherapy for e.g. previous sarcoma or retroperitoneal lymph nodes Genetics, e.g. Li–Fraumeni, hereditary retinoblastoma
Lung	Radiotherapy especially in smokers Potential risk from multiple CT scans for follow-up
Breast	Radiotherapy, e.g. mantle or hemithorax especially if given in late teens or early twenties (up to 4–7 times the standardized mortality ratio)
Uterine	Tamoxifen (risk 1 in 100,000), increased in those with HNPCC
Colorectal	Pelvic or abdominal radiotherapy
Bladder	Pelvic radiotherapy Possibly some alkylating agents (with radiotherapy)

30 years following treatment for Hodgkin's disease. The increased risk of breast cancer in patients treated with mantle radiotherapy for Hodgkin's disease led to the removal of radiotherapy in the treatment of the majority of cases. The relative risk of second malignancy is greatest when treated at a younger age at time of diagnosis and decreases with older age at the time of treatment. In another study, the 15-year cumulative risk of a second malignancy was 11.2% overall, with the greatest number of cases in lung cancer (2.8%), leukaemia (1.5%), colorectal cancer (1.5%) and breast cancer (1.2%).

Infertility

Infertility as a consequence of cancer or its treatment remains a significant issue for young people who have not yet completed their families (Figure 6.2). The risk depends on the gender of the patient and the type of therapy administered as well as the type of cancer (Box 6.3). Overall the fertility of childhood cancer survivors when compared with their siblings is 0.76 for men and 0.93 for women.

20 years of secondary haematological malignancy. Myelodysplastic syndromes have been associated with previous alkylating agents.

The cumulative incidence of any second malignancy increases with time from primary treatment, e.g. from 10.6% at 20 years to 26.3% at

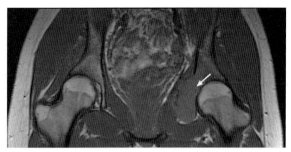

Figure 6.1
Coronal T2 weighted MRI through the pelvis showing abnormal bony texture in the left acetabulum with an irregular margin (arrow) in contrast to the normal right side which shows normal marrow architecture. The left sided mass is an osteosarcoma.

Box 6.3: Risk of infertility in cancer survivors

The greatest risk to fertility in adult survivors is

- Alkylating agents, e.g. ifosfamide
- Procarbazine
- Abdominal/pelvic radiotherapy
- Increasing age, in that women greater than 30 have an increased risk of infertility after chemotherapy (compared with <30) but there is a significant increase in infertility after the age of 40. For example, cyclophosphamide at 5 g/m^2 can cause amenorrhoea in women over 40 but adolescents may continue to menstruate after 20 g/m^2

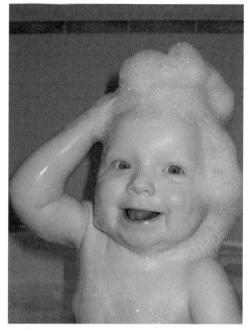

Figure 6.2
Result of successful pregnancy after treatment for cancer!

In the UK, guidelines have been developed by a working party to highlight possible management strategies and risks of infertility with different cancer treatments (Box 6.4). These are available from the Royal College of Radiologist website (http://www.rcr.ac.uk/publications.aspx?PageID=149&PublicationID=269).

Infertility in men commonly occurs after alkylating agents or radiotherapy to the gonadal region or after total body irradiation. For this reason all men who are capable of producing sperm should be offered sperm banking. Sperm aspiration may be considered for those unable to ejaculate e.g. pelvic Ewing's which has affected the sacral nerves. Some men will retain their fertility. This can occur up to 2 years after treatment is completed. Retrograde ejaculation can occur in men who have had bilateral retroperitoneal lymph node dissection e.g. following chemotherapy for a testicular tumour with residual lymph node masses.

Fibrosis of the uterus can occur following pelvic radiotherapy and may cause growth restriction of a developing foetus even if the patient becomes pregnant.

Premature ovarian failure can occur in response to pelvic (or spinal) radiotherapy or certain (but not all) chemotherapy agents. The risk of menopause is associated with the type of therapy rather than the type of cancer. The highest risk for women is those who had radiotherapy below the diaphragm combined with alkylating agents. High-dose treatments (including total body irradiation) and alkylating agents will usually render a woman infertile. Even in those cases where fertility is preserved after treatment, the timing of the menopause is likely to be several years earlier than the patient's peers.

Treatment with anthracyclines as a young adult may require an echocardiogram during pregnancy as cardiac function may be impaired with increased cardiac output requirements due to the developing foetus.

There appears to be no significant increase in congenital abnormalities in the offspring of survivors, nor any increase in childhood cancers in

Box 6.4: Fertility options for women

Currently options are limited for women who require intensive treatment or pelvic radiotherapy and many are costly and not provided by the NHS. Examples include:

- In some cases ovarian suppression with LHRH (leuteinizing hormone releasing hormone) during treatment, e.g. alongside hormonal treatment for their breast cancer (e.g. tamoxifen) rather than removal of the ovaries, allows preservation of fertility for some women.

- Frozen embryos can be successful but the woman needs to be well enough to defer treatment for a few weeks to complete an IVF cycle and egg retrieval. Problems associated with this include the need for a long-term partner to donate sperm to create the embryos, which is often not the case for younger patients. An additional problem is that if the father later withdraws consent for the embryos to be implanted they must be destroyed.

- Oocyte removal after an IVF cycle has also been used, without immediately creating an embryo. Frozen eggs have now given rise to a very few pregnancies and the process is still experimental but the technique is improving so should be discussed if available.

- Research is ongoing using extracted frozen immature eggs which do not require the time delay of a fertility treatment cycle but have yet to be proven to be a reliable option.

- Still in the experimental stages is the storage of ovarian tissue which can later be reimplanted into the patient after treatment.

- Surrogacy can be considered if the woman remains fertile but the uterus is unable to carry a full-term pregnancy due to surgery or radiotherapy.

- Egg donation may be a possibility with or without surrogacy.

- Adoption can always be considered.

Box 6.5: Timing of pregnancy after cancer treatment

Timing of pregnancies for women after treatment for cancer is problematic. If the patient remains fertile they will be advised to start their families earlier rather than later. However, as the risk of relapse occurs in the first few years after treatment for most cancers, and the general advice is to wait at least 2 years after completion of treatment. However a large study showed no increase in rates of relapse for breast cancer patients who became pregnant within a few years of diagnosis.

Patients still on maintenance therapy such as tamoxifen should be advised that pregnancy is not recommended whilst taking these drugs due to the risk for the developing baby.

Box 6.6: Risk factors for hormone induced bone loss and fracture

- Treatment with hormone manipulation, e.g. aromatase inhibitor or anti-androgen
- Smoking
- Heavy alcohol use
- Family history
- Bone metastases
- Increasing age

the offspring, including after bone marrow transplantation (Box 6.5).

Bone late effects

Bone growth is affected by steroids, chemotherapy or radiotherapy (Box 6.6). In addition hormonal manipulation with aromatase inhibitors or anti androgen therapy can have profound consequences on bone loss. Osteopenia occurs frequently at the end of treatment with combination chemotherapy. In ER positive breast cancer where patients may have chemotherapy followed by an aromatase inhibitor, the hormonal treatment compounds the osteoporotic effect of the chemotherapy such that calcium supplementation or bisphosphonates are frequently required to prevent fractures. To minimize the risk of fractures from significant osteoporosis patients should be screened for osteoporosis prior to commencing hormonal treatment using a risk assessment and bone mineral density scan. Patients should be reassessed after 6–12 months on hormonal therapy. Those at significant risk should be advised about calcium in their diet and/or prescribed calcium supplements. At very high risk or after a fracture, bisphosphonates (orally or intravenously) should be prescribed.

Osteoradionecrosis can occur after high-dose radiotherapy particularly to the head and neck region. Pre-treatment dental assessment and corrective procedures are important in preventing this side effect.

Osteonecrosis is a known complication of treatment for leukaemia, lymphoma or bone marrow transplantation and is thought to be due to high-dose steroids. It tends to occur most in weight bearing bones e.g. femur such that arthroplasty of the hip joint may be carried out in up to 20% patients with femoral head osteonecrosis. Osteonecrosis of the jaw is a recognized complication of treatment with zolendronic acid. Patients should see a dental surgeon prior to starting treatment and zolendronic acid should be stopped and further dental assessments made if there is any suspicion of dental abscess.

Neurological

Neurological damage can occur either centrally to the brain itself or to the peripheral or autonomic nerves depending on the tumour and treatment given. For those with CNS tumours, cranial radiotherapy may be given in combination with chemotherapy which can produce combined peripheral and central neurological deficits.

Certain chemotherapeutic agents are known to be neurotoxic such as platinums and vinca alkaloids. The risk is greater with increasing age, particularly over the age of 50 and unless specifically assessed during treatment, the damage may be permanent and debilitating. Painful peripheral neuropathies are most commonly associated with these drugs, especially vincristine. For cisplatin, the symptoms and signs of peripheral neuropathy can progress even after treatment has finished which highlights the importance of detecting deterioration.

Example box 6.2:

A 17-year-old man with medulloblastoma (Figure 6.3A) was treated successfully with combined chemo-radiotherapy followed by further chemotherapy. Although one of his presenting signs was of unsteadiness this deteriorated significantly part way through his chemotherapy such that he was unable to stand or walk unaided. Recurrence was suspected but the MRI (Figure 6.3B) showed no signs of this but showed scarring consistent with previous radiotherapy. On examination of the nervous system, there had been no change in the central features. However, a significant peripheral neuropathy had developed with loss of proprioception below the ankles and wrists. Unfortunately, although his MRI shows no evidence of recurrence 5 years later he has been left unable to walk out of the house unaided and is unable to work due to his peripheral neuropathy (Box 6.7).

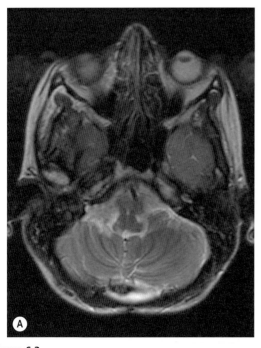

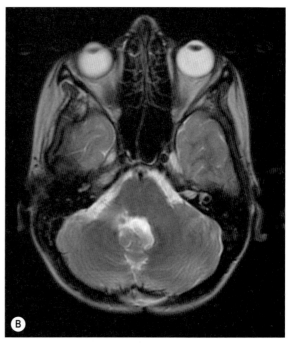

Figure 6.3
MRI FLAIR sequence showing medulloblastoma in right cerebellum prior to radiotherapy (A) and MRI of brain after radiotherapy when the patient presented with worsening neurological symptoms (B).

Hearing loss due to damage to the auditory nerve can occur with platinums, especially cisplatin, so that audiometry should be performed prior to and after treatment.

Neurocognitive impairment can also occur and the risk is greatest amongst survivors of ALL and CNS tumours. Many of these patients are treated at a young age so the impact of neurocognitive impairment reduces their chance of further education or employment. The effects are worse in those treated under the age of 5 and in females.

Gastrointestinal

Following radiotherapy to the pelvis, or abdomen, acute toxicity to the bowel is well known due to inflammation of the intestinal organs. Late toxicity is often underestimated but accounts for significant morbidity (Box 6.8). Intermittent subacute bowel obstruction also occurs. All these symptoms can have a range of causes so referral to a gastroenterologist is recommended for appropriate investigation. Rectal bleeding in particular must not be ignored as this may represent a second malignancy, especially in those who have had pelvic radiotherapy.

Cardiological

Cardiac toxicity can take several forms following treatment including cardiac failure, arrhythmias and increased risk of myocardial infarction (Table 6.2). The major risk factors are mediastinal or left chest wall radiotherapy, anthracyclines and vincristine. Asymptomatic arrhythmias are common. Children treated with anthracyclines have reduced left ventricular wall thickness and reduced left ventricular function which can continue to deteriorate many years after treatment. Treatment with angiotensin converting enzyme inhibitors has been shown to improve left ventricular function in the short term but did not prove effective in symptomatic patients in the longer term.

From the available literature it is difficult to make recommendations on the management and follow up of cardiac and pulmonary complications. It would seem prudent however to reduce other known cardiac risk factors (smoking cessation, and blood pressure and cholesterol control) as part of the suggested lifestyle modifications after treatment.

Pulmonary

Long-term pulmonary toxicities are wide ranging and account for a significant amount of morbidity and later mortality. The types of damage that can occur include fibrosis (from radiotherapy or bleomycin), pneumonitis (radiotherapy, gemcitabine), asymptomatic abnormalities of lung function tests (radiotherapy and combination chemotherapy) or lung cancer (especially after radiotherapy and chemotherapy in patients who continue to smoke). Patients given hemithorax radiotherapy for metastatic Wilms' tumours in childhood are at particular risk.

Endocrine

Endocrine abnormalities can occur in any endocrine organ. The most frequently affected are those who have received radiotherapy close to the pituitary or thyroid (Table 6.3). Hormonal replacement may be necessary for these patients as the hormones involved have significant systemic functions. Abnormalities do not occur immediately after treatment, particularly those from the pituitary or thyroid, so they should be screened for starting at least 1 year post treatment or earlier with symptoms. Adrenal insufficiency should always be considered in patients who have received high-dose steroids, particularly during a period of infection.

Endocrine input is essential in the assessment of late effects in the follow-up clinic.

Obesity

Obesity is a significant problem for survivors of cancer, especially those treated in childhood. The risks are greatest for those treated with cranial radiotherapy, females and those aged 0–4 years at diagnosis. Survivors of ALL have the greatest risk, thought to be due to a combination of

cranial prophylaxis with radiotherapy and the high doses of corticosteroids used.

Chronic health conditions

In addition to specific toxicities the overall health of an individual is likely to be affected after treatment for cancer. Chronic health conditions can include overall health, or any of the above medical conditions which have a chronic effect on an individual's health. It also includes symptoms of chronic fatigue which can cause limitations of everyday life and persist for many years after treatment is complete. In a study of childhood survivors, chronic health conditions occurred in almost all patients with 27.5% experiencing severe or life-threatening health effects. Multiple chronic conditions were also more frequent with 37.6% experiencing at least 2 and 23.8% experiencing at least three significant co-morbidities.

Causes of death after cancer treatment

The main cause of death following a diagnosis of cancer is the cancer itself even after surviving over 5 years from diagnosis. After recurrence the greatest risk of death is from a second malignancy followed by pulmonary then cardiac problems. In one study the standardized mortality ratio was 19.4 for second malignancy, 8.2 for cardiac death and 9.2 for pulmonary death with other causes at 3.3. The risk of death was greatest for women, those diagnosed before age 5 and those with an initial diagnosis of leukaemia or

Table 6.2: Major cardiac problems associated with cancer treatments

Nature of cardiac problem	Causative agent(s)
Arrhythmias (many asymptomatic with impact unknown)	Radiotherapy, multiple chemotherapy agents e.g. anthracyclines, taxanes
Cardiac failure	Radiotherapy Anthracyclines Trastuzumab
Coronary artery disease and myocardial infarction	Supra diaphragmatic radiotherapy Anthracyclines Vincristine

Note:
hypercholesteralaemia is common after chemotherapy

Table 6.3: Overview of most common endocrine abnormalities and their cause

Endocrine organ affected	Hormones affected	Causative agent
Pituitary	Growth hormone TSH FSH/LH	Radiotherapy to brain (pituitary region)
Thyroid	Thyroxine	Radiotherapy to neck or upper chest >15 Gy (scatter effect)
Gonads	Testosterone Oestrogen	Radiotherapy Alkylating agents, radiotherapy to pelvis/TBI
Adrenals	Cortisol	High-dose steroids (mostly haematological malignancies)

CNS tumour. Given the recent change in treatment to reduce mediastinal radiotherapy (a major cause of these sequelae in Hodgkin's disease) it is hoped that these will reduce in the future.

Psychological impact of cancer diagnosis and treatment

Following a diagnosis with cancer patients and their families make psychological adjustments to cope with the treatment and potential outcome. Stress is, not surprisingly, very common and occurs in over 95% of patients. The majority of these will have anxiety and mild depression which may not require treatment. However some will have more significant psychological symptoms and needs including depression, post-traumatic stress disorder, suicidal ideation and various psychoses.

In survivors of childhood cancer there is a greater degree of some aspects of psychological distress in the parents than in the patient themselves. Parents were more concerned about their child's health and thought more often of the cancer and its diagnosis than the patient.

Suicidal ideation and previous attempts at suicide have been shown to be present in up to 12.83% of childhood cancer survivors. Standardized mortality ratios for deaths as a result of suicide in cancer patients are in the order of 1.35–2.9 compared with the general population. Risk factors include male sex, older age, higher disease stage, poor prognosis, poor performance status, alcoholism, other psychiatric illness, fatigue, pain, loss of function and previous or family history of suicide attempts. Lack of family or social support also correlates with increased suicide risk.

Mental health issues must not be underestimated and addressing them throughout treatment will aid with patients seeking help if necessary, even many years later. Recognizing that this is a potential problem and consequence of losses associated with cancer and its treatment allows it to be seen as a normal process which, like the rest of oncology supportive care, should be appropriately managed.

Relationships

On average cancer survivors are less likely to be married and have a higher incidence of divorce than their peers.

Social consequences

When compared with age matched controls cancer survivors have a lower income. They are more likely to have difficulties obtaining life and health insurance or a mortgage after surviving cancer.

Further reading

Ganz PA. Cancer survivorship. Today and Tomorrow. Springer Press. 2007. ISBN-10: 0-387-34349-0.

Mertens A, Yasui Y, Neglia J et al. Late mortality in Five-year survivors of childhood and adolescent cancer: The childhood cancer survivor study. J Clin Oncol 2001;13:3163–3172.

Expert guidance on fertility: The effects of cancer treatment on reproductive functions. Guidance on management. Report of a Working Party. Available from: http://www.rcr.ac.uk/publications.aspx?PageID=149&PublicationID=269.

Helpful websites

The USA National Action Plan for Cancer Survivorship: http://www.cdc.gov/cancer/survivorship/pdf/plan.pdf

SEER survival data: http://seer.cancer.gov/csr/1975_2005/

Palliative care

TV Ajithkumar

Introduction

Palliative care is the active holistic care of patients with advanced progressive illness and includes areas other than oncology. Apart from, managing pain and other symptoms, palliative care is aimed at delivering psychological, social and spiritual support to patients and their family to achieve the best quality of life. Development of cancer palliative care and hospices has gained momentum in the UK since the opening of the World's first hospice in London in 1967 by Cicely Saunders and colleagues. Today, palliative care and end-of-life care are growing areas of research worldwide. This chapter deals mainly with symptom management in cancer patients and a detailed discussion of the principles of multidisciplinary palliative care is beyond the scope of this chapter.

Pain management

Pain control is an important component of cancer management and uncontrollable pain is the major fear for many cancer patients. More than 80% of patients with advanced cancer suffer pain and around 20% of pain in cancer patients may be attributed to surgery, radiotherapy and chemotherapy. Pain control involves two important steps: assessment of pain and management of pain.

Assessment of pain

It is important to assess the multidimensional nature of pain. Intensity of pain, location, duration and factors that modify pain should be assessed. There are various tools to assess the pain and the commonly used ones are shown in Box 7.1.

Management of pain

The management of pain includes analgesics as well as non-pharmacological measures. The World Health Organization (WHO) analgesic ladder (Figure 7.1) has been the gold standard in the management of pain and has been shown to eliminate pain in 80% of patients. The remaining 20% have complex pain which may require specialist interventions. Measures used in complex pain include neuro-anaesthetic interventions, palliative surgery, radiotherapy, chemotherapy, physiotherapy, occupational therapy, and psychosocial care.

Analgesics

Commonly used analgesics are given in Table 7.1. Strong opioids are started at a low dose and titrated according to the clinical need (Box 7.2). Morphine is the strong agent of choice and oral administration is preferred. Transdermal preparations are useful only in stable pain. Some agents may only be prescribed by specialists in palliative care medicine or anaesthetia.

Opioid side effects, toxicity and management

All patients feel some degree of drowsiness when starting or increasing their dosage. This usually wears off 3–5 days after being on a stable dose. Constipation is inevitable and 30–50% patients develop nausea and vomiting; these symptoms should be managed prophylactically. Intolerable side effects necessitate switching to an alternative opioid (Figure 7.2).

Opioid toxicity usually manifests pseudo-hallucinations (shadows at the peripheries of the field of vision), myoclonic jerks, cognitive impairment, and visual and auditory hallucinations.

DOI: 10.1016/B978-0-7234-3458-0.00012-9

Box 7.1: Numerical rating score (NRS) – Wong-Baker FACES Pain Rating Scale.*

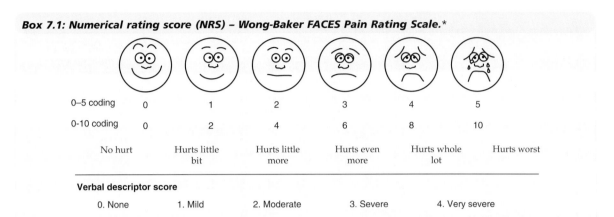

0–5 coding	0	1	2	3	4	5
0-10 coding	0	2	4	6	8	10
	No hurt	Hurts little bit	Hurts little more	Hurts even more	Hurts whole lot	Hurts worst

Verbal descriptor score

0. None	1. Mild	2. Moderate	3. Severe	4. Very severe

*From Hockenberry MJ, Wilson D: Wong's essentials of pediatric nursing, ed. 8, St. Louis, 2009, Mosby. Used with permission. Copyright Mosby.

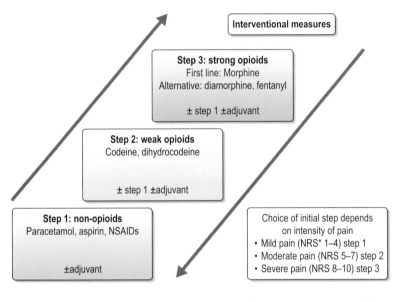

Figure 7.1
The WHO analgesic ladder. *NRS – numberical rating score using 10 point coding.

Initial management includes adequate hydration (dehydration is often a precipitant of toxicity), reduction of opioid and haloperidol (1.5–3 mg oral) for cognitive impairment. If the patient has persistent toxicity without adequate analgesia, opioid switching is needed (Figure 7.2). Though there is no best choice, oxycodone and hydromorphone are the usual alternatives. Naloxone is a short acting opioid antagonist used intravenously for reversing accidental severe opioid overdose.

If pain is relieved rapidly, for example after a nerve block, opioids can be stopped abruptly in many patients without any side effects. However, up to 10% may experience a withdrawal syndrome due to physiological dependence which is managed by reducing doses of opioids over a few days.

Adjuvant analgesics

Adjuvant analgesics (Table 7.2) are a useful complement to regular analgesics in complex pain. These include anticonvulsants, antidepressants, antispasmodics, bisphosphonates, steroids, muscle relaxants and N-methyl-D-aspartate antagonist (ketamine).

Complex pain

Neuropathic pain is often difficult to control. Agents useful to control neuropathic pain are shown in Table 7.2. Amitryptyline along with regular analgesics is the first line management. If

Table 7.1: Analgesics in pain management

Drug	Dose	Precaution	Relative effectiveness compared with oral morphine
Step 1			
Paracetamol	1 g 4-hourly oral	Hepatotoxicity	
Diclofenac	50 mg 4–6-hourly	GI and renal toxicity	
Other NSAIDS		GI and renal toxicity	
Step 2			
Codeine	60 mg 4-hourly oral	Max 240 mg daily	0.1
Dihydrocodeine	60 mg 4-hourly oral	Max 360 mg daily	0.1
Tramadol	50–100 mg 4-hourly	Max 400 mg daily Confusion in elderly	0.1–0.25
Step 3			
Oral morphine: immediate release	Starting dose 2.5–10 mg 6-hourly	Hallucinations and confusion	1
Parenteral morphine	Starting dose 5–10 mg	Accumulate in renal efficiency	
12-hour sustained release – MST continues	12-hourly; dose calculated based on oral morphine requirement		
24-hour release – MXL			
Diamorphine	Parenteral		3
Oxycodone: Immediate release (Oxynorm) Sustained release (Oxycontin)	Starting dose 20 mg	Less hallucination and confusion compared with morphine	1.5–2
Hydromorphone: Immediate release (Palladone) Sustained release (Palladone SR)	Starting dose 8 mg		7.5
Fentanyl: Transdermal Transmucosal Buccal Nasal	12–100 mcg/h over 3 days	Takes 48 hours to reach steady state. Used only for stable pain and relatively safe in renal failure	+4 (12 mcg/h equal to morphine 40 mg/d)
Buprenorphine:			
Oral	0.4 mg		75
IV	0.3–0.6 mg		100
Transdermal	17.5–35 mcg/h		+4 (calculated with conversion from mg/day morphine to mcg/h)
Methadone	10 mg	Useful in neuropathic pain/can be used in renal failure	4 if daily morphine is <90 mg, 8 if 90–300 mg and 12 if >300 mg

Box 7.2: Titration of opioid dose

Step 1
- Start with immediate release opioid (e.g. oral morphine 2.5–10 mg depending on age and intensity of pain) 4 hourly.
- Break through analgesia (immediate release) is given at the same dose as regular dose.

Step 2
- Calculate total analgesic requirement (after 48–72 hours).

Step 3
- Start controlled release preparation at the equivalent daily dose of immediate release (e.g. if oral morphine requirement is 120 mg/day, MST started as 60 mg 12-hourly).
- Breakthrough analgesia is the same analgesia at one-sixth of the regular total daily dose (e.g. oral morphine 20 mg from the previous example).

Step 4
- If patient needs >4 breakthrough doses per day, the baseline controlled release dose needs to be increased by following steps 2 and 3.

pain is not adequately controlled, gabapentin can be either added to amitryptyline or used as substitute. In nerve compression pain steroids or TENS (transcutaneous electrical nerve stimulation) can be considered. Ketamine is useful if these measures fail to control pain. If pain continues to be a problem neuro-anaesthetic interventions such as neural blockade (nerve block, epidural opioids) or neurodestruction (as a last resort) are considered.

Radiotherapy is useful in controlling bone pain. 41% of patients achieve a 50% pain relief within 4 weeks of treatment. Bone pain associated with mechanical instability is difficult to control and often precipitated by movement. In patients with extensive bone metastases, bisphosphonates are shown to reduce skeletal events whereas its analgesic benefit is less clear.

Non-pharmacological interventions

Non-pharmacological interventions such as TENS, acupuncture, relaxation techniques and massage may all be useful.

Nausea and vomiting

Nausea and vomiting are the most common symptoms in cancer management. A thorough clinical assessment including detailed history and examination to establish the cause and severity is important. Possible causes include treatment related (chemotherapy, radiotherapy or other drugs), gastrointestinal pathology (e.g. obstruction), electrolyte abnormalities (e.g. hypercalcaemia), and brain metastases. Investigations are governed by findings from history, clinical examination, and a review of the drug chart and chemotherapy prescription. First-line treatment depends on the possible cause and examples are given in Table 7.3. Levomepromazine (6.25–25 mg subcutaneous per day) and dexamethasone are used as second line treatment.

Constipation

Around 50% of cancer patients will develop constipation, which is due to a number of disease and treatment related causes. Assessment is to evaluate the possible cause(s). Prevention is important, particularly those starting on opioids. Adequate fluid intake should be encouraged except when associated with vomiting related to small bowel obstruction. A combined stimulant/softener is preferred e.g. co-danthramer (2 caps once or twice daily) or movicol is the choice in advanced cancer. Osmotic laxatives are useful in patients who have sufficient oral intake. Rectal preparations are indicated when oral laxatives fail. Glycerol suppositories soften stools while bisacodyl suppositories stimulate the rectum. Resistant cases require an enema.

Diarrhoea

Diarrhoea in cancer patients can be due to chemotherapy (e.g. 5-fluorouracil, docetaxel), pelvic radiotherapy, infection or other medical conditions. Clinical evaluation should be aimed at establishing the cause and severity. Treatment is essentially supportive aimed at improving hydration and correct electrolyte imbalance if any. Infections are treated with appropriate antibiotics. Diarrhoea due to chemotherapy and radiotherapy is treated with dietetic management and loperamide. Octreotide is useful in severe diarrhoea (200–1200 micrograms per day subcutaneously).

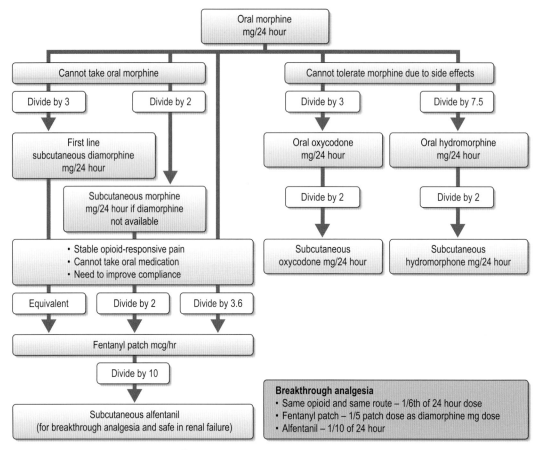

Figure 7.2
Conversion of opioids.

Table 7.2: Adjuvant analgesics

Indication	Drug	Dosage
Neuropathic pain	Dexamethasone	8–16 mg daily
	Gabapentin	100–300 mg (nocte) Titrate to 600 mg TDS
	Amitriptyline	Starting dose 25 mg (nocte) In elderly start at 10 mg
	Pregabalin	150–600 mg
	Carbamazepine	100 mg BD up to 1200 in divided doses daily
	Sodium valproate	200–500 mg nocte
Muscle spasm	Diazepam	2–10 mg daily
	Baclofen	5 mg TDS increased up to max 100 mg daily
Smooth muscle spasm	Hyoscine butylbromide	SC 20 mg stat or SC infusion 60 mg up to 120 mg in 24 hours
Tenesmus	Nifedipine	5/20 mg BD oral

Table 7.3: Agent of choice in nausea and vomiting based on cause

Cause	Treatment – first line anti-emetic
Chemotherapy	Granisetron 1 mg BD PO Ondansetron 8 mg PO BD Dexamethasone 4–8 mg OD PO Metoclopramide 20 mg QDS PO
Radiotherapy	Granisetron 1 mg BD PO Ondansetron 8 mg OD Haloperidol 1.5 mg OD or BD PO
Raised intra-cranial pressure	Cyclizine 50 mg tds PO
Delayed gastric emptying	Metoclopramide 10–20 mg QDS PO Domperidone 10–20 mg QDS PO
Drug induced	Haloperidol 1.5 mg OD or BD PO.
Metabolic e.g. uraemia or hypercalcaemia	Haloperidol 1.5 mg OD or BD PO.

Intestinal obstruction

Intestinal obstruction is common with colorectal and ovarian cancers. Treatment depends on a number of factors. Surgery is the treatment of choice if feasible; however, many patients are only suitable for conservative management. Depending on the level of obstruction, surgical intervention includes bypass surgery, stent or surgical excision. In general surgery is only recommended if there is a single focus of tumour or adhesion causing compression. Multiple areas of involvement or extensive peritoneal involvement is best managed by conservative measures. Conservative management is by bowel rest, nasogastric tube (in case of persistent vomiting), parenteral steroids (to control nausea, bowel oedema and extrinsic compression, control of nausea and vomiting (cyclizine when there is complete obstruction) and metoclopromide (in partial obstruction) and somatostatin analogues to reduce gastrointestinal secretions, promote absorption of fluid and reduce intestinal motility and colic (octreotide 600–800 mcg/day subcutaneously).

Oral infections

Mouth care is important in cancer patients. Immunosuppression and steroids predispose to oral candidiasis, which manifest as white-yellow plaques or as a painful bleeding red area. Treatment is with anti-fungals, e.g. oral fluconazole and may be given prophylactically with high risk treatments. Herpes simplex virus presents as painful, yellow lesions on the oral mucosa. Systemic anti-viral agents and strong opioid analgesics are usually needed. Bacterial infections are treated according to culture results.

Hiccups

Hiccups are a reflex spasm of the diaphragm causing sudden movement of the glottis. Common causes include gastric distension, raised intra-abdominal pressure, high dose steroids and electrolyte imbalance (e.g. hyponatraemia, uraemia). Metoclopramide (10 mg qds PO) is useful in gastric distension. Dimethicone which is an anti-foaming agent which eases flatulence and distension (Asilone 5 ml qds) can be effective. Baclofen (5 mg tds PO) or nifedipine (5 mg tds) can act as smooth muscle relaxants. When these measures fail, chlorpromazine can be used as a central hiccup reflex suppressant (12.5–25 mg daily).

Breathlessness

Breathlessness is the subjective experience of discomfort in breathing. Common causes include disease affecting the lungs, increased intracranial pressure, anaemia and pulmonary embolism. Supportive measures include breathing exercises, a stream of air, either from a fan or through an open window, and treatment of infections, cardiac failure, effusion, COPD and anaemia. Radiotherapy is useful for large tumours and bronchial obstruction. Lymphangitis carcinomatosis is treated with dexamethasone 16 mg daily. Oxygen therapy is useful in patients with SaO_2 <90%. Morphine 5 mg 6-hourly is also useful in breathlessness.

Cough

Cough in cancer patients can be either due to underlying malignancy or due to co-existing non-malignant conditions. Treatment depends on the type of cough and underlying cause. Treatable causes should be appropriately treated. Physiotherapy aids expectoration and repositioning may alleviate the cough (e.g. lying on same side as pleural effusion). Codeine linctus and strong opioids (e.g. oral morphine sulphate) are also beneficial in symptomatic relief.

Haemoptysis

Haemoptysis is managed with oral haemostatic agents (e.g. tranexamic acid), local radiotherapy or bronchoscopic intervention. Massive terminal exanguination requires appropriate sedation.

Depression

Depression is common in cancer patients. In a physically well patient, depression usually manifests as poor appetite, weight loss, and even fatigue. The Hospital Anxiety and Depression Scale (HADS) is useful in diagnosing anxiety and depression. Management is with counselling, psychological interventions and antidepressants. Some cancer centres have a designated psycho-oncology service to assist in the management of these patients. The commonly used antidepressants are:

- Citalopram, an SSRI used as first line treatment of depression at a dose of 20 mg which can be increased to 40 mg.
- Mirtazapine, a noradrenaline and specific serotonin antagonist (NaSSA) given at a dose of 15–45 mg daily.
- Venlafaxine, a serotonin-noradrenergic re-uptake inhibitor (SNRI), the starting dose is 75 mg daily.

Treatment is usually started with one class of agent and if a patient does not respond in 4 weeks, it is changed to another class of antidepressant.

Delirium

Delirium (acute confusional state) is a common psychiatric disorder in cancer patients. Common causes include metabolic abnormalities (hyponatraemia, hypercalcaemia), drug toxicity (opioids, steroids), infection and metastatic brain disease or its treatment. Antipsychotic medications are often needed and the commonly used agent is haloperidol 5–30 mg daily.

Cancer-related fatigue

Cancer-related fatigue has been defined as 'a persistent subjective sense of tiredness related to cancer or cancer treatment that interferes with usual functioning'. The aetiology is multifactorial. Treatment includes relaxation, stress management, regular exercise and psychological interventions.

Cancer cachexia

Cachexia has been defined by a triad of weight loss >10%, reduced food intake (<1500 kcal/day) and systemic inflammation (CRP >10 mg/l). All reversible causes of anorexia should be identified and treated. Nutritional support may be helpful. Progestogens are commonly used to improve appetite and weight. The commonly used agents are megestrol acetate (160–320 mg/day) and medroxyprogesterone acetate (200 mg tds). Steroids may help to improve appetite and give a sense of wellbeing but caution should be used if given for prolonged periods as they can exacerbate proximal weakness.

Symptom cluster

A symptom cluster is defined as three or more concurrent symptoms that are related to each other. Commonly occurring symptom clusters are:

- fatigue, pain and drowsiness
- poor appetite and nausea and anxiety and low mood
- pain, fatigue, low mood and function.

These symptom clusters highlight the importance of treating several symptoms in unison, rather than individually.

End-of-life care

End-of-life care of the cancer patient is most challenging. Management of the primary illness is no longer the priority and the focus of care shifts to optimize symptom control. An important aspect of this is recognition of end-of-life and it is often difficult to make a decision to stop anticancer treatment. This needs a very sensitive approach involving patients, their families and all concerned parties in the care of patients.

In patients with advanced cancer the following signs and symptom suggest that the patient is dying:

- bedbound or immobile
- difficulty managing medication
- confusion
- marked generalized weakness
- drowsy or comatose
- poor appetite and decreased fluid intake.

The Liverpool Care Pathway for the Dying Patient (LCP) is a framework for the care of the dying patient. This framework emphasizes the need to discontinue all inappropriate interventions including monitoring of vital signs, use of IV fluids and antibiotics. All the clinical measures are to improve comfort for the patient. The minimum medications are used to ease distress and pain and medications are given by a syringe driver.

Principles of management of specific symptoms are as discussed previously. Terminal agitation is treated initially with haloperidol and midazolam. Severe uncontrolled agitation may need titrating doses of methotrimeprazine. Respiratory secretions, which produce 'death rattle', should be treated with anti-muscarinic agents such as hyoscine hydrobromide, hyoscine butylbromide and glycopyrronium.

An important psychological aspect of end-of-life care is patient dignity. Place of death should be discussed with the patient and their carers whilst they are still able to make the decision. Although the majority of patients die in hospital many would prefer to die in a hospice or home environment. This may take time to organize so should be considered early in the outcome is poor so that there is sufficient time to make the necessary arrangements.

After death, the death certificate should be issued with appropriate advice on the necessary legal requirements and process of arranging a funeral. Bereavement care is often offered either actively or passively to family members. The family should be offered an opportunity to discuss any unanswered questions which may ease the process of bereavement.

Further reading

Fallon M & Hanks G. ABC of Palliative care. 2nd Edition. Wiley Blackwell, Oxford, 2006.

Part II

Site-specific cancer management

Head and neck cancer

AA Edwards and RL Mendes

Introduction

Head and neck oncology is challenging. It demands a thorough knowledge of head and neck anatomy to guide multi-modality treatment and the treatment itself can lead to significant impairment in important functions such as swallowing, facial expression and speech. Tumours arising within various head and neck subsites can differ in presentation, clinical course and therapeutic options.

Cancers of the head and neck account for around 6% of malignancies worldwide. It is more common among men, with a male-female ratio of 2–3 : 1. Squamous head and neck cancers tend to affect patients between the ages of 40–70 years. The incidence varies geographically – for instance, nasopharyngeal carcinoma is most frequent in the Far East.

Aetiology

The important aetiological factors in squamous cell carcinomas of the head and neck include:

- Tobacco – smoking or chewing tobacco is the strongest risk factor for squamous cell carcinomas (SCC) of the head and neck, with more than 90% of patients having a history of tobacco use.
- Alcohol – increased alcohol consumption is associated with an increased risk of head and neck SCC, and has been shown to have a synergistic effect with tobacco in the development of SCCs.
- Viral infections:
  - Human papilloma virus – About a quarter of head and neck SCC specimens contain HPV and about 90% of these are positive for HPV-16. HPV-16 is particularly associated with oropharyngeal SCC.
  - Epstein–Barr virus has been implicated in nasopharyngeal carcinoma. Plasma levels of EBV DNA before treatment and after radiotherapy have been correlated with outcome and survival.
- Other risk factors:
  - Lower socioeconomic status is associated with SCC of the oral cavity and larynx.
  - Chewing betel quid – a mixture of tobacco, slaked lime and areca nut, wrapped in betel pepper leaf – is popular in India and parts of South East Asia. It is associated the development of oral submucous fibrosis and leucoplakia and is a risk factor for developing carcinoma of the oral cavity.
  - Occupational risk factors include: asbestos (larynx), wood dusts (nasal cavity, nasal sinuses, nasopharynx and larynx), nickel (maxillary sinus) and pesticides (larynx).
  - UV exposure is a risk factor for SCC of the lip.
  - Previous head and neck irradiation increases the risk of subsequent head and neck malignancies.

Pathogenesis and pathology

SCC is thought to develop in a stepwise progression from squamous metaplasia to dysplasia, through carcinoma-in-situ to invasive squamous cell carcinoma. These histological changes are accompanied by molecular alterations which disrupt the regulation of cell proliferation, by inactivating tumour suppressor genes and activating oncogenes.

The majority (90%) of malignant tumours of the head and neck are squamous cell carcinomas. The WHO classification of head and neck cancers is outlined in Box 8.1.

Anatomy

Figure 8.1 shows the anatomical sites in the head and neck. Figure 8.2 demonstrates the anatomical levels of neck nodes and the typical regional lymphatic drainage for head and neck subsites, which are important in planning surgery and radiotherapy. In the unoperated neck, the pattern of lymph node drainage is relatively predictable for different tumour subsites. The risk of occult lymph node metastasis varies according to the primary site and the size of the primary tumour. Clinical assessment of this risk of cervical nodal metastasis dictates subsequent decisions on inclusion of lymph node groups within a neck dissection or radiotherapy target volume during the definitive treatment.

> **Box 8.1: WHO Classification of malignant head and neck tumours**
>
> - Squamous cell carcinoma and variants such as verrucous carcinoma
> - Nasopharyngeal carcinoma
> - Salivary gland tumours – acinic cell carcinoma, mucoepidermoid carcinoma, adenoid cystic carcinoma
> - Adenocarcinoma
> - Lymphoma
> - Small cell carcinoma
> - Carcinoid
> - Sarcoma
> - Metastasis

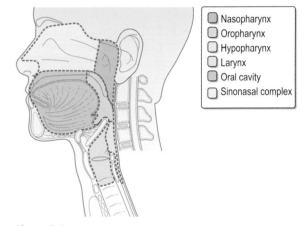

Nasopharynx
Oropharynx
Hypopharynx
Larynx
Oral cavity
Sinonasal complex

Figure 8.1
Anatomy of the head and neck region.

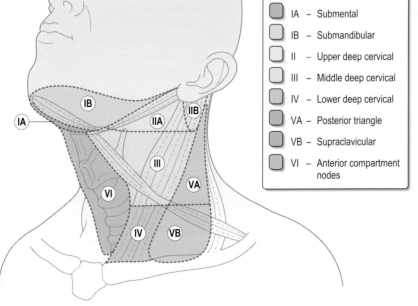

IA – Submental

IB – Submandibular

II – Upper deep cervical

III – Middle deep cervical

IV – Lower deep cervical

VA – Posterior triangle

VB – Supraclavicular

VI – Anterior compartment nodes

Figure 8.2
Anatomical levels of neck nodes.

Presentation

Most patients with head and neck cancer present with local symptoms due to the growth and depend on the site of tumour (see later).

Evaluation of patients with head and neck cancer

Important features in the history for head and neck cancer patients are:

- Duration and intensity of symptoms and signs
- Age
- Socioeconomic status
- Tobacco and alcohol use
- Co-morbid conditions: smoking-related illness, respiratory disease, cardiac disease, diabetes, liver disease, peripheral vascular disease, immunodeficiency, poor nutrition
- History of previous malignancy or pre-malignancy (especially in the head and neck region). In patients with recurrent disease or second malignancy, details of previous surgery and/or radiotherapy should be sought to guide further treatment

Clinical examination

The whole oral cavity and teeth should be inspected carefully (after removing any dentures). The tongue, cheeks, and floor of mouth should be palpated bi-manually. The ears and nose should be examined for mass lesions, discharge or bleeding. The pharynx and larynx should be examined using flexible fibreoptic nasoendoscopy or indirect laryngoscopy and the mobility of the vocal cords assessed. The neck should be palpated for enlarged lymph nodes or thyroid masses. In patients presenting with metastatic carcinoma in a cervical lymph node, an occult primary should be sought, with particular attention paid to the base of tongue, tonsil, nasopharynx and piriform fossae.

Investigations and staging

The objectives of the clinical assessment of a patient with a suspected head and neck cancer are:

- to establish a histological diagnosis
- to stage the disease

- to exclude synchronous tumours of the upper aerodigestive tract
- determine fitness for radical treatments.

Tissue diagnosis

- Fine needle aspiration/core biopsy may be used to sample enlarged lymph nodes.
- Examination under anaesthesia (EUA) with panendoscopy is often used to obtain biopsies to establish a histological diagnosis, and to clinically stage the tumour.

Imaging

- Suspicious cervical nodes may be further characterized by ultrasound examination of the neck.
- CT and/or MRI of the head and neck region are used to assess the extent of the primary tumour and the regional lymph nodes (Figure 8.3). MRI is superior for assessing soft tissue infiltration, cartilage invasion and perineural spread. CT is useful for assessing bone involvement and has the advantage of being better tolerated by patients with swallowing difficulties because of its faster speed of acquisition. USS of the neck also has a role in neck staging.
- CT chest (or chest X-ray) may be needed to rule out pulmonary metastases in locally advanced disease. Chest X-ray, however, may not detect small volume metastatic disease.
- ^{18}FDG PET-CT has a role in assessing suspected tumour recurrence and in detecting occult primary tumours.

Staging

TNM staging is based on the primary tumour size and/or extent, regional lymph node metastasis and distant metastatic spread (Box 8.2).

Management of head and neck cancers

Pre-treatment assessment

Management of head and neck cancers is complex, and needs a multidisciplinary approach. All patients require assessment of performance status, dentition, swallowing and nutrition. Dental assessment is important in minimizing late side effects of radical radiotherapy such

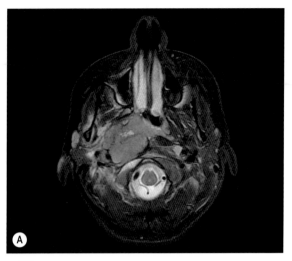
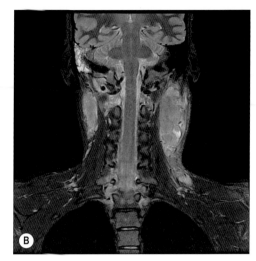

Figure 8.3
MRI of nasopharyngeal cancer.

Box 8.2: A general TNM staging of head and neck tumour

Stage I	T1N0M0	tumour of ≤2 cm
Stage II	T2N0M0	tumour of >2–4 cm
Stage III	T3N0M0	tumour of >4 cm
	T1–3N1M0	ipsilateral single node ≤3 cm
Stage IV	T4N0–1M0	involving adjacent structures
	Any T N2M0	ipsilateral single node >3–6 cm (N2a)
		ipsilateral multiple nodes <6 cm (N2b)
		contralateral or bilateral nodes <6 cm (N2c)
	Any T N3M0	nodes >6 cm
	Any T, any N, M1	Distant metastasis

T4 tumours are divided into T4a (resectable) and T4b (unresectable). Hence stage IV can be IVa (T4a), IVb (T4b) or IVc (M1).

Larynx and pharynx has T staging based on local spread, whereas nasopharynx has separate T and N staging.

---

as dental caries and osteoradionecrosis. Maintaining adequate nutrition is a challenge in patients with head and neck cancer. Patients who are malnourished or at risk of becoming malnourished need dietetic assessment and often intervention is needed. All patients with locally advanced head and neck cancer need a swallowing and language therapy (SALT) assessment prior to radical treatment. Patients are encouraged to stop smoking and minimize alcohol intake during radiotherapy.

Principles of treatment

Early stage disease (stages I–II/T1–2N0M0)

Early stage disease is usually managed with either surgery or radiotherapy. The choice of treatment is based on location of tumour and anticipated morbidity. Radiotherapy results in a local control rate of 85–95% for T1 and 70–85% for T2 lesions. Treatment of the neck should be considered in addition to the treatment to the primary site. Node negative head and neck cancers with a >15–20% risk of occult cervical node metastasis (all cancers except <2 cm lesions in oral cavity and T1 glottic cancers) need elective management of neck nodes – either by a neck dissection or neck irradiation. The level(s) of nodes to be treated depends on the primary site of tumour and T stage, and the choice of treatment modality depends on the treatment of the primary site (Box 8.3).

Locally advanced disease (Stage III–IVb/T3–4N1–3M0)

Patients with locally advanced disease are treated with combined modality treatment. The treatment decision is based on chance of local control and outcome. The options are:

- Surgery followed by postoperative radiotherapy or chemoradiotherapy

Box 8.3: Recommended elective node treatment in stage I–II (T1–2N0) head and neck cancer

Primary site	Nodal irradiation in N0 disease	Selective node dissection in N0 disease
Oral cavity:		
T2 well lateralized	Ipsilateral level I–II	I–III
T2 reaching midline	Bilateral level I–III	
Oropharynx:		
T1 Tonsil	Ipsilateral Ib–II	II–IV
T2 lateralized tonsil	Ipsilateral Ib–IV	
All other N0	Bilateral Ib–V	
Larynx:		
T1–2 Glottic	No nodal radiotherapy	II–IV and if extends below glottis, II–V
T1/2 Supraglottic	Bilateral level Ib–III	
All other N0	Bilateral Ib–V	
Hypopharynx:		
All N0	Bilateral I–V	II–V
Nasopharynx:		
T1N0 squamous carcinoma	No neck irradiation	–
All N0	Bilateral I–V	

- Radical chemoradiotherapy – option for organ preservation
- Nodal dissection followed by chemoradiotherapy

Metastatic disease

The management of patients with distant metastases is essentially symptomatic and supportive. Palliative radiotherapy, surgery and chemotherapy are options in an otherwise fit patient.

Radiotherapy in head and neck cancer (Box 8.4)

Conventional fractionation involves delivering a total dose of 66–70 Gy in 2 Gy daily fraction, 5 days a week. Elective irradiation of the clinically node-negative neck requires a dose of 44–50 Gy in 22–25 fractions.

The indications for postoperative radiotherapy are based on risk factors (Table 8.1). The treatment target is generally the tumour bed and involved neck to a dose of 60–66 Gy in 30–33 fractions (Box 8.4). Consideration may be given to prophylactic nodal irradiation to a lower dose depending on risk.

Alternate fractionation schedule studied in head and neck cancer include hyperfractionation (80.5 Gy in 70 fractions over 7 weeks using two 1.15 Gy fractions per day), accelerated fractionation (68 Gy in 34 fractions giving six fractions per week). The CHART trial failed to improve local control in locally advanced head and neck cancer. Though generally hyperfractionation and acceleration improve local control by a modest amount compared with conventional fractionation, these are not universally adopted in clinical practice because of practicality of delivery and the advent of chemoradiotherapy.

Role of primary chemoradiation (Box 8.5)

A meta-analysis showed that concurrent cisplatin with conventional radiotherapy fractionation results in an absolute 5-year survival improvement of approximately 10% compared with radiotherapy alone. This potential survival benefit needs to be carefully weighed against its increased acute toxicity of adding concurrent chemotherapy to radiotherapy for each individual patient.

Role of postoperative chemoradiation

Two randomized studies (one North American and another European) showed differing benefit and hence its role is not clear.

New treatment approaches

Intensity modulated radiotherapy *(IMRT)* (Figure 8.5) – the role of IMRT in head and neck cancer is evolving, whereby radiation dose can be reduced to critical structures e.g. spinal cord and side effects can be modified, e.g. minimizing salivary gland toxicity with additional scope for increasing the dose to gross disease.

Role of brachytherapy

Brachytherapy using low-dose rate iridium implantation or high-dose rate after loading may be used in a few head and neck subsites at specialist centres. Brachytherapy may be considered for some early tumours of the lip, base of tongue, floor of mouth and anterior tongue, as well as certain small volume tumour recurrences within a previously irradiated site.

Role of chemotherapy

The use of neoadjuvant (induction) and adjuvant chemotherapy in the treatment of locally

Table 8.1: Risk factors for predicting locoregional recurrence in the postoperative setting

	Primary site	Neck nodes
Major risk factors	Positive resection margins	Extracapsular spread
Minor risk factors	Close resection margins (<5 mm)	2 or more involved nodes
	Invasion of soft tissues	More than one lymph node level involved
	Multifocal primary	Involved node >3 cm in diameter
	Perineural invasion	
	Vascular invasion	
	Poorly differentiated	
	T3 or T4 disease	

High risk of recurrence is associated with the presence of one major risk factor or two minor risk factors.

Intermediate risk of recurrence is associated with the presence of one minor risk factor.

Factors of less importance in predicting risk of recurrence include: oral cavity primary site; presence of carcinoma-in-situ or dysplasia at the resection margin; and uncertain surgical or pathological findings.

advanced head and neck cancer has been controversial. A large meta-analysis of trials studying the role of chemotherapy in locally advanced head and neck SCC showed no significant benefit for induction or adjuvant chemotherapy. More recent studies have supported a role for induction chemotherapy in improving laryngeal preservation in locally advanced SCC of the larynx. A study comparing cisplatin-5-FU with docetaxel, cisplatin and 5-FU showed a better survival with three drugs (Box 8.5).

Palliative

Palliative chemotherapy provides a modest benefit in advanced head and neck cancer with objective response rates of 30–40% and median survival around 6 months. Cisplatin/5-FU combinations are most commonly used although capecitabine, taxanes and biological targeting agents are all being studied. Patients who fail to respond to first line chemotherapy should be considered for phase 2 experimental studies. Head and neck cancer provides an ideal template for the study of novel agents as its accessibility permits scrutiny of both tumour control and normal tissue effects. The EXTREME study showed that addition of cetuximab to cisplatin and 5-FU improves overall survival compared to chemotherapy alone.

Role of biological agents

Epidermal growth factor receptor (EGFR) inhibitors have been studied in head and neck cancer. Over 80% of head and neck SCC tumours overexpress EGFR. This is associated with aggressive tumours, resistance to cytotoxic agents and irradiation, hence a poor prognosis. Cetuximab combined with radical radiotherapy is proven to improve both 3-year local control (41% vs. 34%) and overall survival (55% vs. 45%) in locally advanced head and neck SCC compared with radiotherapy alone. Hence NICE recommends the use of cetuximab with radiotherapy in patients with locally advanced head and neck cancer with good performance status in whom platinum-based chemoradiation is contraindicated.

Care during and after treatment

Radiotherapy toxicity is discussed on p. 348. Rehabilitation of the patient after completion of treatment involves input from a multidisciplinary team including clinical nurse specialists, speech and language therapists, dietitians, physiotherapists, occupational therapists, dental surgeons, dental hygienists and prosthetic specialists.

Box 8.4: Radical radiotherapy in head and neck cancer

Radical radiotherapy
- Position – All patients supine with the head in the neutral position, except nasopharyngeal cancer and parotid tumours and tumours of the ear (neck extended). Mouth bite for oral cavity, nasal cavity and sinus tumours will facilitate normal tissue sparing.
- Immobilization – customized shell
- Localization – CT planning
- Target volume definition:
  - GTV – all radiologically visible tumour
  - CTV – with 1–2 cm margin depending on the anatomic area. CTV may need editing in the areas of anatomical barriers to spread
  - CTV – Figure 8.2 shows anatomical boundaries of nodes and Box 8.2 shows nodes need to be treated for N0 disease. For node positive disease, patients generally receive radiotherapy to bilateral level I–V nodes; the exceptions beings well lateralised T2N1 tongue tumours and T1–2N1 tonsil tumours when just the ipsilateral level I–V nodes may be treated
  - PTV – depends on the method of immobilization and ranges from 3–5 mm
- Radiation dose:
  - Phase I (see Figure 8.4)
    - Photons – 44 Gy in 2 Gy per fraction with a lateral parallel opposed beam to the primary tumour and upper neck nodes
    - Photons – 44 Gy in 2 Gy per fraction to anterior neck split with cord and lung shielding
  - Phase II
    - Photons – 22–26 Gy in Gy per fraction with lateral opposed beam moved anterior to spinal cord
    - Photons – 0–6 Gy in 3 fractions to anterior neck split
    - Electrons – if posterior neck nodes, need treatment. A total dose of 44–50 Gy to elective nodes and 66–70 Gy to involved nodes is delivered
  - Bolus is indicated if:
    - there is skin involvement
    - close superficial margin
    - primary electron treatments e.g. pinna
    - postoperative tracheostome site
- Monitoring
  - Follow-up to assess and treat toxicity
  - Haemoglobin should be maintained above 12 g/dl
- Tolerance dose of organs at risk in Gy (at 2 Gy per fraction)
  - Lens 8–10 Gy, cornea 40 Gy, retina 50 Gy, optic nerve 50 Gy, optic chiasm 50 Gy, spinal cord and brain stem 44–48 Gy, hypothalamus 44 Gy

Postoperative radiotherapy
- CTV – surgical bed and areas at risk+1–2 cm
- PTV – dependent on set up error
- Dose – 60–64 Gy in 30–32 fractions to areas at risk 44–50 Gy in 25 fractions to elective nodes

Treatment of recurrent disease

The common pattern of recurrence is loco-regional. The options for managing recurrent disease depend on the initial treatment. Patients who were treated initially with surgery, may be considered for salvage surgery, radiotherapy or palliative chemotherapy or best supportive care.

Patients who developed recurrent disease following previous radical radiotherapy or chemoradiation would be considered for salvage surgery.

The management options for advanced, recurrent or metastatic head and neck cancer depend on factors such as co-morbid conditions, previous treatment, performance status, patient preferences and the nature of their symptoms.

Advanced head and neck cancer can have a devastating impact on personal appearance and vital functions such as speech and swallowing. Quality of life is of paramount importance when deciding management in recurrent disease.

Box 8.5: Systemic treatment in head and neck cancer

Cisplatin with concurrent radiotherapy
- Cisplatin 100 mg/m^2 IV 3-weekly on days 1, 22 and 43 (if GFR is >50 ml/min). This is the regimen employed in the EORTC and RTOG trial of postoperative chemoradiotherapy.
- Cisplatin 40 mg/m^2 (max 70 mg) IV weekly for 6 courses (if GFR is <55 and >40 substitute with carboplatin AUC 5 and no platinum if GFR <40). This regimen is also used in some UK centres.

Cetuximab (when concurrent cisplatin is contraindicated).

The initial dose is 400 mg/m^2 IV followed by weekly doses are 250 mg/m^2 for 2–8 weeks.

Neoadjuvant chemotherapy
- Docetaxel 75 mg/m^2 IV day 1
- Cisplatin 100 mg/m^2 day 2
- 5-Fluorouracil 1000 mg/m^2/day days 1–4

Cycle duration 3 weeks.

Maximum 3 courses, assessment after 2 courses.

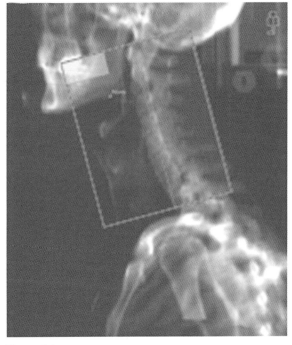

Figure 8.4
Illustration of phases of radiotherapy in locally advanced laryngeal cancer: Phase I treatment volume (green rectagle) includes posterior triangle nodes and during phase II, spinal cord is shielded (red shade). Note shielding of oral mucosa (yellow shade) to minimise mucositis.

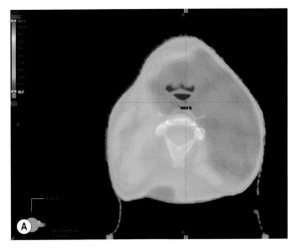
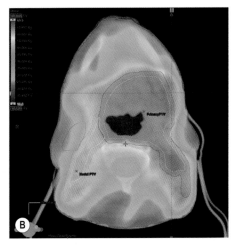

Figure 8.5
An axial CT slice of the neck shows an IMRT plan with (A) concave isodose patterns around the spinal cord, sparing it from the high-dose region and (B) another plan shows sparing of parotid.

Prognosis

The overall 5-year survival for head and neck cancer is around 50%. Prognosis is adversely affected by cervical node involvement. The number of involved lymph nodes, the extent of involved nodal levels and the presence of extracapsular spread all impact overall survival.

Follow-up

Ninety percent of recurrences occur in the first 2 years. A second primary tumour is the leading cause of death of patients successfully treated for early cancers of the head and neck, e.g. lung cancer or other head and neck cancers. Patients are followed up for 5 years to detect recurrent disease and second primary tumours, and in order to manage late morbidity following treatment.

Management of specific cancers

Tumours of the eye

Malignant tumours of the eyelids include basal cell carcinoma and squamous cell carcinoma, which are managed similarly to skin cancers (p. 237).

Malignant melanoma is the most common primary intraocular tumour in adults, which behaves similarly to melanoma elsewhere. In localized disease, treatment is by surgical excision and management of advanced disease is the same as melanoma arising from skin (p. 231).

A variety of malignant tumours, such as sarcomas and lacrimal gland cancers, can arise in the orbit. Sarcomas are managed with exenteration of the eye, with adjuvant radiotherapy with or without chemotherapy (p. 254). Lacrimal gland tumours are treated with complete surgical excision if possible and radiotherapy is indicated for inoperable tumours and for close/positive margins postoperatively.

Cancers of pinna

Management of basal cell carcinomas and squamous cell carcinomas is dealt within Chapter 14 (p. 231).

Cancers of external ear canal and middle ear

Cancers of the external ear canal have a high risk of local recurrence and are therefore treated with an aggressive surgical approach. Middle ear tumours are usually squamous cell carcinoma and evaluation should include high resolution CT scan to assess the extent of disease. Treatment is with radical surgery followed by postoperative radiotherapy. Small tumours may be treated with radical radiotherapy alone. 5-year survival rate is around 10% for advanced disease and 80% for early disease.

Tumours of the nose, nasal cavity and paranasal sinuses

Malignant tumours from this region are a diverse group. 50% of sinonasal tumours arise from the maxillary sinus, 25% from the ethmoid and 25% from the nasal cavity. Squamous cell carcinoma accounts for 50% of these cancers and the remainder include adenocarcinoma, adenoid cystic carcinoma, melanoma, olfactory neuroblastoma and undifferentiated carcinoma.

Clinical features and evaluation

Presentation can be complex, often with features of infection and inflammation, resulting in advanced disease at presentation. Symptoms depend on the site of origin and include epistaxis and nasal obstruction for nasal tumours, eye signs for ethmoidal tumours, unilateral cheek swelling, trismus, oro-antral fistulas and problems wearing dentures for maxillary tumours. Around 5% of patients have neck node disease which indicates a poor prognosis.

Evaluation includes history and examination including eye and cranial nerves I–VI, endoscopy and biopsy and imaging. CT scan is useful in local staging and MRI scanning is beneficial particularly to assess skull base and orbital involvement.

Management

The treatment approach is usually a combination of total surgical excision followed by postoperative radiotherapy. The surgical approach varies with the location of tumour. Patients with clinically involved lymph nodes need node dissection. In those with clinically negative nodes, an elective node dissection may be indicated for patients with high risk of nodal spread (e.g. soft palate). Patients with inoperable loco-regional disease can be treated with radical chemoradiotherapy.

Prognosis

With the combined approach the reported 5-year survival rates are around 30–50%.

Salivary gland tumours

Salivary gland tumours are a heterogeneous group of tumours which usually present in the sixth decade of life. These can arise from the major (parotid, submandibular and sublingual) and also the minor salivary glands of the oral cavity and oropharynx. Around 20% of parotid, 50% of submandibular and 80% of sublingual and minor gland tumours are malignant. The most frequent malignant tumour is mucoepidermoid, followed by adenoid cystic, adenocarcinoma, acinic cell carcinoma and squamous cell carcinoma.

Presentation and evaluation

A common presentation is painless swelling. Pain, nerve palsies, nodal metastasis and fixity of mass can occur in malignant lesions. Minor salivary gland tumours often present as painless submucosal masses.

Clinical assessment includes detailed examination of the mass, oral cavity and oropharynx, assessment of facial nerve and other cranial nerves and examination of regional nodes.

FNA is useful to establish diagnosis. Imaging with CT and/or MRI helps to assess the anatomical extent of the tumour and lymph node status.

Management

The aim of treatment is complete surgical removal with minimal morbidity. This involves total parotidectomy for parotid cancers and wide surgical excision of tumours in other glandular tumours. Neck dissection is needed in those with enlarged nodes but as the risk of nodal recurrence is low in node negative patients it is not routinely advised. A selective neck dissection may be advised in high-grade aggressive tumours.

Postoperative radiotherapy is indicated in cases of close or positive margins, high-grade tumour, advanced disease and those with cartilage, bone, muscle, or perineural involvement. The radiotherapy target volume encompasses the tumour bed with adjacent nodal areas.

Pleomorphic adenoma is a benign tumour of the parotid gland with a long natural history and variable chances of local recurrence. Radiotherapy may be indicated for patients with high risk of recurrence after first surgery and after second and subsequent recurrences.

Prognosis

Overall 5-year survival of T1–2 tumours is 60–75% while that of T3–4 is less than 50% with postoperative radiotherapy. Poor prognostic features include high grade tumour, nodal metastasis, and perineural invasion.

Nasopharyngeal cancer

Nasopharyngeal cancer (NPC) is common in south-east Asia. Factors such as Epstein–Barr virus infection, genetic predisposition and diets including salty fish are thought to increase the risk of NPC in south-east Asia. Smoking also increases the risk. Most of the cancers are variants of squamous cell carcinoma.

Presentation and evaluation

The majority of patients present with a neck node mass (70%). Other presenting symptoms depend on the direction of spread of the local tumour. For example spread through the Eustachian tube can result in unilateral middle ear problems and postero-lateral spread leads to cranial nerve involvement. Multiple cranial nerves can be involved in NPC which include III, IV, VI and IX–XII.

Evaluation is to assess local tumour spread including cranial nerve involvement and nodal involvement. All levels of neck nodes can be involved in NPC. Local staging is with endoscopic examination which also helps to obtain tissue biopsy. CT of the head and neck is obtained. MRI is better in demonstrating soft tissue and submucosal involvement.

Management

Concurrent chemoradiotherapy is the treatment of choice. The target volume for radiotherapy encompasses both the primary tumour site and the bilateral neck nodes. Neck dissection may be indicated for nodal recurrence after radiotherapy.

Prognosis

Stage is the most important prognostic factor. Overall 5-year survival is around 80% for stage I disease and 30% for stage IV disease. Poor prognostic factors include skull base involvement, advanced age, and supraclavicular node involvement.

Oral cavity

Oral cavity tumours account for 30% of all head and neck cancers. Anatomically the oral cavity is divided into lip, anterior two-thirds of tongue, buccal mucosa, floor of mouth, gingival, retromolar trigone and hard palate. The commonest site is lip followed by the lateral border of tongue and floor of mouth. 90% of cancers are SCC.

Presentation and evaluation

Early cancers present as a white or red patch which can progress to an ulcerative lesion. Other presenting features include difficulty in eating and ill fitting dentures.

Evaluation includes detailed history, examination of the lesion including palpation to assess local deep tissue infiltration. Trismus indicates pterygoid muscle involvement with retromolar lesions. Cranial nerve examination and regional nodal examination should also be performed.

Management

Early cancers (T1–2N0) of the lip and oral cavity are curable either by surgery or by radiotherapy. The choice is dictated by anticipated cosmetic outcome and availability of local expertise. In patients with positive margin or deep tumour (>5 mm), postoperative radiotherapy minimizes the risk of local recurrence.

The majority of advanced cancers (T3–T4N+) are treated with a combination of surgery and radiotherapy.

Prognosis

The prognosis depends on the stage and site of the tumour. Early lip cancers have cure rates of 90–100% with surgery or radiotherapy. Tumours without lymph node involvement have a survival rate 65–90% depending on the site of the lesion.

Oropharynx

Anatomical divisions of the oropharynx include the tongue base, the faucial arch, the tonsil and tonsillar fossa, and the pharyngeal wall. The majority of tumours are SCC (85%) and NHL can also occur in the tonsils (10% of tumours). The most frequent sites are the tonsils and tongue base.

Presentation and evaluation

Presenting features include painful swallowing, sore throat, muffled speech and referred ear ache. Up to 20% patients present with neck nodes which can be cystic mimicking a branchial cyst.

Evaluation includes history, examination of the upper aerodigestive tract and neck and a flexible nasal endoscopy. Biopsy of the primary is essential as well as FNA of suspicious nodes. MRI is indicated for loco-regional staging.

Management

Early disease is usually treated with radiotherapy, which results in better function compared with surgery.

Patients with advanced disease need a combined approach with neck dissection followed by chemoradiotherapy if the lesion is midline or involving both sides. Patients with lateralised lesions may be considered for radical resection with reconstruction followed by postoperative radiotherapy. Alternatively, these patients can be treated with primary chemoradiotherapy which may give local control rates comparable to surgery and less morbidity.

Prognosis

Prognosis depends on site and stage. With primary radiotherapy the local control rate is >80% for early stage disease.

Hypopharynx

The anatomical divisions of the hypopharynx are pyriform fossa, postcricoid, and posterior pharyngeal wall. More than 95% of cancers are epithelial, predominantly SCC. The most frequent site is pyriform fossa (60%) followed by postcricoid (30%) and posterior pharyngeal wall (10%).

Hypopharyngeal cancers are aggressive with diffuse locoregional spread and early metastasis. 60% of patients present with locoregional disease and 15–25% have distant metastasis. The most common site of metastasis is lung (80%) followed by liver and bone.

Presentation and evaluation

Presenting features include progressive dysphagia, odynophagia, hoarseness and a neck mass. Some patients present with a metastatic neck node from an occult primary.

Evaluation includes endoscopy and biopsy. Local staging is with CT and MRI.

Management

Most patients present with locally advanced disease. Surgery involves total pharyngolaryngectomy with reconstruction, which is associated with significant morbidity. An alternative treatment is chemoradiotherapy (with or without neo-adjuvant chemotherapy) which improves the chances of laryngeal preservation. Patients with early disease can be treated with radical radiotherapy.

Prognosis

Overall prognosis is generally poor (5-year survival of 15–65%).

Laryngeal cancer

Laryngeal cancer is the most common malignancy within the head and neck. 90% are SCC. The anatomical divisions are glottis, supraglottis and subglottis. Glottic cancers often present as T1 disease and have the best prognosis.

Presentation and evaluation

Hoarseness is the most common presentation. Other features include pain, dysphagia, and odynophagia and referred earache. Presentation as metastatic neck node can occur in supraglottic tumours.

Management

Early stage disease (T1–T2N0) is generally managed with either surgery or radiotherapy. Preservation of the voice is an important factor in determining treatment. In early stage disease both conservation surgery and radiotherapy offer similar survival. Radiotherapy is preferable where the extent of surgery will result in poor voice.

Advanced stage patients are treated with an organ preserving approach using chemoradiotherapy, provided there is no breach of the cartilages of the larynx. Surgical management involves a total laryngectomy, with permanent tracheostomy. Voice rehabilitation is an essential component of treatment in patients who undergo a total laryngectomy. The options of voice rehabilitation include voice prosthesis, oesophageal speech and an electrolarynx.

Prognosis

Glottic cancers have the best prognosis with local control rates of 90% for T1, 75% for T2 and 60% for selected T3 tumours. In patients who recur, salvage surgery yields a 5-year cancer specific survival of 95–100% for T1 and 85–90% for T2 tumours.

Uncommon tumours of head and neck

These tumours include adenoid cystic carcinoma, sarcomas and paragangliomas. Adenoid cystic carcinoma is characterised by perineural invasion and late recurrences including lung metastasis. Surgery followed by radiotherapy is the treatment of choice.

Sarcomas are treated with surgical excision followed by postoperative radiotherapy if high grade or close/positive margins (p. 254).

Paragangliomas arise from neuroectodermal tissue and the most frequent sites are carotid body and jugulo-tympanic region. Surgery is the treatment of choice and in patients who decline surgery, radiotherapy is an option.

Further reading

Argiris A, Karamouzis MV, Raben D, Ferris RL. Head and neck cancer. Lancet. 2008;371:1695–1709.

Grégoire V, Levendag P, Ang KK et al. CT-based delineation of lymph node levels and related CTVs in the node-negative neck: DAHANCA, EORTC, GORTEC, NCIC,RTOG consensus guidelines. Radiother Oncol. 2003;69:227–236.

Machtay M, Moughan J, Trotti A t al. Factors associated with severe late toxicity after concurrent chemoradiation for locally advanced head and neck cancer: an RTOG analysis. J Clin Oncol. 2008;26:3582–3589.

Baujat B, Audry H, Bourhis J et al. Chemotherapy in locally advanced nasopharyngeal carcinoma: an individual patient data meta-analysis of eight randomized trials and 1753 patients. Int J Radiat Oncol Biol Phys. 2006;64:47–56.

Emami B, Lyman J, Brown A et al. Tolerance of normal tissue to therapeutic irradiation. Int J Radiat Oncol Biol Phys. 1991;21:109–122.

Rivera F, García-Castaño A, Vega N, Vega-Villegas ME, Gutiérrez-Sanz L. Cetuximab in metastatic or recurrent head and neck cancer: the EXTREME trial. Expert Rev Anticancer Ther. 2009;9:1421–1428.

Corry J, Peters LJ, Rischin D. Optimising the therapeutic ratio in head and neck cancer. Lancet Oncol. 2010;11:287–291.

Dirix P, Nuyts S. Evidence-based organ-sparing radiotherapy in head and neck cancer. Lancet Oncol. 2010;11:85–91.

Bernier J, Bentzen SM, Vermorken JB. Molecular therapy in head and neck oncology. Nat Rev Clin Oncol. 2009;6: 266–277.

Cancers of the thorax

9

TV Ajithkumar and HM Hatcher

Lung cancer

Epidemiology

Lung cancer is the most common cause of death from cancer in the industrialized world. There are 37,000 new patients per year in the UK and 170,000 per year in USA. Lung cancer is rarely diagnosed below 40 years, but the incidence rises steeply thereafter with a peak at 75–84 years. The median age at diagnosis is 60 years. The life time risk is 1 in 13 in men and 1 in 20 in women in the UK. Lung cancer is responsible for 25% of all cancer deaths in the UK and 28% in USA.

Aetiology

Smoking

Smoking accounts for up to 92% of lung cancer deaths in men and 80% in women. The age-adjusted relative risk of developing lung cancer for people who smoke more than 20 cigarettes per day is 20 times that compared with life-long non-smokers. This risk remains the same until approximately 5 years after smoking cessation and even 15–20 years after stopping smoking there is 2–3 times the risk of developing lung cancer, compared to life-long non-smokers.

Passive smoking causes an average 24% increase in the incidence of lung cancer compared to non-smokers living with non-smoking partners. Passive smoking causes about 3% of the lung cancers.

Environmental and occupational hazards

It has been suggested that up to 15% of cases in men (5% in women) may be attributable to occupational factors in conjunction with smoking.

- Asbestos increases the incidence of mesothelioma as well as lung cancer, particularly in smokers.
- Radon, a radioactive gas released from granite rock, accounts for around 2000 lung cancer deaths (6% of total) per year in the UK.
- Other industrial carcinogens include uranium, arsenic, nickel and vinyl chloride.

Other risk factors

- Lung diseases – previous tuberculosis, silicosis and fibrosing alveolitis may increase the risk of lung adenocarcinomas (called 'scar carcinomas').
- Genetic factors – relatives of patients with lung cancer have a two-fold higher risk of developing lung cancer than the general population. An increased lung cancer risk is observed in carriers of mutations of the TP53 gene and retinoblastoma (RB) gene and in xeroderma pigmentosum, Blooms's syndrome and Werner's syndrome.
- Previous malignancies – long-term survivors of lung cancer are at risk of developing a second lung cancer. The risk of lung cancer is also increased in breast cancer patients who had radiotherapy and are smokers.

Pathogenesis and pathology

Pathogenesis

Lung cancer arises in the mucosa of the bronchi or more rarely in the lung parenchyma. It has been hypothesized that invasive lung cancer is the endpoint of a multi-step process as a result of cumulative genetic abnormalities involved in the regulation of epithelial cell growth and division caused by carcinogens in tobacco smoke.

© 2011, Elsevier Ltd
DOI: 10.1016/B978-0-7234-3458-0.00014-2

Pre-invasive lesions

The two well-known pre-invasive lesions are atypical adenomatous hyperplasia (AAH) and diffuse idiopathic pulmonary neuroendocrine cell hyperplasia (DIPNECH). AAH manifests as localized ground glass areas of less than 5 mm on high resolution CT scan and progresses to invasive adenocarcinoma at an unknown rate. DIPNECH manifests as small nodules and thickened bronchiolar walls associated with a mosaic pattern of air trapping on CT scan, and is a precursor of pulmonary carcinoid.

Malignant lesions

Box 9.1 shows a classification of lung tumours, which is based on light microscopic assessment of patterns of differentiation. The most important distinction is between small cell carcinoma (SCLC: 15–25% of lung cancers) and other carcinomas, collectively called non-small cell carcinoma (NSCLC). These subgroups behave differently in their presentation, natural history and response to treatment.

Small cell carcinoma (SCLC)

SCLC is a highly malignant neuroendocrine tumour and typically presents as large central masses with atelectasis and extensive mediastinal lymphadenopathy. Two-thirds of the patients have detectable metastases at diagnosis and there is a high risk of brain metastases. Microscopically these tumours consist of small round cells with round or oval nuclei and nuclei and scant cytoplasm. Immunohistochemically these stain for cytokeratin as well as neuroendocrine markers (e.g. neuron specific enolase).

Box 9.1: Malignant tumour of lung

- Squamous cell carcinoma and variants
- Small cell carcinoma
- Adenocarcinoma and variants including bronchoalveolar carcinoma
- Large cell carcinoma and variants
- Adenosquamous carcinoma
- Carcinomas with pleomorphic, sarcomatoid and sarcomatous elements
- Carcinoid tumours
- Carcinomas of salivary gland type
- Unclassified

Non-small cell lung carcinoma (NSCLC)

NSCLC consist of the following types:

- Squamous cell carcinoma – which accounts for 30% of lung cancer, presents with large central lesions with associated atelectasis, pneumonitis and hilar and mediastinal lymphadenopathy. Cavitation is seen in up to 10% of cases. Microscopically these tumours show presence of keratin production and/or intercellular bridges.
- Adenocarcinoma (30–35%) – the proportion of adenocarcinoma has been increasing over time with a relative decrease in squamous cell and small cell carcinomas, and this trend is expected to continue. Adenocarcinoma usually presents as small peripheral lesions with a high propensity for nodal and distant spread. A variant of adenocarcinoma called bronchoalveolar carcinoma grows diffusely and has a characteristic appearance on chest X-ray mimicking slowly progressive or non-resolving 'pneumonia'. Histological diagnosis is based on presence of neoplastic gland formation or intracytoplasmic mucin. Immunohistochemical staining with TTF-1 (thyroid transcription factor-1 which is expressed by lung adenocarcinoma and thyroid cancer) helps to distinguish metastastic adenocarcinoma (TTF-1 negative) from lung carcinoma.
- Large cell carcinoma (10–20%) tends to be a relatively large peripheral lesion and has high propensity for regional lymph node and distant metastasis. Microscopically this tumour is diagnosed by exclusion of all other types of lung cancer.

Other neuroendocrine tumours

These tumours have immunohistochemical (e.g. chromogranin) or electron microscopic (neurosecretory granules) evidence of neuroendocrine differentiation. They represent 2% of lung tumours and have heterogeneous behaviour.

- Typical carcinoid can occur centrally or peripherally, are not linked to smoking and have an excellent prognosis. Microscopically these tumours are composed of polygonal cells arranged in distinct organoid, trabecular or insular growth pattern. There will be <2 mitotic figures per 10 HPF and no necrosis.

- Atypical carcinoid shows morphological features of carcinoid with 2–10 mitotic figures per 10 HPF and/or necrosis. These are thought to be intermediate in behaviour between typical carcinoid and SCLC. There is no evidence that there is progression from typical carcinoid to atypical carcinoid and SCLC.
- Large cell neuroendocrine carcinoma has a worse prognosis than atypical carcinoid. These tumours have features of neuroendocrine tumour but do not meet the criteria of carcinoid, atypical carcinoid or small cell carcinoma. There will be prominent necrosis and more than 10 mitotic figures per 10 HPF.

Presentation

More than 90% of patients are symptomatic at presentation of which approximately 30% are due to tumour, 30% are due to non-specific systemic symptoms (anorexia, weight loss or fatigue) and 30% due to metastatic disease. Five percent of patients are asymptomatic and are detected incidentally.

Respiratory symptoms

Cough is the most common presenting symptom (70%), followed by dyspnoea (60%), chest pain/discomfort (50%) and haemoptysis (41%).

Other symptoms

Symptoms due to compression of recurrent laryngeal nerve (hoarse voice), phrenic nerve (breathlessness), brachial plexus (shoulder pain and/or arm pain, sensory changes and muscle wasting in the distribution of C8 and T1–2 nerves) and sympathetic plexus (Horner's syndrome) can occur. Four percent of lung cancer patients present with superior venacaval obstruction (SVCO) and is most common with small cell lung cancer. Pleuritic chest pain and pleural effusion occurs in pleural involvement. Pericardium involvement can present with pericardial effusion and rarely, tamponade. Rarely, dysphagia due to massive nodal disease compressing the oesophagus can occur.

Bone pain is the presenting symptom in up to 25% patients. Liver involvement usually leads to pain if there is massive metastasis. Clinical adrenal insufficiency is rare. Brain metastases at diagnosis occur in up to 10% and present with features of raised intracranial tension, focal neurologic deficits, fits and mental and personality changes.

Paraneoplastic syndromes occur in up to 10% of patients. Box 9.2 lists the paraneoplastic syndromes. SCLC is the most common type associated with paraneoplastic neurologic syndromes.

Box 9.2: Paraneoplastic manifestations of lung cancer

Nervous system
Multifocal encephalopathy[1]
Cerebellar degeneration[1]
Limbic encephalitis[1]
Extrapyramidal syndrome[1]
Stiff-person syndrome[1]
Opsoclonus-myoclonus[1]
Optic neuritis[1]
Sensorimotor polyneuropathy[1]
Lambert–Eaton syndrome[1]
Chronic gastrointestinal pseudo-obstruction[1]

Endocrine
Syndrome of inappropriate ADH secretion (SIADH)[1]
Humoral hypercalcaemia of malignancy[2]
Ectopic Cushing's syndrome[1,3]
Ectopic hCG syndrome[4]
Growth hormone excess[3]

Cardiovascular
Thromboplebitis[2]
Arterial thrombosis
Marantic endocarditis

Musculoskeletal and dermatological
Hypertrophic osteoarthopathy[2,5]
Clubbing[2,5]
Dermatomyositis
Acanthosis nigricans[5]
Erythema gyratum repens
Acquired hypertrichosis lanuginosa[2]
Pruritus[2,5]
Raynaud's syndrome

Haematological
Haemolytic anaemia
Red cell aplasia
Thrombocytosis

Others
Nephrotic syndrome
Hypouricaemia

Commonly seen in [1]small cell lung cancer, [2]squamous cell carcinoma, [3]carcinoid, [4]large cell carcinoma, [5]adenocarcinoma.

Hypercalcaemia either due to excess parathyroid hormone (PTH) or PTH-related peptides is common in squamous cell carcinomas (15%). Hyponatremia occurs in up to 10% of patients, which is either due to syndrome of inappropriate secretion of ADH (SIADH) or to atrial natriuretic factor. SIADH is commonly associated with SCLC.

Signs

A normal physical examination does not exclude lung cancer.

> **General:** cachexia, finger clubbing, anaemia, enlarged supraclavicular lymph node, features of SVCO and Horner's syndrome (in upper lobe tumours).
>
> **Chest:** reduction of breath sounds over a lobe, signs of lobar collapse, inspiratory crackles over a lobe, unilateral wheeze, features of pleural effusion, rib tenderness.
>
> **Other systems:** bone tenderness, hepatomegaly, features of brain metastasis, peripheral neuropathy and proximal myopathy.

Investigations and staging (Figure 9.1)

Evaluation of a patient with suspected lung cancer is to:

- establish histologic type
- define extent of disease (staging)
- assess fitness to undergo the best appropriate treatment.

Imaging

Chest X-ray (Figure 9.2A) may show lung lesion with or without lymphadenopathy. There can be associated lung collapse, pleural effusion, synchronous nodules or pericardial effusion. Bone metastases or bony destruction due to direct invasion can also been seen.

Contrast enhanced CT scan of chest, including upper abdomen (3–10% patients show asymptomatic liver and/or adrenal metastasis – Figure 9.2B&C) should be performed prior to further diagnostic investigations including bronchoscopy.

Lymph nodes of >1 cm in short axis diameter, a central low intensity suggesting necrosis and rounding of the contour of a hilar node where it meets the lung margin suggest malignant lymph nodes. CT is not reliable in assessing lymphadenopathy, to distinguish T3 from T4 disease and in demonstrating chest wall invasion, which all are important in making treatment decision.

CT scan is useful in assessing resectability. Encasement of proximal pulmonary arteries/veins, gross mediastinal involvement by tumour, widespread mediastinal lymphadenopathy and distant metastasis on CT scan suggest an unresectable tumour (96% accuracy). Tumour invasion of central pulmonary artery and vein, involvement of main stem bronchus and tumour extension across the major fissure (anywhere on the left side, above the minor fissure on right), all suggest the need for pneumonectomy for complete resection.

CT scan of brain is done if there is clinical suspicion of brain metastasis or patient is planned to undergo curative treatment.

Bone scan is indicated if there is bone pain or isolated raised alkaline phosphatase.

Tissue diagnosis

Flexible bronchoscopic biopsy can be obtained in 60–70% of lung cancers (central tumours). Sampling using multiple techniques (biopsy, brushings and washings) gives the highest diagnostic yield (sensitivity of 83–88%).

CT guided percutaneous needle aspiration/biopsy – is useful in peripheral tumours. Core biopsies improve the sensitivity compared with aspirates. Complications include bleeding and pneumothorax.

Fine needle aspiration is suitable for sampling lymph nodes, skin nodules and liver and adrenal metastases. Pleural effusion requires aspiration, biochemical analysis and cytology together with multiple pleural biopsies.

Sputum cytology has wide variation in sensitivity (10–97%) and should be reserved for patients with central tumours who are unable to tolerate or unwilling to undergo bronchoscopy or other invasive procedures.

Staging

Stage determines prognosis and guides treatment. TNM staging of lung cancer is given in Box 9.3. Small cell lung cancer can also be staged using a simple staging classification (Box 9.4).

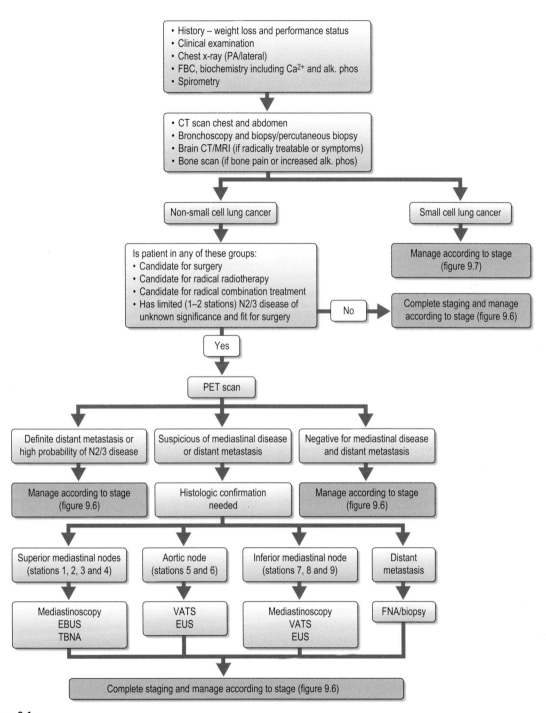

Figure 9.1
Evaluation of lung cancer.

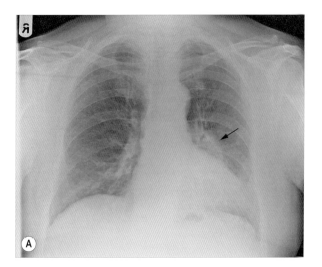

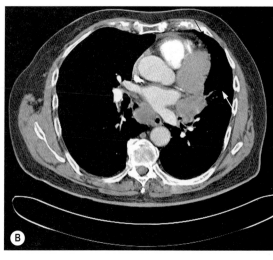

Figure 9.2
Imaging in lung cancer.

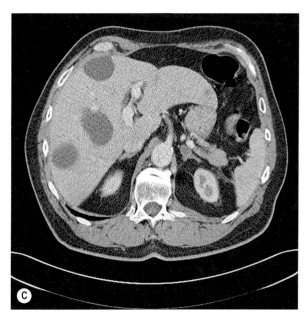

SCLC can be classified as TNM staging or using the simplied.

Mediastinal staging in non-small cell lung cancer

Accurate distinction of stages II, IIIA and IIIB is important in deciding optimal surgical treatment in the potentially operable patients. Stage II disease is treated with lobectomy or pneumonectomy with mediastinal sampling or dissection. Stage IIIA disease may be treated with neoadjuvant chemotherapy followed radical surgery or radical chemoradiotherapy, whereas IIIB disease is unresectable. This necessitates both an accurate distinction of T3 from T4 tumours and an accurate staging of nodal status. A classification of mediastinal nodes is shown in Figure 9.3.

Methods of mediastinal staging
Positron emission tomogram (PET) (Figure 9.4) – PET is scan based on the principle of differential uptake of 2-[fluorine-18]-fluoro-2-deoxy-D-glucose (FDG) by cancer cells. FDG is metabolized at a higher rate by tumour cells than normal cells and the areas of increased activity can be detected by a scanner. FDG-PET has higher sensitivity (87% vs. 68%), specificity (91% vs. 61%) and accuracy (82% vs. 63%) at detecting mediastinal disease than CT scan. PET also has a high negative predictive value in exclusion of N2/N3 disease, which helps to omit further mediastinal staging in case of a negative PET. Overall, there is 20% improvement in accuracy of PET over CT for mediastinal staging of NSCLC.

PET also detects distant metastases. The incidence of extra thoracic metastases on PET which are not suspected by CT scan is 9 to 11%. CT false-positive adrenal nodules have been correctly identified as negative on FDG-PET.

One of the limitations of PET is false-positive 'hot spots' in the mediastinum due to inflammatory processes (in up to 13 to 17%). It is less

Box 9.3: Staging of non-small cell lung cancer

Stage Ia

T1N0 — Tumour ≤3 cm diameter

Stage Ib

T2aN0M0 — Tumour >3 cm or ≤5 cm OR
Tumour of ≤5 cm with involvement of visceral pleura, main bronchus ≥2 cm distal to the carina or partial atelectasis

Stage IIA

T2bN0M0 — Tumour >5 cm or ≤7 cm
T1-T2aN1M0 — Metastasis in ipsilateral hilar or peribronchinal nodes

Stage IIB

T2bN1M0
T3N0M0 — Tumour of >7 cm OR
Tumour invading chestwall, diaphragm, phrenic nerves, mediastinal pleura or parietal pericardium OR
Tumour <2 cm from carina, atelectasis of entire lung or nodule in the same lobe

Stage IIIA

T4N0-1M0 — Tumour invading mediastinal structures or nodule in different ipsilateral lobe
T1-3N2M0 — Metastases in ipsilateral mediastinal and/or subcarinal nodes

Stage IIIB

T4N2M0
anyT N3M0 — Metastases in contralateral hilar or mediastinal nodes
Metastases in scalene or supraclavicular nodes

Stage IV

M1a — contralateral lung nodule/pleural nodule/malignant effusion
M2b — distant metastasis

Box 9.4: Staging of small cell lung cancer

Limited stage (stage I-III)
Tumour confined to the hemithorax of origin, the mediastinum, and the supraclavicular nodes, that can be encompassed within a tolerable radiation therapy port.

Extensive stage (stage IV)
Tumor that is too widespread to be included within the definition of limited-stage disease above. Patients with distant metastases (M1) are always considered to have extensive stage disease.

accurate when the lesion is <1 cm and in tumours of low metabolic activity such as carcinoid and bronchoalvelolar carcinoma.

PET scan is recommended for all NSCLC patients being considered for radical treatment. Patients with no lymphadenopathy on CT scan but with PET scan positive nodal disease needed mediastinoscopy prior to definitive treatment as 50% of patients can have false positive PET scan.

MRI scan – has limited role in staging. This may be useful to evaluate vascular and vertebral body invasion and to assess integrity of brachial plexus in Pancoast's tumour.

Endobronchial ultrasound (EBUS) – EBUS is able to penetrate up to 5 cm and can identify lymph nodes and vessels. It is helpful in visualizing paratracheal (stations 2 & 4) and peribronchial lymph nodes (see Figure 9.3) and enables EBUS guided transbronchial needle aspiration (Figure 9.5). Sonographic features of malignant lymph node are round shape, sharp margins and hypoechoic texture. The advantage of EUS over CT and PET is that it can characterize lymph nodes smaller than 1 cm. It can also determine the depth and extent of tumour invasion of tracheobronchial lesions and helps to define the relationships to the pulmonary vessels and the hilar structures. EBUS has been found to predict the lymph node staging correctly in 96% of cases, with a sensitivity of 95% and specificity of 100%.

Endo-oesophageal US (EUS) with fine needle aspiration is useful to assess sub-aortic (station 5), subcarinal (station 7), and paraoesophageal (station 8) lymph nodes as well as the upper retroperitoneum, which are not accessed by mediastinoscopy. It is envisaged that EUS-FNA and EBUS will not replace but will complement surgical techniques like mediastinoscopy.

Transbronchial needle aspiration (TBNA) – TBNA using a flexible fibre optic bronchoscope has a sensitivity of 78% and high specificity (approaching 100%) for identifying mediastinal metastases. However, the diagnostic yield is operator dependent.

Mediastinoscopy is generally regarded as the gold standard for preoperative mediastinal evaluation. CT scan is helpful in guiding selection of patients for mediastinoscopy prior to surgery. Cervical mediastinoscopy allows better access to contralateral lymph nodes. It is useful in evaluat-

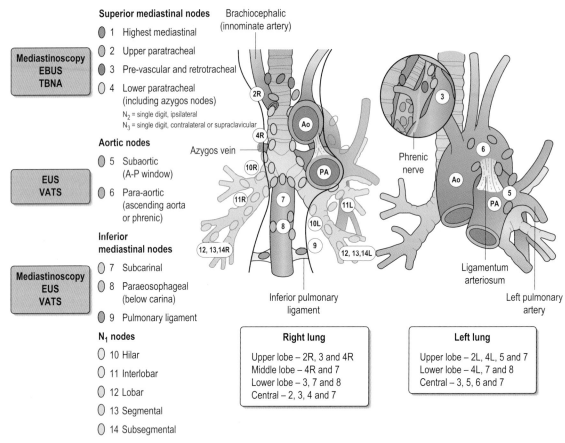

Figure 9.3
The classification of mediastinal nodes, patterns of nodal spread and method of choice of staging.

ing paratracheal (2 & 4), scalene and inferior mediastinal nodes (7, 8 & 9). It is not useful in evaluating aortic nodes (5 & 6). Mortality rates from mediastinoscopy are negligible, but morbidity rates especially arrhythmias are reported to be 0.5–1%. It has to be borne in mind that up to 30% of patients with lung carcinoma who have a negative mediastinoscopy prove to have mediastinal nodal metastasis at surgery.

Video-assisted thoracoscopy (VATS) is useful to evaluate aortic (5 & 6), paraoesophageal (8) and pulmonary ligament nodes (9). It is also useful in assessing the pleural cavity and obtaining pleural biopsies.

Management of lung cancer

Patients presenting with symptoms suggestive of lung cancer need urgent evaluation (Figure 9.1)

and referral to a team specializing in the management of lung cancer. Treatment depends on type of lung cancer (NSCLC vs. SCLC), stage, performance status, co-morbidities and cardiopulmonary reserve.

Non-small cell lung cancer (Figure 9.6)

Stage I–II

Patients presenting with stage I–II disease are generally treated with curative intent if performance status is good (0–1) and pulmonary function are adequate. The treatment options include:

- Surgery alone (if excision complete).
- Surgery followed by radiotherapy (in case of microscopic residual disease).
- Surgery followed by chemotherapy (in selected cases of IB & II).

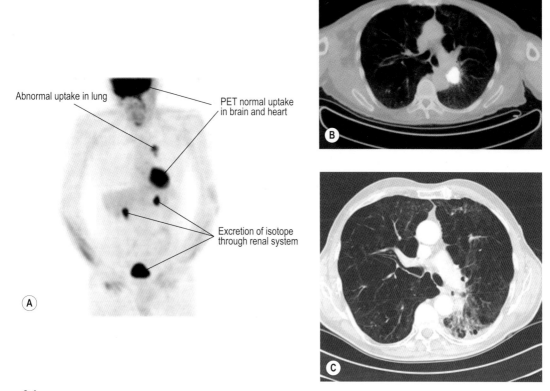

Figure 9.4
PET scan in lung cancer.

- Radical radiotherapy (in patients who are unfit or unwilling for surgery).

Radical surgery

Surgery offers the best prospect of cure in stage I–II disease, but only 10–20% of patients are suitable for surgery. Surgery is aimed at complete resection of the tumour and its intrapulmonary lymphatics. Patients need careful preoperative evaluation as they are often frail and frequently have cardiopulmonary morbidity due to chronic smoking. Spirometry is required in all patients. If the FEV1 is less than 1.5 L for lobectomy and less than 2 L for pneumonectomy, full lung function tests are required. Table 9.1 shows minimal pulmonary function required for different curative treatments. All patients require an ECG and patients with murmurs should have echocardiogram. Patients with known ischaemic heart disease should have detailed cardiologic assessment.

A complete anatomical resection is achieved by one of the following procedures:

- Lobectomy is the most common procedure which carries a postoperative mortality of 2–4%.
- Pneumonectomy is indicated if the tumour invades hilar structures (e.g. main bronchi, main pulmonary artery) and has a higher mortality rate (6–8%).
- Wedge or segmental resection is useful in patients with peripheral tumours and impaired lung function but carries a high rate of local recurrence (3–5 times) and a lower survival (reduce survival by 5–10%).
- Bronchoplastic or 'sleeve' resection is designed to spare lung tissue as an alternative to pneumonectomy. This procedure is used to resect endobronchial lesions at or adjacent carina to preserve distal tissue.

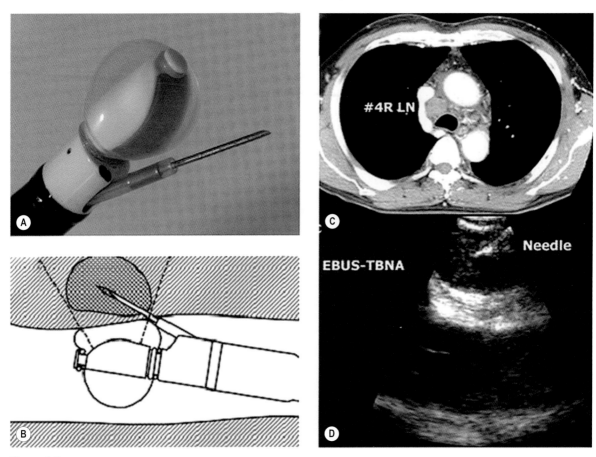

Figure 9.5
Endobronchial ultrasound (A) and its use for FNA (B) of an enlarged lower paratracheal node (C&D).

Radical radiotherapy (Table 9.2)

Patients with medically inoperable stage I/II are treated with radical radiotherapy if lung function is adequate (Table 9.1). In the only randomized trial, radiotherapy was inferior to surgery (4-year survival 7% vs. 23%). After conventional radical radiotherapy (60 Gy in 30 fractions over 6 weeks), 2-year survival is about 20%. A UK MRC study showed that 2-year survival is better (20 vs. 29%) with continuous hyperfractionated accelerated radiotherapy (CHART). This radiotherapy regime consists of 54 Gy in 36 fractions over 12 continuous days giving three fractions per day with a minimum interval of 6 hours between each fraction.

An evolving technique of stereotactic radiotherapy typically delivers high doses of radiotherapy in 3–5 fractions using precise method of tumour localization and radiation delivery. Early results suggest a 2-year local control of >90% in patients with stage I tumours with <5% significant toxicity.

Postoperative treatment

Radiotherapy

There is no proven role for postoperative radiotherapy after complete surgical resection of stage I–II lung cancer. There is some suggestion that routine radiotherapy in N0–N1 disease significantly decrease survival. Hence radiotherapy may be offered in incomplete resection and/or unexpected N2 disease (improve local control with no effect on survival) if performance status and residual lung function permits. However, further studies are needed to define the exact role of radiotherapy in the adjuvant chemotherapy era.

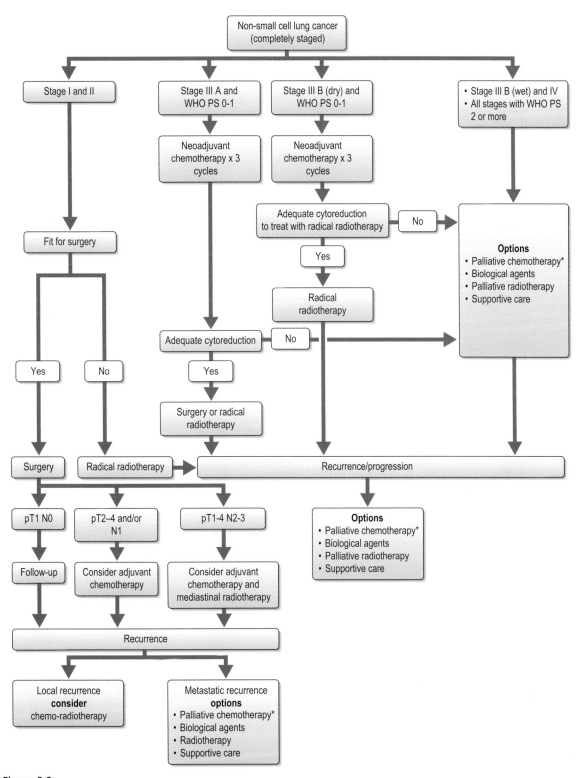

Figure 9.6
Management of non-small cell lung cancer. *palliative chemotherapy is considered only in patients with good performance status (0-2).

Table 9.1: Minimal pulmonary function for curative treatment

Test	Pneumonectomy	Lobectomy	Radical radiotherapy
FEV_1	≥2 L	≥1.5 L	Stage I & II: >1 L* Stage III: >1.5 L$^\text{S}$
FEV_1/FVC	≥50	≥50	
FEF 25–75	≥0.6 L	≥0.6 L	–
PCO_2	35–45 mmHg	35–45 mmHg	–
PO_2	>60 mmHg	>60 mmHg	–
Predicted postoperative FEV_1	≥1 L or 40%	≥1 L or 40%	–
MVO_2	>15 ml/kg/min	≥15 ml/kg/min	–

*For peripheral tumours and small tumours (planning volume <150 cm^3) >0.7 L.
$^\text{S}$For small tumours >1 L.

Table 9.2: Radiotherapy in lung cancer

Indication	Technique	Target volume	Dose*
Incomplete resection	CT-planned conformal	Known area of residual tumour identified by surgical clips + 1–2 cm margin	50 Gy/20 fractions (microscopic) 55 Gy/ 20 fractions (macroscopic)
Postoperative N2 disease	CT-planned conformal	Whole mediastinum + 1–1.5 cm margin	50 Gy/20 fractions or 60 Gy/30 fractions
Radical radiotherapy – stage I & II	CT planned conformal	Radiological mass with 1–2 cm margin	55 Gy/20 fractions or 64 Gy/32 fractions or 'CHART'
Radical radiotherapy – stage III	CT-planned conformal	Radiological residual mass with 1–2 cm margin	55 Gy/20 fractions or 64 Gy/32 fractions or 'CHART'
Palliative	Conventional	Radiological disease +1–2 cm margin	39 Gy/13 fractions 10 Gy in single
Thoracic radiotherapy – small cell cancer	CT-planned conformal	Pre-chemotherapy tumour if feasible with adjacent mediastinal nodes + 1.5 cm margin	40 Gy/15 fractions

*V20 (volume of normal lungs receiving 20 Gy) should be less than 34% and spinal cord dose should be <38–40 Gy with 4 weeks' treatment and <44 Gy with 6 weeks' treatment.

Chemotherapy (Box 9.5)

In randomized trials, there is no survival benefit with adjuvant chemotherapy for stage IA. In stage IB and II, an early meta-analysis showed a 5% overall survival benefit with postoperative cisplatin-based combination chemotherapy. This has been supported by several recent trials of cisplatin combinations. The NCIC JBR 10 and ANITA trials both used vinorelbine and cispla-

tin. 5-year overall survival in NCIC JBR 10 trial was increased from 54 to 69% in stage IB and II disease. In the ANITA trial overall survival was not significantly different in stage IB (62% vs. 63%) but was statistically significant in stage II (52% vs. 39%) resected NSCLC. More heterogeneous trials which have allowed a wider range of tumour stages, more variety in chemotherapy combinations within the trial and less stand-

Box 9.5: Chemotherapy regimes in lung cancer

Non-small cell carcinoma

- Cisplatin 80 mg/m² IV Day 1 + vinorelbine 30 mg/m² IV Days 1&8. Cycle repeated 3 weekly.

This regime is used in adjuvant chemotherapy trials.

- Carboplatin (AUC 5) IV Day 1 + vinorelbine 25 mg/m² IV Days 1 & 8. Cycle repeated 3 weekly.
- Carboplatin (AUC 5) IV Day 1 + gemcitabine 1200 mg/m² IV Days 1 & 8. Cycle repeated 3 weekly.
- Carboplatin (AUC 5) IV Day 1 + paclitaxel 175 mg/m² IV Days 1 & 8. Cycle repeated 3 weekly.

The above three regimes are equally effective.

- Docetaxel 75 mg/m² IV Day 1. Cycle repeated 3-weekly. Used as second-line chemotherapy.

Small cell lung cancer

- Carboplatin (AUC 5–6) + etoposide – is the usual first line regime.
- CAV (cisplatin, adriamycin and vincristine).
- ACE (Adriamycin, cyclophosphamide and etoposide.
- CAV & ACE are not given with concurrent radiotherapy as adriamycin causes 'radiation recall'.
- Oral topotecan.

ardized surgical eligibility have provided less obvious benefits in survival (ALPI and European BIG lung trial). The IALT trial did however show a benefit in survival and the trial was closed early when the planned interim analysis showed a significant impact on survival with a median follow-up of 56 months. In summary, fit patients with resected stage IB–II should therefore be offered four courses of a cisplatin combination chemotherapy within 12 weeks of surgery.

Stage III

Stage IIIA (T1–3, N2 M0/T3 N1 M0)

Patients with stage IIIA comprise a complex and heterogeneous group with varied treatment outcome. The result of surgery alone is poor and the expected 5-year survival is between <10 and 40%; it is dependent on the extent of mediastinal nodal involvement.

The treatment of choice is radical chemoradiotherapy if good performance status (0–1). Patients with small volume N2 disease can be considered for surgery after neoadjuvant chemotherapy or chemoradiotherapy.

The treatment options are:

- Radical chemoradiotherapy (for T1–3N2 disease with PS 0-1).
- Surgery alone or with postoperative radiotherapy and/or chemotherapy (for unexpected N2 disease after resection).
- Neoadjuvant chemo-radiotherapy or chemotherapy followed by surgery (for T3 N1 and small volume N2 disease, both with PS 0–1).
- Radical radiotherapy (if chemotherapy contraindicated, radical RT feasible & PS 0–1).
- Palliative chemotherapy (not suitable for radical radiotherapy and PS 2 or less).
- Symptomatic treatment and palliative radiotherapy (PS 2 or more).

The IALT trial and meta-analysis showed at least a 5% survival advantage with adjuvant chemotherapy in resected stage IIIA disease. Similarly, the ANITA trial also showed statistically significant improved survival with adjuvant vinorelbine and cisplatin in completely resected stage IIIA disease (42% vs. 26%).

Stage IIIB (T4 any N, M0/ any T N3 M0) without malignant effusion

Treatment options are:

- Radical chemoradiotherapy (if PS 0–1 and disease can be radically irradiated).
- Neoadjuvant chemoradiotherapy or chemotherapy followed by surgery (selected group with good PS).
- Radical radiotherapy (small radically treatable disease, PS 0–1, chemotherapy contraindicated).
- Palliative chemotherapy (not suitable for radical treatment and PS not >2).
- Symptomatic and supportive care.

In young fit patients with stage IIIB disease due to involvement of adjacent structures, neoadjuvant chemotherapy or chemoradiotherapy can be used to downstage the tumour and aim for surgical resection. There is a trend towards increased survival at least in the first 2 years for these patients particularly when chemotherapy is given concurrently with radiotherapy. Trials have examined dose and scheduling and concluded that full dose chemotherapy concurrently with radiotherapy was most beneficial.

Stage IIIB with malignant effusion/stage IV

Patients with malignant effusions (IIIB) or metastatic disease (IV) are incurable and both carry a similar prognosis. The treatment aim is palliative with the intention of improving symptoms as much as disease control. Treatments will be greatly affected by patient fitness as these patients will often be frail and suffer several co-morbidities. Many trials have examined the role of chemotherapy versus best supportive care in this group. Overall chemotherapy has a response rate of 20–40% with a duration of 6 months and a median overall survival of less than 1 year. The survival benefit from chemotherapy is in the range of 6–8 weeks. Response rates for an individual reflected overall survival in a meta-analysis. Frequent assessment prior to chemotherapy with CXR is recommended to assess response.

Chemotherapy has been associated with symptomatic benefits such as reduced palliative radiotherapy requirements, reduced analgesia, weight stabilization and maintenance of performance status. Toxicity was frequently seen, worse with combination chemotherapy but quality of life studies showed that these were not perceived as worse compared with patients not on chemotherapy.

In general, chemotherapy has a greater benefit in fit patients of good performance status (WHO 0 or 1). In these patients combination chemotherapy (a platinum and other agent such as vinorelbine or gemcitabine) can be offered. A recent study has shown that a combination of cisplatin and pemetrexed improves overall survival in patients with locally advanced or metastatic adenocarcinoma (12.6 vs. 10.9 months) and large cell carcinoma (10.4 vs. 6.7 months) compared with cisplatin and gemcitabine. In the less fit or elderly single agent treatments, palliative radiotherapy, biological agents or appropriate trials can be considered.

Recently phase III studies have shown that maintenance treatment with pemetrexed and erlotinib are useful in patients who had not progressed after first line chemotherapy.

Palliative radiotherapy

A significant number of patients may need radiotherapy to palliate symptoms. There will be a subgroup of patients with large localized NCSLC which cannot be encompassed in a radical radiotherapy field or with co-morbidity. An MRC study showed that for such patients with performance status 0–1, high-dose palliative radiotherapy (39 Gy in 13 fractions, if no spinal cord in the field or 36 Gy in 12 fractions, if cord in the radiotherapy field) results in better 2-year survival (13% vs. 9%) compared with 17 Gy in two fractions. Patients who need relief of local symptoms due to primary tumour or metastases are treated with palliative radiotherapy. This is either 10 Gy single fraction (PS >2), or 17 Gy in two fractions (PS 2). The side effects of large fractions include nausea, acute chest pain and fever.

Relapsed pre-treated NSCLC

In the small number of stage IIIB/IV patients who have received previous platinum-based chemotherapy and relapse whilst still fit, second line chemotherapy can be considered. Docetaxel has shown good activity and improved median survival of 3 months over best supportive care in this subset of patients. Re-irradiation is an option if >6 months after previous radiotherapy and it is possible to avoid spinal cord.

Erlotinib has shown a survival advantage of 2 months and improved symptom control when used in combination with chemotherapy. In the UK, erlotinib is recommended as a clinically and cost-effective alternative to docetaxel for the second line treatment of NSCLC.

New agents

Understanding some of the molecular mechanisms in NSCLC has led to the development of new targeted therapies. The mechanisms of these are common to several malignancies (see Appendis, p. 370). The most successful agents in NSCLC are those targeted against the epidermal growth factor receptor (EGFR). Two oral drugs which inhibit the tyrosine kinase domain of the EGFR are erlotinib (Tarceva™) and gefitinib (Iressa™). Toxicity with these drugs is unlike standard chemotherapy drugs and includes a characteristic rash which often reflects drug activity, diarrhoea and pneumonitis (reported in gefitinib in a Japanese study). The patients most likely to benefit from these drugs are female, those with an adenocarcinoma (especially bron-

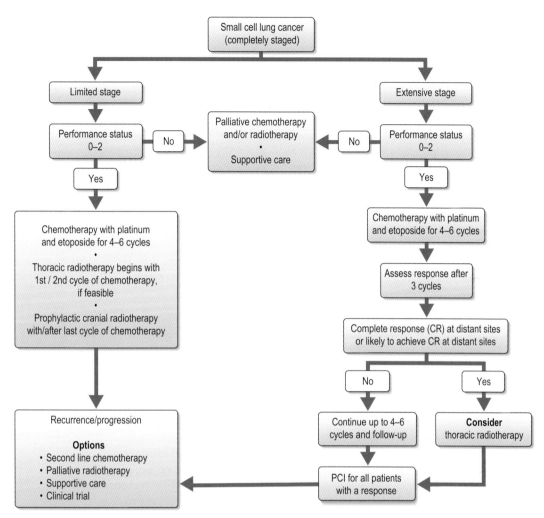

Figure 9.7
Management of small cell lung cancer.

choalvelolar subtype), be non-smokers and be Asian. At the molecular level, increased EGFR protein expression, gene amplification and the presence of EGFR mutations in the tyrosine kinase domain increase patient response. A recent comparative study of gefitinib with a combination of carboplatin and paclitaxel (IPASS study) has shown that gefitinib results in a better progression free survival in patients with EGFR+ tumours.

A randomized study (E4599) showed that a combination of bevacizumab (anti-VEGF) with chemotherapy improves survival by 2.3 months in patients with untreated advanced non-squamous cell lung cancer.

Small cell lung cancer (Figure 9.7)

Small cell lung cancer (SCLC) accounts for 20% of lung cancer. Up to 60% have extensive stage disease at diagnosis.

Limited stage disease

The standard treatment for patients with good performance status (0–2) and no significant co-morbidity is combination chemotherapy with platinum regime with concurrent thoracic radiotherapy and prophylactic cranial radiotherapy.

In 5–10% of patients with SCLC limited to lung, diagnosis is established only after resection. These patients need adjuvant chemotherapy as there is high likelihood of development of distant metastasis. Role of surgery in early stage disease is not well established. Surgery following complete or partial response to chemotherapy is not beneficial.

Chemotherapy (Box 9.5)

Chemotherapy remains the mainstay of treatment of small cell lung cancer. Randomized trials have shown that multiple agent chemotherapy is better than single agent in terms of response rate and survival.

Meta-analysis showed that cisplatin regime results in higher response rate (69% vs. 62% p < 0.001) and lower risk of death at 12 months (OR 0.80 CI 0.69–0.93; p = 0.002) for both localized and extensive SCLC. Platinum based regime has less mucosal toxicity, less myelosuppression and is easier to combine with radiotherapy than anthracycline-based regimes. Though there is no conclusive evidence that carboplatin-etoposide is similar in efficacy to cisplatin-etoposide, the former regime is easier to administer and the current clinical practice resides with using cisplatin where survival is the primary aim and carboplatin where palliation is the primary aim.

There is no established role for maintenance chemotherapy and patients are treated with 4–6 courses of chemotherapy. Dose intensification leads to increased toxicities with no survival advantage over standard dose chemotherapy.

Radiotherapy

Thoracic radiotherapy

Thoracic radiotherapy is indicated for patients with limited stage SCLC. A meta-analysis showed that addition of radiotherapy reduced the risk of death by 14% which is equivalent to 5% absolute increase in 3-year survival. In terms of intra-thoracic control, there is 25% absolute improvement with addition of radiation at an expense of 1.2% absolute increase in the risk of treatment related mortality. Interruption of radiotherapy results in lower survival (median survival 14 vs. 16 months). Patients who continue to smoke during radiotherapy also have a lower survival (median survival 14 vs. 18 months).

While the optimal dose and fractionation of radiotherapy remains unclear, most clinicians use 40 Gy in 15–20 fractions over 3 weeks which is given concurrently with 1st, 2nd cycle of chemotherapy if feasible or at the end of the chemotherapy. Some others use a radiotherapy regime of 50 Gy in 25 fractions. One study shows that twice-daily concurrent radiotherapy is better than once daily radiotherapy.

Prophylactic cranial irradiation (PCI)

Brain metastases are present at the time of diagnosis of small cell lung cancer in up to 10% patients. Another 40–50% of patients develop brain metastases during the course of illness suggesting that brain metastases are a common cause of treatment failure.

A meta-analysis of PCI for patients with SCLC in complete remission showed that PCI reduces the risk of brain metastasis by 54%, the risk of death is reduced by 16%, contributing to an increase in 3-year survival of 5.4% (20.7% vs. 15.3%). There is no evidence of differential benefit with age or radiation dose. Though, optimal timing of PCI is not clear, it is recommended that PCI should be administered without delay after primary treatment. There is no conclusive data on optimal dose of radiotherapy. 30 Gy in 10 fractions over 2 weeks is the commonly used regime in the UK. Other regimes include 20 Gy in 10 fractions, 30 Gy in 15 and 36 Gy in 18 fractions. Since there is some concern about the risk of long term neurological toxicities such as cognitive impairment and ataxia, PCI may be avoided in patients older than 70 years and those with cerebrovascular disease.

Extensive stage

Chemotherapy is the main modality of treatment and a recent Cochrane review showed that in patients with extensive SCLC chemotherapy prolongs survival. One of the regimes shown in Box 9.5 is used.

In patients with extensive disease who achieve complete response at extra-thoracic sites after primary chemotherapy, thoracic radiotherapy improves survival to a similar extent as that of limited stage disease. A recent randomized study has shown that patients with extensive SCLC (aged 18–75 years) who had a response to chemotherapy, would benefit from PCI. Patients who received PCI has a lower risk of brain metastases (1-year risk of 15% vs. 40%), and better 1-year survival (27% vs. 13%). The commonly used radiotherapy regime in this study is 20 Gy in five fractions.

Second-line chemotherapy

The median survival following relapse after first-line chemotherapy is approximately 4 months. There are two groups: the sensitive group who have previously responded and who have had a relapse-free-interval of at least 3 months and the resistant group who do not fit in the sensitive group. The sensitive group may be re-induced with same type of first-line chemotherapy. Of patients with sensitive disease 30–40% respond to second-line chemotherapy (median survival 6 months), while less than 10% of patients with resistant disease will respond to chemotherapy. The commonly used second line chemotherapy regimes are CAV or oral topotecan (Box 9.5).

Prognostic factors and survival

In general, performance status is the best predictor of outcome in lung cancer. In early stage NSCLC, tumour staging and nodal status are important prognostic factors.

In advanced stage NSCLC, females have better prognosis. Significant weight loss (>10% within last 3 months) and large cell histology indicate poor prognosis. An early response to treatment implies a longer survival.

Good performance status, female gender and limited stage predict prolonged survival in small cell lung cancer.

5-year survival by non-small cell lung cancer by stage is as follows:

Stage I	60–80%
Stage II	25–40%
Stage IIIa	10–40%
Stage IIIb & IV	<5%

30–40% of limited stage SCLC patients survive 2 years median survival 18–20 months). Median survival of extensive stage SCLC is 10–12 months.

Special situations

Superior sulcus tumour

Superior sulcus tumour (Pancoast's tumour) typically presents as T3/T4 lesion. Accurate staging is important in the optimal management of these tumours. Recent studies indicate that a subgroup of patients without distant metastasis can be managed with combined modality approach. A recent phase II study of concurrent chemoradiotherapy (two cycles of combination chemotherapy with cisplatin and etoposide and radiotherapy to primary tumour and supraclavicular fossa giving 45 Gy in 25 fractions) reported a complete resection of tumour in more than three-fourths of the patients and an overall 5-year survival of 44%. In this study, surgery was done 3–5 weeks after chemoradiotherapy and additional two courses of chemotherapy were given postoperatively.

Selected series of radical radiotherapy (60–66 Gy) alone report a 5-year survival of up to 40%.

In summary, patients with operable tumours and good performance status (0–1) are treated with chemoradiotherapy followed by surgery and postoperative chemotherapy. Patients with medically inoperable or locally advanced tumours with good PS are treated with either radical radiotherapy or chemoradiotherapy. Patients with metastatic disease or with poor PS are treated symptomatically.

Carcinoid tumours

Localized carcinoid tumour is treated with surgery. Typical carcinoids are low-grade malignancies which are usually treated with excision, with parenchyma-sparing sleeve or bronchoplastic resections indicated whenever possible. Atypical carcinoids are aggressive malignancies, and radical surgical resection is indicated. Locoregional failure rates of 8% have been reported for typical carcinoids and 23% for atypical carcinoids. Role of adjuvant treatment is unknown. Up to 64% of patients with atypical carcinoid can develop systemic metastases at a median time of 17 months after diagnosis.

Combination chemotherapy using the regimes as in SCLC is used to treat metastasis carcinoid.

Mixed small and non-small cell lung cancer

A small proportion of patients (2%) present with mixed small and non-small cell lung cancer. There is no clear recommendation for management of these tumours exists. Hence treatment should be individualized based on the stage of the disease and general condition of patients. Although, there is no role for surgery for pure small cell lung cancer; patients with localized mixed tumours may be candidates for aggressive surgery or chemo-radiotherapy (similar to NSCLC as it requires higher dose of radiotherapy for optimal long term control). Patients with poor performance status or metastatic disease are treated with palliative measures.

Lung cancer in never smokers

Never smokers are those who have smoked less than 100 cigarettes in their lifetime. Studies suggest that environmental tobacco smoke is a common cause of these cancers. Other risk factors may also contribute. Women are more commonly affected than men. Adenocarcinoma is more common, particularly the bronchoalveolar carcinoma subtype. Treatment is essentially the same as that of smokers. However, recent data suggest that this group of patients have a higher response rate and better survival with EGFR tyrosine kinase inhibitors such as erlotinib and gefinib (see IPASS study, p. 102).

Multiple primary lung cancer

2–4% patients can present with multiple primary lung tumour which can be either synchronous (detected simultaneously) or metachronous (detected after an interval). However it is often difficult to distinguish this from a metastasis from the lung tumour. Patients with multiple primary cancers are managed as two individual tumours.

NSCLC with solitary metastases

A small subset of patients present with isolated extrathoracic metastasis either after radical treatment or at presentation. Studies show that in patients with good performance status, resection of the lung tumour and metastasis with or without systemic treatment result in improved survival.

In patients with synchronous isolated adrenal metastases, this approach results in a 5-year survival of 10–23%, whereas in those with isolated metachronous adrenal metastasis occurring >6 months after initial curative treatment, the 5-year survival is around 38%. Of those with recurrence in <6 months, none survive for 2 years.

In patients with synchronous isolated brain metastases with complete resection of all disease, the reported 5-year survival is 21%. Hence synchronous brain metastasis in a fully staged (including PET scan) resectable stage I–II lung cancer patient with good performance status is treated with resection or radiosurgical ablation with complete excision of the primary tumour. They also need systemic treatment as well as whole brain radiotherapy (WBRT) after resec-

tion (conflicting results). Patients with metachronous brain recurrence after a curative resection are also considered for resection ± WBRT or radiosurgery.

Palliative care issues

Despite recent advances in treatment, many patients with SCLC and NSCLC will progress and eventually die of their disease. Patients with advanced disease can present with a number of problems which require specialist services.

- Bone metastases are very common and can result in pain and spinal cord compression (p. 328). Pain can be improved using radiotherapy with a single 8 Gy fraction or 20 Gy in five fractions for spinal cord compression.
- Haemoptysis: invasion of vessels by expanding tumours can result in haemoptysis which can be significant. Palliative radiotherapy (10 Gy single fraction) may alleviate the bleeding but other measures can be used, e.g. cryotherapy.
- Superior vena cava obstruction can occur and should be treated as an emergency (p. 337). Steroids should be given in the first instance and radiotherapy (20 Gy in five fractions) is successful at reducing symptoms in 60%.
- Hypercalcaemia can be due to bone metastases or the production of a PTH like peptide. It should be tested for regularly in advanced lung cancer to prevent it presenting as an emergency (p. 339). It is treated with hydration, bisphosphonates and treatment of the underlying cancer if that is possible.
- Stridor is a rare but distressing symptom caused by compression of the proximal airways, usually by tumour or lymph nodes. Initial supportive care includes assessment of the airway by otolaryngologist, steroids and oxygen (p. 339). If severe, heliox, a mixture of helium and oxygen where the small particle size of helium facilitates delivery of the oxygen, can be given. Treatment of the compressive lesion (e.g. radiotherapy to the nodal mass) may be the only option to prevent progression of stridor.
- Breathlessness is the most common symptom in advanced NSCLC and can be debilitating. Investigations should be done to rule out significant pleural effusion and pulmonary

emboli as these are both treatable. Assuming the breathlessness is due to tumour progression and no further active treatment is possible, simple measures such as the use of a fan, teaching relaxation techniques and the cautious use of oral morphine, which causes dilatation of smooth muscle walls in blood vessels leading to an improvement in symptoms, can be helpful. Overall lung cancer patients often have an array of palliative care needs such that specialist in symptom control should be involved at an early stage.

Follow-up

Role of follow-up in patients after curative treatment for NSCLC remains controversial. For patients with potentially curative re-treatment, it is reasonable to cover routine follow-up 3–6 monthly for 2 years and 6–12 monthly thereafter, with clinical examination and radiological evaluation. The role of routine follow-up after treatment for SCLC is less clear.

Some evidence suggests that continued smoking adversely affects the overall prognosis and hence discouraged.

Mesothelioma

Introduction

Mesothelioma is an aggressive tumour arising from the cells of pleura and peritoneum. Currently just over 2000 new cases are diagnosed in the UK annually and the number of cases is expected to peak in 2015. In the USA, 2000 new cases are diagnosed annually and the incidence is declining. Widespread use of asbestos after World War II correlates with the anticipated increase in Europe within the next 15 years. The median age at diagnosis is 60 years and males are five times more commonly affected than females.

Aetiology

Mesothelioma is the most strongly linked cancer to occupation. It is estimated that 80–90% of mesothelioma cases or deaths in men are caused by occupational exposure to asbestos. The latency period after exposure ranges from 15–50 years. Shipbuilding and construction are the industries which used to involve high exposure of asbestos. Smoking does not increase the risk of mesothelioma. However, smoking combined with asbestos exposure increases the risk of lung cancer.

Pathogenesis and pathology

Pathogenesis

Amphiobile (blue and brown) asbestos is strongly linked to mesothelioma. It is postulated that the thin and long fibres of amphiboles when inhaled could penetrate and scratch the pleural surfaces. The chromosomal changes caused by fibres as they pierce the mitotic spindle as well as free radical formation from the fibres cause malignancy. The possibility of relationship between simian virus 40 (SV40) and mesothelioma is still debatable. Recent studies suggest a possible genetic susceptibility to asbestos-induced carcinogenesis.

Pathology

There are four histological subtypes of mesothelioma:

- Epithelial (40%) – associated with pleural effusions and better prognosis.
- Sarcomatoid (20%) – 'dry' mesothelioma.
- Mixed (35%).
- Undifferentiated (5%).

The important histopathological diagnosis is adenocarcinoma, which is differentiated immunohistochemically. Mesothelioma is positive for calretinin, WT1 (Wilms' tumour 1) antigen, epithelial membrane antigen (EMA) and cytokeratin 5/6 and negative for cytokeratin 7, 8, 18 & 19, TTF-1, BER-EP4 (mostly), CEA and MOC. The converse is diagnostic of adenocarcinoma.

Presentation

The usual presentations are exertional dyspnoea, chest pain or pleural effusion. Weight loss, fatigue, cough and paraneoplastic fever are also common. Right hemithorax (65%) is more often affected than left (35%) and 3% cases are bilateral.

Investigations and staging

Imaging

Chest X-ray and CT scan (Figure 9.8) are the initial methods of imaging. Chest X-ray shows evidence of pleural thickening, pleural effusion and volume loss. CT scan shows unilateral pleural effusion, nodular pleural thickening and tumour encasement of the lung ('rind like'

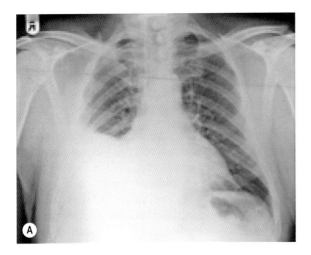

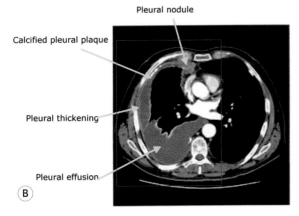

Pleural nodule

Calcified pleural plaque

Pleural thickening

Pleural effusion

Figure 9.8
Imaging of mesothelioma.

appearance – seen in 70% of cases) leading to contraction of hemithorax. Calcified plaques are found in 20% of patients. Chest wall invasion leads to obliteration of extrapleural fat planes, invasion of intercostal muscles, displacement of ribs, or bone destruction.

PET scan is helpful in distinguishing benign from malignant pleural masses and to detect extrathoracic and nodal disease. Recent studies report increasing usefulness of PET scan in defining prognostic group and to assess response to chemotherapy.

Tissue diagnosis

Histopathological diagnosis should be made in all cases using cytological analysis of pleural fluid or pleural biopsy done either under radiological guided or by VATS. A cell block prepared from at least 500 ml of pleural fluid is often helpful.

Staging

The recommended staging system is the International Mesothelioma Interest Group (IMIG) staging system, which is based on clinico-pathological tumour variables and nodal classification that of lung cancer (Table 9.3).

Management

There is no standard of care and only a minority of patients (10–15%) are eligible for any potentially curative treatment. The majority of patients (85–90%) presents with advanced disease with medial survival of less than 12 months and 5-year survival of ≤1%. Suitable patients with stage I and II disease may be treated with radical surgery or multimodality treatment aimed at long-term survival.

Surgery

There are no randomized data on the benefits of surgery. Radical treatment involves resection of the entire parietal and visceral pleura en bloc with underlying lung, ipsilateral pericardium and diaphragm called extrapleural pneumonectomy (EPP). Historical series suggest 5-year survival of 10–20% with EPP. The MARS trial (Mesothelioma and Radical Surgery) is aimed to determine whether EPP is better than no surgery in terms of survival and quality of life. However the majority of patients are not suitable for such extensive surgery. It has a reported morbidity up to 60% and mortality of 3.4% in expert hands.

Palliative surgery involves pleurectomy or decortication. It is an option for palliation of breathlessness caused by effusion when standard treatment options failed. The exact benefits of these procedures are not well-defined.

Radiotherapy

Mesothelioma is not a radiosensitive tumour. However, radiotherapy is still used in the following settings:

- Prophylaxis of thoracic tract seeding – to avoid mesothelial cell seeding down the tracts after thoracoscopies and drains. There is no convincing evidence for this indication (three small trials; one showed benefit and two did not). Radiotherapy dose is 21 Gy/3 fractions over a week using electrons.

Table 9.3: IMIG staging system for mesothelioma

Stage	
Ia	
T1aN0M0	Limited to parietal pleura; no involvement of visceral pleura.
Ib	
T1bN0M0	Limited to parietal pleura: scattered foci involving visceral pleura.
II	
T2N0M0	Ipsilateral pleura with (i) involvement of diaphragmatic muscle or (ii) confluent visceral pleural tumor or extension from visceral pleura into the lung parenchyma.
III	
T3N0M0	Ipsilateral pleura with involvement of the endothoracic fascia, or extension into mediastinal fat or solitary resectable extension of chest wall or non transmural involvement of pericardium.
T1–3N1M0	Ipsilateral bronchopulmonary or hilar nodes.
T1–3N2M0	Ipsilateral mediastinal or internal mammary nodes/subcarinal nodes.
IV	
T4N0M0	Diffuse or multiple chest wall involvement; transdiaphragmatic extension to peritoneum; direct extension to contralateral pleura; mediastinal organ extension; extension to spine; extension to internal surface of pericardium or involvement of myocardium.
Any T, N3M0	Contralateral mediastinal nodes; contralateral internal mammary nodes or any supraclavicular nodes.
Any T, Any N, M1	Distant metastases present.

- Palliative radiotherapy –to relieve pain.
- Adjuvant radiotherapy following EPP – no randomized trial data. One phase II trial reported reduced local recurrence and prolonged survival.

Chemotherapy

Although chemotherapy is used a part of multimodality treatment, many regimes have poor response to treatment and severe toxicity. Many chemotherapy studies using single or combination regimens showed an objective response rate of <20% with no impact on survival. A systematic study suggested cisplatin as the most active single agent. The antifolate agent, pemetrexed, which inhibits enzyme thymidylate synthetase, represents the recent advance in chemotherapy. A recent randomized study of 456 patients with PS 0–1, cisplatin with pemetrexed vs. cisplatin alone showed a superior response rate (41.3 vs. 16.7%; $p < 0.001$), median survival (12.1 vs. 9.3 months; $p = 0.02$), and time to progression (5.7 vs. 3.9 months; $p = 0.001$). Neutropenia was the commonest toxicity in the combined arm. The recommended dose of pemetrexed is 500 mg/m^2 given IV on day 1 followed by cisplatin 75 mg/m^2 of each 21 day cycle for 4–6 cycles. There are no data on benefit of chemotherapy beyond six courses.

In elderly patients, carboplatin is often substituted for cisplatin and data from phase II studies suggest similar efficacy.

Palliative care

Recurrent pleural effusion is a debilitating problem. Talc pleurodesis seems to give the best results with low morbidity. Alternate option is PleurX catheters with repeated drains.

Management of other symptoms follows the same principle of any advanced cancer.

Prognostic factor and survival

There are two prognostic predictive models: EORTC and Cancer and Leukaemia group-B (CAL-B). EORTC system (Table 9.4) distinguishes patients with mesothelioma as good (median survival 10.8 months) and poor (5.5 months) prognostic groups, where as CAL-B distinguishes six groups with median survival ranging from 1.4 months to 13.9 months. Table 9.4 shows the EORTC prognostic index.

Medicolegal implications

Mesothelioma is a notifiable disease. Patients diagnosed to have mesothelioma are automatically eligible for some benefits and allowances.

Table 9.4: EORTC prognostic index of mesothelioma

Prognostic factor		Score
Sex	Male	+0.60
Performance status	1 or 2	+0.60
Histological diagnosis	Possible or probable	+0.52
Sarcomatous type	Yes	+0.67
WBC count	$>8.5 \times 10^9$/L	+0.55

Calculate total score by adding all the individual scores which can be 0–2.94

Outcome measures	Good prognosis (total score ≤1.27)	Poor prognosis (total score >1.27)
Median survival	10.8 months	5.5 months
1-year survival	40%	12%
2-year survival	14%	0%

Peritoneal mesothelioma

Mesothelioma can also arise from peritoneal and pericardial cavities. Malignant peritoneal mesothelioma consists of up to 10–15% of all mesotheliomas and presents with abdominal symptoms due to ascites and tumour mass. The majority of patients present with diffuse peritoneal mesothelioma which is characterized by multiple nodules involving the entire peritoneal surface. Tissue diagnosis is by biopsy and it is important to rule out associated pleural disease.

Treatment options include systemic chemotherapy, cytoreductive surgery with or without intraperitoneal chemotherapy and radiotherapy. Patients with good PS (0–1) with diffuse disease and no extraperitoneal spread are considered for maximal cytoreduction and intraperitoneal hyperthermic chemotherapy. The chemotherapy agent used is mitomycin C. A systematic review reported a median survival ranging from 34–92 months and a 5-year survival ranging from 29% to 59% with this approach. The perioperative morbidity varied from 25% to 40% and mortality ranged from 0% to 8%.

Other patients with good PS and inoperable tumours may be considered for chemotherapy with cisplatin and pemetrexed (reported median survival 13.1 months). Surgery alone may be adequate for indolent well-differentiated tumours and multicystic mesothelioma variants (both variants are common in young women and arise from the pelvic peritoneum).

Patients with poor performance status are treated with symptomatic and supportive care. The overall median survival is around 12 months.

New agents and future direction

Since the success of pemetrexed, there have been attempts to improve survival with targeted agents. Most mesotheliomas overexpress EGFR and there have been phase II trials with two EGFR small molecules, gefitinib and erlotinib. Gefitinib showed limited activity in less than 10% and erlotinib did not produce any responses. TKIs which act on the VEGF pathway have also been examined (p. 372). Both sorafneib and vatalanib have shown a small number of responses in pretreated patients. However, bevacizumab, the monoclonal antibody against VEGF, showed no improvement in survival or response when compared with chemotherapy alone in a randomized trial.

There is some interest in the antineoplastic ribonuclease, rapirnase, which is isolated from frogs' eggs. In 81 patients who had evaluable disease and progressed after chemotherapy, there were four partial responses, two minor responses and 35 patients achieved stable disease with a median overall survival of 6 months.

Thymoma

Introduction

Thymoma is an epithelial tumour arising from the thymus accounting for nearly half of all primary mediastinal tumours. It presents with a spectrum of manifestations and has a wide ranging prognosis from benign to highly malignant.

The peak incidence if thymoma occurs at 40–60 years, with no predilection for gender. There is no known aetiological factor.

Pathology

WHO classification (Box 9.6) which correlates with prognosis, is based on the histological assessment of morphology of the neoplastic epithelial cells and the non-neoplastic lymphocytic component.

Box 9.6: WHO classification of thymoma

Type	Description	Characteristics	10-year survival
A	Medullary thymoma	4–7% of thymoma; 17% associated with myasthenia; epithelial cells are spindle or oval with a few lymphocytes	100
AB	Mixed thymoma	28–34%; 16% associated with myasthenia; foci with type A thymoma admixed with foci rich lymphocytes	100
B1	Predominantly cortical thymoma	9–20%; 57% associated with myasthenia; tumour resembles normal functional thymus with large number of cells	83
B2	Cortical thymoma	20–36%; 71% associated with myasthenia; scattered plump cells with vesicular nuclei and distinct nucleoli with heavy population of lymphocytes	83
B3	Well differentiated thymic carcinoma	10–14; 46% associated with myasthenia; epithelial cells are round or polygonal admixed with a minor component of lymphocytes	35
Carcinoma	Thymic carcinoma – various subtypes Thymic neuroendocrine tumors	Histologic features not specific to thymus but those of carcinomas of other organs	28
	Combined thymic epithelial tumours	At least 2 distinct areas each corresponding to one hisological thymoma and/or thymic carcinoma; commonest combination B2&B3	–
New entities	Micronodular thymoma	1–5%; not usually associated with myasthenia; good prognosis	–
	Biphasic metaplastic thymoma	Males common; not associated with myasthenia; good prognosis	–
	Hepatoid carcinoma	Features that of hepatoid carcinoma	–
	Carcinoma with t(15;19) translocation	Aggressive cancer with survival only a few weeks	

Presentation

Nearly 50% are asymptomatic with diagnosis being made incidentally. Common symptoms include chest pain, cough, dyspnoea, dysphagia, hoarseness, respiratory tract infections and superior vena caval obstruction. Various paraneoplastic syndromes can be associated with thymoma. About 30–40% of thymoma patients have myasthenia gravis and conversely, 10–15% of patients with myasthenia have underlying thymoma.

Investigations and staging

Imaging

In chest X-ray, large tumours are seen as mediastinal widening or anterior mediastinal mass (Figure 9.9A). The typical appearance in CT scan is a well-defined homogenous anterior mass lesion (Figure 9.9B) within a well-defined fibrous capsule. MRI scan is useful to evaluate mediastinal, cardiac and pericardial spread when CT findings are unequivocal.

Tissue diagnosis

CT guided FNA is less reliable. CT-guided core biopsy can be safely performed for large tumours. When CT guided biopsy is inconclusive or when not feasible, anterior mediastinotomy is the next choice. Although VATS helps to provide a tissue diagnosis, a theoretical risk of pleural seeding exists. For small tumours excisional biopsy is advisable.

Staging

Thymoma is staged according to Masaoka staging (Box 9.7), which is a postoperative staging. Invasion is the most important prognostic factor.

Management (Figure 9.10)

Successful treatment of thymoma depends on complete surgical resection. The majority of thymomas confined to the thymus are amenable to curative resection. Stage-wise management of thymoma is shown in Figure 9.10.

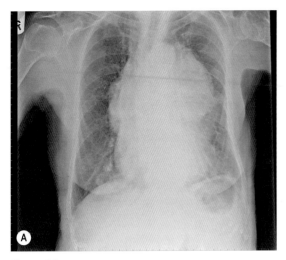
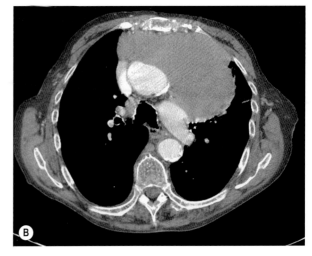

Figure 9.9
Imaging in thymoma.

Box 9.7: Masaoka staging of thymoma

Stage	Description
I	Macroscopically completely encapsulated with no microscopic capsular extension
IIa	Microscopic invasion through the capsule
IIb	Macroscopic invasion into mediastinal fat or pleura
III	Invasion into adjacent structures (pericardium, lung or great vessels)
IVa	Pleural or pericardial metastases
IVb	Lymphatic or haematogenous metastases

Early stage (stage I and II)

Surgery

En bloc surgical resection through a median sternotomy is the treatment of choice. Patients with myasthenia gravis or suspected to have myasthenia should have appropriate preoperative measures to avoid postoperative myasthenic crisis. Recurrence after complete excision of a stage I thymoma is less than 2%. 30% people will have invasive disease at surgery; still a complete resection can be achieved in the majority of these cases. However, recurrence of completely resected invasive thymoma is approximately 30% with median time of local recurrence around 3.8 years.

Radiotherapy

There is no proven role for radiotherapy in stage I disease. Previously, radiotherapy was considered as a standard adjuvant for stage II disease, as radiotherapy may reduce the risk of relapse from 26% to 5% in invasive disease. However, more recent studies challenge this approach as the most common mode of failure is pleural recurrence rather than mediastinal. Hence some recommend radiotherapy only if the resection margin is <1 mm and suggest histology should also be taken into account.

Chemotherapy

A subgroup of patients with pleural disease (IIb) are at risk of pleural relapse. These patients cannot be considered for radiotherapy because of the extensive radiation field, and hence may be considered for adjuvant chemotherapy.

Locally advanced disease (stage III and IVA)

If stage III or IVA with limited pleural disease is suspected preoperatively, patients should be treated with neoadjuvant treatment. This can be either chemotherapy alone (PAC) or chemoradiotherapy (EP with 45 Gy of radiation) (see below). Surgery is done 4–6 weeks after neoadjuvant treatment. Patients who haven't had radiotherapy preoperatively, should be considered for postoperative radiotherapy (Box 9.8) provided the area of risk can be encompassed in a radical radiotherapy portal and pulmonary function tests are adequate.

Metastatic disease

Patients are treated with palliative chemotherapy if general condition permits. Otherwise treatment is essentially symptomatic and supportive.

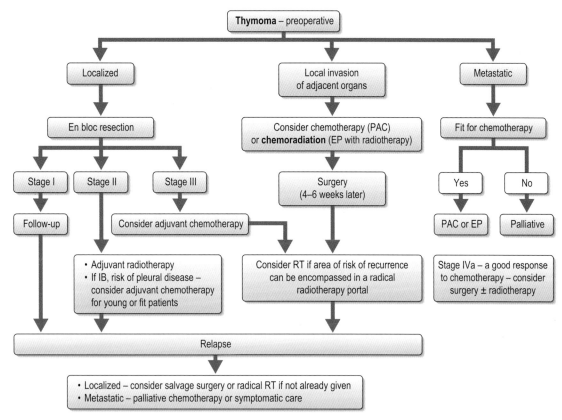

Figure 9.10
Management of thymoma.

Chemotherapy

Patients who fail surgery and/or radiotherapy or who present with metastatic disease are candidates for chemotherapy (Box 9.9). However, there are no randomized trials of chemotherapy in thymoma. Studies showed that a combination of cisplatin, doxorubicin and cyclophosphamide (CAP) resulted in an overall response of 50%, medial duration of response of 12 months and median survival of 38 months. Another combination regime of etoposide and cisplatin (EP) showed a response rate of 56% with median response of duration of 3.4 years and median survival of 4.3 years. Hence CAP and EP remains the standard chemotherapy combination for thymomas and thymic carcinoma.

Salvage treatment

Often disease recurrence is limited to the thorax. These patients should be considered for re-resection as they may have similar 5-year survival

as those with no recurrence. In one series the reported 5-year survival is 51% and those who had complete resection had a better survival of 64%.

Patients who may relapse with metastatic disease may be managed according to the fitness of the patient and prior treatment. Fit patients who haven't had any previous chemotherapy are treated with platinum based regime (PAC or EP). Patients who relapse 12 months after a previous platinum-containing regime, may be rechallenged with the same regime while treatment of patients who relapse within 12 months of initial platinum regime remains investigational. In patients who are chemotherapy refractory and showing demonstrable uptake on In-labelled octretide scan, may be candidates for treatment with somatostatin analogues plus prednisolone. The commonly used regime is either octreotide 1.5 mg/day subcutaneously, or lantreotide 30 mg intramuscularly every two weeks with prednisolone daily until progression.

Box 9.8: Radiotherapy in thymoma

Target volume
- GTV – defined by visible tumour and/or surgical clips on postoperative scan
- PTV = GTV + 1.5–2 cm

Critical organs
- Lung, heart and spinal cord

Energy
- 6 MV

Field arrangement
- Single anterior
- Un-equally weighted (2:1) or (3:2) Antero-posterior
- Anterior wedge pair
- Multiple field

Dose
- Complete excision/microscopic disease – 50 Gy in 20–25 fractions over 5 weeks
- Macroscopic disease – 55 Gy in 20 fractions or 60 Gy in 30 fractions
- Preoperative – 45 Gy in 20 fractions

Special situation
- Patients with lupus erythematosus may need dose modification to minimize late toxicity

Box 9.9: Chemotherapy in thymoma

CAP
- Cisplatin (50 mg/m^2), doxorubicin (50 mg/m^2), and cyclophosphamide (500 mg/m^2) given on day 1.
- Repeated every 21 days for a maximum of eight cycles, if stable or responsive disease after 2 cycles.

EP
- Cisplatin 60 mg/m^2 given on day 1 and etoposide 120 mg/m^2 on days 1, 2, and 3.
- Cycles repeated every 3 weeks for a maximum of eight cycles

Palliative care

Management of palliation of symptoms follows the same principles as that of any other advanced cancer. The common issues are dyspnoea due to pleural effusion and locally advanced tumour.

Prognostic factor and survival

Prognosis is dependent on clinical stage and histology and the most important prognostic factor is the completeness of resection. Presence of myasthenia does not influence the survival while autoimmune diseases such as red cell aplasia, hypogammaglobulinemia and lupus erythematosus appear to have a poor prognosis. 10-year survival of non-invasive (stage I) thymoma ranges between 67–80%, while those for invasive (stage II–IV) ranges from 35–53%. 5-year survival rates are: 93% for stage I, 86% for stage II, 70% for stage III and 50% for stage IV.

Up to 28% patients are reported to develop second primary cancer and the most common is colorectal. The reason for this association is unknown.

Follow-up

Patients should be monitored up to 10 years, since late metastases are not unusual. Follow-up should be in the form of clinical examination, blood tests and CT staging at appropriate interval.

Future direction

There is an evolving role for somatostatin analogues and radiotargeted therapy. Monoclonal antibodies such as gefinitib and cetuximab are reported to have therapeutic benefits in thymoma.

Further reading

Herbst RS, Heymach JV, Lippman SM. Lung cancer. N Engl J Med. 2008;359:1367–1380.

Bonomi PD. Implications of key trials in advanced nonsmall cell lung cancer. Cancer. 2010;116:1155–1164.

Puglisi M, Dolly S, Faria A et al. Treatment options for small cell lung cancer – do we have more choice? Br J Cancer. 2010;102:629–638.

Tassinari D, Drudi F, Lazzari-Agli L et al. Second-line treatments of advanced non-small-cell lung cancer: new evidence for clinical practice. Ann Oncol. 2010;21:428–429.

Dempke WC, Suto T, Reck M. Targeted therapies for non-small cell lung cancer. Lung Cancer. 2010;67:257–274.

Stahel RA, Weder W. Improving the outcome in malignant pleural mesothelioma: nonaggressive or aggressive approach? Curr Opin Oncol. 2009;21:124–130.

Ceresoli GL, Zucali PA, Gianoncelli L et al. Second-line treatment for malignant pleural mesothelioma. Cancer Treat Rev. 2010;36:24–32.

Falkson CB, Bezjak A, Darling G et al. The management of thymoma: a systematic review and practice guideline. J Thorac Oncol. 2009;4:911–919.

Breast cancer

10

TV Ajithkumar and HM Hatcher

Introduction

Breast cancer is the most common female malignancy in the UK and USA. In the UK, 30,000 new cases and 15,000 deaths occur each year due to breast cancer. In the USA, there are 192,000 new cases and 43,300 breast cancer deaths every year. The life-time risk of developing breast cancer for a woman is 1 in 12 in the UK and 1 in 8 in the USA.

Aetiology

The reported risk factors include hormonal, genetic, dietetic and radiation. Table 10.1 shows these risk factors and protective factors for breast cancer. The effect of hormones, notably oestrogen, is the most significant aetiological factor in breast cancer. Genetic factors in breast cancers are dealt with in Chapter 5 (p. 47). BRCA1 mutation associated cancers tend to occur at an early age, are highly aggressive and are typically negative for oestrogen (ER), progesterone (PgR) and human epithelial growth factor receptor 2 (HER2/neu ('Triple negative'). BRCA2 mutations account for 1% of breast cancers which are often ER and PgR positive.

Other risk factors include:

- Previous breast cancer – increases the risk of a contralateral breast cancer (0.5–1% per year).
- Prior radiation – to the breast or part of breast increases the risk of cancer (RR 3) (e.g. Mantle radiotherapy for Hodgkin's disease).
- Some benign conditions of the breast (e.g. atypical hyperplasia).

Pathogenesis and pathology

Breast cancer arises from the epithelial cells lining the terminal duct lobular unit. Development of invasive breast cancer is thought to be due to a multi-step process. WHO classification of breast cancer is shown in Box 10.1.

Precursor lesions

Lobular carcinoma-in-situ is considered as a precursor of invasive lobular cancer, but in most cases, it does not progress to the invasive stage. It is regarded as a marker for either lobular or ductal carcinoma.

Atypical ductal hyperplasia is characterized by intraductal epithelial proliferation with some of the features of DCIS. These increase the risk of invasive cancer 4–5 times.

In ductal carcinoma-in-situ (DCIS) malignant epithelial proliferation is confined to a duct with no stromal invasion. It accounts for 3–5% of palpable breast cancer and 15–20% of screen detected cancer. It is graded according to the appearance of cell nuclei. Low-grade micropapillary DCIS can occur as a multicentric tumour whereas high-grade comedo carcinoma DCIS can be associated with invasive tumour in the same quadrant.

Microinvasive carcinoma is focus of invasive cancer of <1 mm in maximum extent.

Malignant breast lesions

- Invasive ductal carcinoma: 70–80% of all invasive carcinomas are classified as invasive ductal carcinomas, which are thought to arise from DCIS. They occur most commonly as 'ductal no special type' (ductal NST). Ductal

DOI: 10.1016/B978-0-7234-3458-0.00015-4

Table 10.1: Risk factors of breast cancer

	Relative risk
Early menarche (before 11 years)	3
Late menopause (after 54 years)	2
First pregnancy after 40 years	3
Nulliparity	3
HRT	1.7
Oral contraceptive	1.2
One maternal first degree relative	1.5–2
Two first degree relatives	3–5
First degree relative diagnosed before 40 years	3
Bilateral breast cancer	4
Alcohol	1.3
Protective factors	
Artificial menopause before 35 years	0.5
Increased parity	0.5–0.8
Age at first pregnancy less than 30 years	0.6–0.8
Breast feeding	0.8

Box 10.1: Modified WHO classification of breast cancer

Precursor lesions
Lobular carcinoma-in-situ
Intraduct proliferative lesions
    Atypical ductal hyperplasia
    Ductal carcinoma-in-situ
Microinvasive carcinoma
Intraductal papillary neoplasms
    Papilloma
    Atypical papilloma
    Intraduct papillary carcinoma
    Intracystic papillary carcinoma

Malignant lesions
Invasive ductal carcinoma (NST) and subtypes
Invasive lobular carcinoma
Tubular carcinoma
Invasive cribriform carcinoma
Medullary carcinoma
Mucinous carcinoma
Neuroendocrine tumours
Metaplastic carcinoma
Sarcoma

NST is a diagnosis of exclusion. Other special subtypes of ductal carcinomas include:

- Tubular carcinoma: 1–2% of breast cancer.
- Medullary carcinoma: 4–9% of breast cancer.
- Mucinous carcinoma: 2%.
- Papillary carcinoma: 1–2%.
- Invasive lobular carcinoma – constitutes 10–15% of invasive cancers. These tumours infiltrate diffusely leading to a discrepancy between imaging findings and histologic tumour size.
- Other cancers: include lymphoma, sarcoma, melanoma and metastasis.

The postoperative pathology report should include: number of tumours, maximum diameter of largest tumour, histologic type and grade, circumferential excision margin and minimal margin, vascular invasion, number of nodes retrieved, number of nodes involved and extent of involvement (e.g. micrometastasis or metastasis), presence of DCIS and immunohistochemical status of ER and PgR and HER2. Patients with an ambiguous HER2 (2+) status on immunohistochemistry, require fluorescent in situ hybridization (FISH) to look for gene amplification (Box 10.2).

Molecular profiling has identified five subtypes of breast cancer: luminal A, luminal B, HER2+, normal breast-like and basal-like. The luminal tumours are ER+ whereas others are ER–. The outcome of these types is different. The role of molecular profiling in routine clinical practice is evolving but it is possible in the future that these subtypes will be treated differently.

Surgical anatomy of breast and lymphatics (Figure 10.1)

The adult breast extends from the second rib superiorly to the sixth rib inferiorly and from the lateral edge of the body of the sternum medially to mid-axillary line laterally. There are

Box 10.2: Grading and scoring systems in breast cancer

Nottingham grading of breast cancer

Characteristics	Score 1	Score 2	Score 3
Degree of tubule formation	>75%	10–75%	<10%
Nuclear pleomorphism	Mild	Moderate	Severe
Mitoses/10 HPF	Score of 1–3 based on the diameter of high power field and mitotic frequency		

Grade I: score 3–5
Grade II: score 6–7
Grade III: score 8–9

ER and PgR scoring systems

McCarty's Semi quantitative H scoring (total score 0–300).
(Percentage of stained cells multiplied by a number, 0–3, reflecting the intensity of staining).

Negative	score ≤50 (–)
Weakly positive	51–100 (+)
Moderately positive	101–200 (++)
Strongly positive	201–300 (+++)

Her-2/neu scoring

Immunohistochemical scoring
Score 0–1+: Negative

2+: Borderline – needs further testing

3+: Positive

FISH score
<2.0, not amplified: Negative
>2.0, amplified: Positive

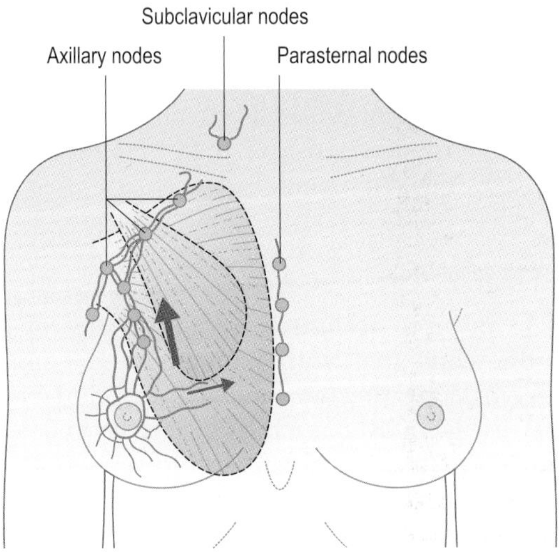

Figure 10.1
Surgical anatomy of breast and lymphatic drainage.

approximately 20–30 axillary lymph nodes which are surgically defined as:

- Level I – nodes inferior to pectoralis minor (12–14 in number).
- Level II – nodes posterior to pectoralis minor (6–8 in number).
- Level III – nodes superior to the pectoralis minor (2–4 in number).

Internal mammary nodes (3–5 nodes on either side) lie 2–3 cm from the sternal edge from the 3rd to 5th to intercostal space at a depth of 4–6 cm depending on the body habitus.

More than 75% of all lymphatic drainage passes through the axillary nodes and the remainder through the internal mammary nodes. There is a higher risk of internal mammary node involvement with medially located tumours and in those with extensive axillary nodes. Apical axillary node involvement leads to blockage of lymphatics and subsequent retrograde spread of cancer to supraclavicular nodes (see Figure 10.1).

Presentation

Many patients with early breast cancer are detected during screening by mammography.

The usual presentations are painless lump (65–75%), distortion of the breast (5%) and nipple discharge (2%). A small proportion of patients present with isolated axillary lymphadenopathy. Some patients present with metastatic manifestations such as bone pain, respiratory symptoms and features of liver metastases and brain disease.

Signs

Breast examination may reveal a non-tender, well or ill-defined lump with or without fixity to the skin or chest wall. The skin may be dimpled, invaded, reddened, indurated or with nodular irregularity.

Axillary and supraclavicular lymph nodes may be enlarged. Hepatomegaly, pleural effusion and spinal tenderness (usually thoracic and lumbar) can occur in metastatic disease.

Initial assessment

'Triple' assessment of patients with suspected breast cancer includes a combination of clinical

All patients
- Age, menopausal status, performance status
- Previous breast disease, co-morbidities which affect treatments (cardiac/diabetes/systemic sclerosis), history of blood clots, other medications and allergies
- Family history (breast cancer, ovary, prostate, sarcoma)

New patient with local disease
- Size and location of tumour
- Nodal status
- Receptor status
- Patient anxieties about body image and thoughts about reconstruction if appropriate
- Planned surgery

New patient with metastatic disease
- Location and extent (bulk) of metastatic disease
- Receptor status
- Any signs of impending emergencies which affect treatment (e.g. SVCO, SCC)
- Any signs of life-threatening visceral involvement

Patient with local relapse
- Previous stage and date of original diagnosis
- Details of previous treatments and treatment related complications and time since completion of original treatment
- Receptor status
- Duration of current symptoms/signs hormone status
- Staging at time of local relapse (current staging)

Patient with metastatic relapse
- Previous stage and date of original diagnosis
- Details of previous treatments and treatment related complications and time since completion of original treatment
- Receptor status
- Duration of current symptoms/signs hormone status
- Current staging
- Any signs of impending emergencies which affect treatment (e.g. SVCO, SCC)
- Any signs of life-threatening visceral involvement

examination, breast imaging (mammography and/or ultrasound) and pathologic evaluation (core biopsy). With this approach, a definite diagnosis of breast cancer can be made in 99% of cases.

Clinical examination

Clinical examination helps to elicit physical signs, accurately document the site of lesion, and contributes to tumour and nodal staging.

Breast imaging

Mammogram

The commonest mammographic abnormality of DCIS is micro-calcification (in 50% cases). Other features include asymmetric density and mass. High-grade DCIS is associated with linear and branching calcification, whereas low-grade DCIS is associated with fine and granular calcification. Invasive cancer appears as a speculated mass (Figure 10.2). Although calcification can occur in various conditions, a linear small (<1 mm in diameter), non-uniform size and clustered calcification is suggestive of malignancy.

Mammogram has a low sensitivity in breasts with considerable fibroglandular tissue, particularly in young women and those on hormone replacement therapy (HRT). The evolving digital mammography has the benefits of better imaging of dense breast and computer-assisted detection.

Ultrasound

Ultrasound examination of the breast helps to distinguish between solid and cystic lesions of more than 1 cm in size. Malignancy appears as a hypoechoic lesion with associated distortion of the surrounding tissues and an acoustic shadow on the breast tissue below it (Figure 10.3). It is also useful to assess axillary nodal status as well as to aid in guided FNA and core biopsy. Ultrasound is less sensitive than mammography for early detection and hence is not used for screening.

MRI scan

MRI can more accurately define the size of the tumour compared with mammography and is better in delineating intraductal disease and multifocal disease. MRI has a high sensitivity in detecting cancers (almost 100%) and lower sensitivity in detecting DCIS (80%), but has a higher false positivity. MRI is more useful for young women who have dense breast tissue (Figure 10.4). MRI is particularly useful in screening women less than

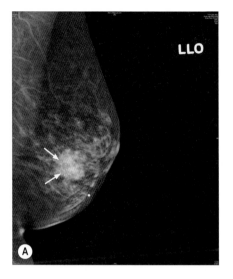

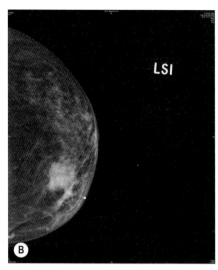

Figure 10.2
Mammogram. Mediolateral oblique (MLO) view (A) shows an irregular lesion in the breast with specks of calcification (arrows). Craniocaudal (superioinferior) view (B) conventionally represents the outer or lateral aspect of breast at the top of the film and medial aspect at the bottom of the film and hence the mass is in the medial aspect of breast.

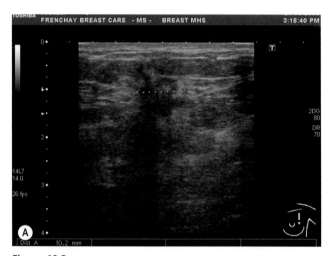

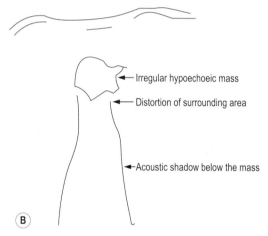

Figure 10.3
Ultrasound in breast cancer.

40 years with a high risk of breast cancer, to rule out multifocal disease prior to conservation, imaging women with implants and to distinguish scars from tumour recurrence.

Pathological diagnosis

Pathological diagnosis may be obtained by core biopsy or open surgical biopsy. Core biopsy can be obtained by conventional or vacuum assisted means such as Mammotome. Vacuum assisted core biopsy yields a larger sample and may in some cases allow complete removal of the target abnormality in the breast. Clinically impalpable lesions may necessitate image localization using mammography or ultrasound and hook wire replacement before open biopsy.

Investigations after triple assessment

Most patients with early stage disease without clinical evidence of metastatic disease will proceed to surgery after preoperative assessment. Patients who require neoadjuvant systemic treatment prior to definite surgical management need staging investigations including:

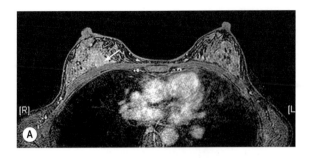

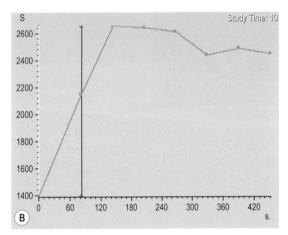

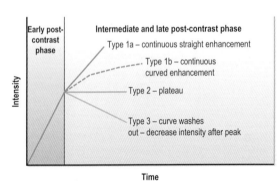

Type 1 – mostly benign (83%) and 9% malignant
Type 2 – 11% benign and 35% malignant
Type 3 – typical malignant (57% malignant and 5% benign)

Figure 10.4
MRI showing breast cancer and different time–intensity curves. Breast lesion near the chest wall (A) shows a time-intensity curve which washes out (B) after the early peak suggesting malignancy. C shows different types of dose–intensity curves.

- Full blood count, liver function, renal function tests and serum alkaline phosphatase.
- Chest X-ray and CT scan of chest and abdomen – to rule out distant metastasis.
- Bone scan.

Box 10.3: Staging of breast cancer

Stage 0
- Tx – primary tumour cannot be assessed.
- T0 – no evidence of primary tumour.
- Tis – carcinoma-in-situ and Paget's disease with no tumour

Stage I (T1N0M0)
- T1 – tumour 2 cm or less in its greatest dimension
- N0 – no regional lymph node metastasis
- M0 – no distant metastases

Stage II

IIA (TxN1M0, T1N1M0, T2N0M0)
- T2 – tumour larger than 2 cm but not larger than 5 cm
- N1 – ipsilateral non-fixed lymph node metastasis

IIB (T2N1M0, T3N0M0)
- T3 – tumour more than 5 cm

Stage III

IIIA (Tx-2N2M0, T2-3N1-2M0)
- N2 – ipsilateral fixed axillary node or ipsilateral internal mammary lymph nodes

IIIB T4N0-2M0
- T4 – tumour of any size with direct extension to:
  - T4a – Extension to chest wall
  - T4b – oedema (including peau d'orange) or ulceration of the breast skin, or satellite skin nodules confined to the same breast
  - T4c – both T4a and T4b
  - T4d – inflammatory breast cancer

IIIC (any T, N3 M0)
- N3 – metastasis to ipsilateral supraclavicular lymph nodes or infraclavicular lymph nodes or metastasis to the internal mammary lymph nodes with metastasis to the axillary lymph nodes.

Stage IV (any T, any N, M1)
- M1 – distant metastasis

Postoperatively, patients with ≥4 positive lymph nodes and T4 disease also need the above investigations. In those with less than four positive nodes, normal biochemistry and no symptoms suggestive of metastasis, the incidence of metastasis is 2–4% and hence routine staging is not advised.

Staging

TNM staging of breast cancer is given in Box 10.3.

Management of carcinoma-in-situ

Ductal carcinoma-in-situ (DCIS)

Treatment is aimed at preventing local recurrence, particularly of invasive cancer. After biopsy alone, 40% will progress to invasive cancer. Surgical management of unicentric DCIS includes conservative surgery and simple mastectomy. These choices should be discussed with patients. Those who undergo mastectomy can be considered for immediate reconstruction. There is no recommended optimal margin for DCIS; a margin of >10 mm is adequate and <1 mm in inadequate (NICE recommends 2 mm). Patients with a persistent positive margin after repeat surgical excision, widespread DCIS (involving two or more quadrants), suspicious microcalcification throughout the breast and those likely to have an unacceptable cosmetic result with conservative surgery are considered for simple mastectomy. Axillary staging and dissection are unnecessary for patients with pure DCIS. Some series report up to 2% incidence of axillary node metastasis due to an unrecognized invasive cancer.

Randomized studies show that postoperative radiotherapy (45–50 Gy in 1.8–2 Gy per fraction) reduces breast recurrence (both in situ and invasive) with no effect on survival and irrespective of prognostic factors. However, in a subgroup with <10 mm, low/intermediate grade DCIS with adequate margin, radiotherapy may be safely omitted (<10% local recurrence at 10 years). Though there is no randomized study looking at the benefit of tumour bed boost radiotherapy, it may be considered if further excision to obtain a wider margin is likely to compromise cosmetic results.

Two studies evaluated the benefits of tamoxifen in DCIS. NSABP B-24 showed that tamoxifen reduced local recurrence of DCIS and invasive cancer (11% vs. 7.7%, p = 0.02) whereas UKCCCR trial showed that tamoxifen had no beneficial effect in reducing local recurrence when combined with whole breast radiotherapy (15 vs. 13%, p = 0.42). In the absence of radiotherapy tamoxifen reduced the risk of DCIS recurrence (10 vs. 6%, p = 0.03) but not invasive recurrence.

There is no universally accepted recommendation for adjuvant hormones. Current studies evaluate various hormonal agents (e.g. IBIS II).

With mammographic follow-up, breast cancer disease free survival in DCIS approaches 100%.

Women with DCIS in one breast are at risk of a contralateral tumour occurring at a rate of 0.5–1% per annum.

Lobular carcinoma-in-situ (LCIS)

LCIS comprises 30–50% of carcinoma-in-situ, associated with invasive cancer in 10% and are frequently bilateral (35–60%). It is usually undetectable clinically and cannot be seen on mammogram due to the lack of central necrosis. One-third of people develop invasive cancer in the same or contralateral breast over 20 years. However, the issue of whether LCIS is a direct precursor of invasive lobular carcinoma has yet to be resolved.

Isolated LCIS following biopsy is managed with close observation. The rate of progression to cancer after biopsy alone is approximately 1% per annum. Mastectomy is generally reserved for patients with the highest risk of invasive recurrence such as young age, diffuse high-grade lesions and significant family history. Tamoxifen is being increasingly used as prophylactic treatment which has shown to reduce the invasive recurrence by 56%.

LCIS associated with DCIS or invasive cancer is managed according to the dominant malignant histology. There is no need for further surgery to obtain a clear margin for LCIS.

Management of early stage invasive cancer (Figure 10.5)

After triple assessment, initial treatment options for early stage (non-inflammatory T1–2N0–1M0) include:

- Conservative surgery with axillary surgery.
- Mastectomy with axillary surgery.
- Neoadjuvant chemotherapy followed by conservative surgery (when primary surgery is likely to result in unacceptable cosmesis).

Surgery

Surgery is aimed at removal of the primary breast tumour and staging and/or treating the axilla.

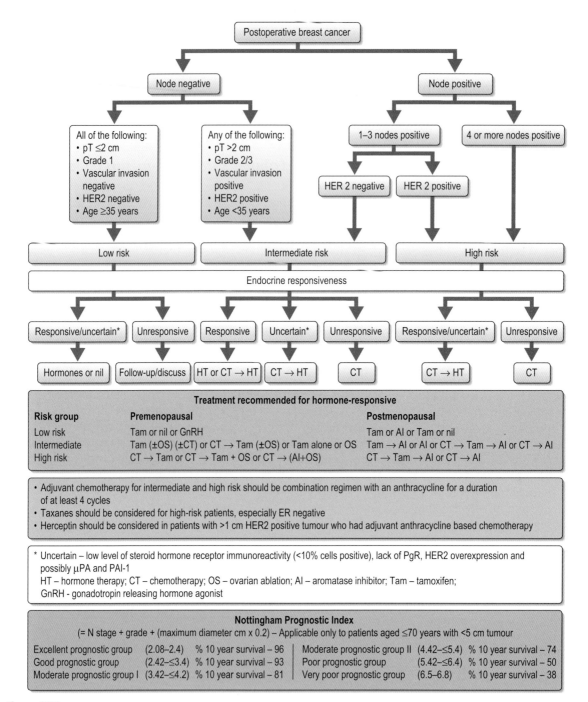

Figure 10.5
Adjuvant systemic treatment in breast cancer (based on St. Galen International consensus 2007).

- Prior radiotherapy to the breast or chest wall (can't give more radiotherapy)
- Radiotherapy during pregnancy (risk of radiation to the foetus)
- Diffuse suspicious or malignant appearing microcalcification (difficult to obtain clear margin)
- Widespread disease that cannot be completely excised with satisfactory cosmesis through a single incision (result in negative margin and/or poor cosmesis)
- Persistent positive pathological margin (can't obtain clear margin of >1 mm)
- Active connective tissue disease involving skin (scleroderma and lupus) (due to increased risk of radiation toxicity, if patient insists on conservation, radiotherapy is given at a reduced dose)
- Tumours of >5 cm (may result in poor cosmesis; however conservation can be attempted after neoadjuvant chemotherapy)
- Focally positive disease with extensive intradual component (focally positive disease without extensive intraductal component can be treated with higher dose of radiotherapy)
- Women ≤35 years or premenopausal with BRCA1/2 mutation (higher risk of recurrence)

Primary breast surgery can be either conservative (wide local excision – WLE followed by radiotherapy) or mastectomy. Conservative surgery followed by postoperative radiotherapy offers a better cosmetic outcome than mastectomy. However, not all patients are suitable for breast conservation (Box 10.4).

Breast surgery

WLE aims to remove the cancer with at least >1 mm circumferential microscopic disease free margin. The clinico-pathological factors that increase the risk of local recurrence after WLE include:

- Positive margin (<1 mm). The risk of recurrence is 16–21% with a positive margin compared with 2–5% with a negative margin and hence all patients need re-excision if technically feasible.
- Age ≤35 years (2–3 times increased risk of local recurrence).
- Extensive intraductal component (defined as an infiltrating ductal cancer where >25% of the tumour volume is DCIS and DCIS extends beyond the invasive cancer into the surrounding normal breast parenchyma).
- Lymphovascular invasion – increases the risk of recurrence by 1.5 times.
- Grade (grade I tumours have 1.5 times less risk of recurrence than grade II–III).

Mastectomy: involves complete removal of the breast from the pectoral fascia. Risk factors for chest wall recurrence after mastectomy include tumour of >5 cm, more than 4 nodes involved, margin <1 mm. Grade 3 and vascular invasion are not independent risk factors for recurrence.

Breast reconstruction after mastectomy

Reconstruction can be done at the same time as mastectomy (immediate) or at a later date (delayed). Immediate reconstruction can be offered to patients with diffuse DCIS and early breast cancer who may not require postoperative radiotherapy (radiotherapy to a reconstructed breast can result in poor cosmetic outcome). Delayed reconstruction is appropriate when postoperative radiotherapy is planned and there is concern about tumour clearance.

Methods of reconstruction include:

- Tissue expanders – initially the expander is placed in the pocket deep to pectoralis muscle, which is later replaced with a permanent implant containing silicone gel or saline after a few months. Complications include infections, failure of expansion and capsular contracture (particularly after radiotherapy).
- Autologous tissue – using either a pediculated flap (e.g. latissimus dorsi flap) or a free flap (free transverse rectus abdominis – TRAM flap).

Axillary surgery

Axillary surgery includes sentinel node biopsy (SNB) alone, SNB followed by axillary dissection or axillary dissection alone. SNB is not done in cases of high risk of axillary node involvement (e.g. palpable axillary node >3 cm or T3 or T4 tumours, multicentric tumours), previous history of surgery to breast or axilla, during pregnancy or lactation (contraindication of dye and radioisotope) and after neoadjuvant systemic treatment outside of clinical trials (role not defined), where dissection is the norm.

For SNB the sentinel node is localized by preoperative intradermal injection of technetium labelled colloid and lymphoscintiscan or by intraoperative injection of blue due or using both techniques. Sentinel node biopsy has >95% detection rate.

Patients who are sentinel node positive will undergo axillary clearance. A current study (ALMANAC) is evaluating the role of axillary radiotherapy in patients who are sentinel node positive.

Adjuvant radiotherapy
(Boxes 10.5 and 10.6)

A meta-analysis suggests that adjuvant radiotherapy results in a reduction of local recurrence by two-thirds and improves 15-year survival by 5%. It also suggested that at 15 years one breast cancer death is avoided for every four local recurrences prevented.

After conservative surgery

Radiotherapy reduces the risk of local recurrence after breast conservation (5-year local recurrence of 7% with radiotherapy and 26% without radiotherapy) and is the current standard after WLE. However, one study showed that in patients over 70 years with good prognostic factors (less than 2 cm tumour, grade 1 or 2, ER positive, node negative and no lymphovascular invasion) omission of radiotherapy may not compromise survival.

Addition of radiotherapy to the tumour bed (boost) after whole breast radiotherapy has shown to reduce local recurrence (10-year local recurrence rate of 6.2% with boost and 10.2% without boost p < 0.001). On multivariate analysis, age was the only significant predictor of local recurrence and the greatest benefit was seen in those aged <40 years. Boost radiotherapy did not improve 10-year overall survival. Many centres now follow a risk adapted policy for boost.

Postmastectomy radiotherapy
(Boxes 10.5 and 10.6)

There is ongoing debate on the role of radiotherapy after mastectomy. Chest wall recurrence is thought to arise from tumour that has involved dermal lymphatics. Patients with a tumour of ≥5 cm size and ≥4 positive lymph nodes are at

---

Box 10.5: Radiotherapy in breast cancer

Indications

Whole breast
- After breast conservation for invasive cancer
- After breast conservation for DCIS (except low risk of recurrence)

Tumour bed boost
- All patients <40 years
- 40–50 years with high risk features
- Patients with <1 mm margin and further surgery is not contemplated

Postmastectomy chest wall
- T3/T4 tumour
- ≥4 positive nodes after dissection

Supraclavicular fossa
- ≥4 positive nodes after dissection

Position
- Supine with arm abducted (for CT plan)
- Supine with angled breast boards (conventional)

Localization
- Simulator or CT planning
- Target volume

Clinical target volume (CTV)
- Whole breast – entire breast tissue and subcutaneous tissue excluding muscles, rib cage and skin
- Chest wall – skin including scar extending up to deep fascia excluding muscles and rib cage
- Tumour bed – 1.5–2 cm around surgical cavity or haematoma
- SCF nodes – SCF node, infraclavicular nodes and apical nodes

Planning target volume
- 1 cm margin around CTV

Dose
Whole breast, chest wall and supraclavicular fossa
- 50 Gy in 25 fractions/40 Gy in 15 fractions

Tumour bed boost
- 16 Gy in 8 fractions (EORTC study)
- 9 Gy in 3, 10 Gy in 5, 12.5 Gy in 5 etc

---

high risk of chest wall recurrence (20–30%) and routine postoperative chest wall radiotherapy is advised. This results in less local recurrence (6% vs. 23%) and improvement of 15-year survival by 5%. Postmastectomy radiotherapy may be considered in cases of T1 tumour with 1–3 positive nodes or T2 tumours with features of biological aggressiveness (ER−, HER2+, grade 3 and high proliferative index).

Box 10.6: Radiotherapy side effects

Acute
- Fatigue
- Skin erythema (100%) and inframammary fold desquamation (10%)

Late
- Swelling and induration of breast (30%)
- Telangiectasia (1% severe)
- Asymptomatic lung changes (1%)
- Sarcoma (<1% risk at 30 years)
- Lymphoedema (3–40% depends on the extent of axillary surgery)
- Brachial plexopathy (1%)

Patients with ≥4 involved nodes after axillary dissection are at risk of supraclavicular recurrence (>15%) and hence supraclavicular radiotherapy is advised. Axillary radiotherapy is not recommended after axillary dissection as there is 30–40% risk of significant lymphoedema and the risk of isolated axillary recurrence without radiotherapy is only 1–4%. However, it may be considered in rare instances of residual macroscopic disease in the axilla or positive dissection margin.

Adjuvant systemic treatment

Adjuvant systemic therapy is aimed at preventing recurrences by eradicating micro metastatic disease which is presumed to be present at the time of diagnosis. Adjuvant systemic treatment is recommended when there is a significant reduction in calculated risk of recurrence with an acceptable level of treatment related toxicity. However, the optimal strategy for advising systemic treatment has not yet been determined.

Hormone receptor status and HER2 status are the most important determinants in the choice of systemic treatment. Patients with ER+ tumours may receive hormones alone or a combination of endocrine treatment and chemotherapy. Patients with ER– tumours are considered for adjuvant chemotherapy alone. However, there are no clear guidelines on the threshold of benefit above which adjuvant chemotherapy is advised. Some experts justify adjuvant chemotherapy for patients with <90% 10-year survival and others use an absolute survival benefit of at least 3–5% at 10 years with chemotherapy. Several decision

making tools (e.g. adjuvant online – https://www.adjuvantonline.com and Nottingham prognostic index) have been developed to help to make adjuvant treatment decisions. According to the 2007 St. Gallen Consensus adjuvant chemotherapy is generally recommended for intermediate and high-risk patients (Figure 10.5). Patients with HER2+ tumours of >1 cm and/or nodal involvement are considered for adjuvant trastuzumab (see later, p. 128).

Adjuvant chemotherapy

A meta-analysis suggest that 6 months of anthracycline based combination chemotherapy reduces yearly death from breast cancer by about 38% in women younger than 50 years and by 20% for women aged 50–69 years (absolute risk reduction at 5 years of approximately 3% for DFS and OS). A recent meta-analysis showed that addition of a taxane to anthracycline-based chemotherapy results in an absolute risk reduction at 5 years of 5% for DFS (17% relative reduction in relapse) and 3% for OS (15% relative reduction in death) for high risk early breast cancer. Subgroup analysis showed that the DFS benefit was present irrespective of ER status, number of lymph nodes involved, age, menopausal status and HER-2 status. However, it is uncertain whether all subgroups, particularly those with node-negative disease, derive such benefit from adjuvant taxanes.

A practical approach is to use anthracycline based chemotherapy (e.g. FEC or Epi-CMF) for patients without high-risk early breast cancer and taxane-anthracycline chemotherapy for high risk patients needing chemotherapy (Figure 10.5). In the UK, anthracyclines-taxane combination is licensed to use in patients with node positive breast cancer. Box 10.7 shows the commonly used chemotherapy regimes in breast cancer

Adjuvant endocrine therapy (Figure 10.5)

The Early Breast Cancer Trialists' Group overview of adjuvant tamoxifen has shown that tamoxifen for 5 years results in a 41% proportional reduction in recurrence and 34% proportional reduction in mortality in oestrogen receptor positive breast cancer patients irrespective of age, menopausal status, and administration of

Box 10.7: Chemotherapy regimes in breast cancer

Adjuvant/neoadjuvant

CMF
- Cyclophosphamide 100 mg/m^2 po days 1–14
- Methotrexate 40 mg/m^2 IV days 1 and 8
- 5 FU 600 mg/m^2 IV days 1 and 8
- Folinic Acid Rescue 15 mg 6-hourly × 6 doses po days 2 and 9. Start 24 hours post MTX

28-day cycle × 4–6 cycles

Epi-CMF (efficacy based on preliminary results from the NEAT study, ASCO 2003)
- Epirubicin 100 mg/m^2 IV bolus 21-day cycle for 4 cycles
- CMF as below for 4 cycles for 4 cycles

FEC
- 5 FU 600 mg/m^2 IV day 1
- Epirubicin 60–75 mg/m^2 IV day 1
- Cyclophosphamide 600 mg/m^2 IV day 1

21-day cycle. For 6 cycles

FEC100
- Epirubicin 100 mg/m^2 IV day 1
- 5 FU 500 mg/m^2 IV day 1
- Cyclophosphamide 500 mg/m^2 IV day 1

21-day cycle. For 6 cycles

FEC-D

FEC given 3 weekly for 3 cycles (as above) followed by docetaxel 100 mg/m^2 IV on D1 every 21 days for 3 cycles.

TAC
- Docetaxel 75 mg/m^2 IV day 1
- Adriamycin 50 mg/m^2 IV day 1
- Cyclophosphamide 500 mg/m^2 IV day 1

21-day cycle for 6 cycles

EC-T (EC given 3 weekly for 4 cycles followed by T given 3 weekly for 4 cycles)
- Epirubicin 90 mg/m^2 IV day 1 once in 3 weeks
- Cyclophosphamide 600 mg/m^2 IV day 1 once in 3 weeks
- Docetaxel 100 mg/m^2 IV day 1 once in 3 weeks

Docetaxel
- Docetaxel 100 mg/m^2 IV day 1

21-day cycle for 6 cycles

AC
- Doxorubicin 60 mg/m^2 IV day 1
- Cyclophosphamide 600 mg/m^2 IV day 1

21-day cycle for 4–6 cycles (there is controversy regarding optimum duration)

Palliative
- Capecitabine 1250 mg/m^2 PO twice daily 1-14 given 3 weekly until progression, intolerable toxicity or patient/clinician choice to stop

And many others including the previous regimes!

Weekly treatments in bone marrow failure

(If bone marrow recovers the patient may be switched to a 3-weekly regimen)

Weekly Epirubicin
- Epirubicin 20 mg/m^2 IV day 1 every week for 12 weeks

Weekly docetaxel
- Docetaxel 30–40 mg/m^2 IV weekly for up to 12 weeks

Weekly paclitaxel
- Paclitaxel 80–100 mg/m^2 IV weekly up to 12 weeks

chemotherapy. There is also a proportional reduction of contralateral breast cancer by 47%.

In premenopausal women tamoxifen (20 mg daily for 5 years) or tamoxifen combined with ovarian function ablation achieved either by bilateral oophorectomy or gonadotropin releasing hormone agonists (GnRH) for at least 2 years are standard recommendations. Aromatase inhibitors (AIs) are not indicated for premenopausal women (see below). A study of GnRH agonist, goserelin for 2 years (ZIPP) showed that in women who weren't given tamoxifen, goserelin resulted in 14% less cancer related events and prevented 8.5 deaths whereas when given with tamoxifen, goserelin results in 2.8% fewer events and 2.6% less death compared with patients received only tamoxifen.

In postmenopausal women the adjuvant hormone options are:

- Tamoxifen for 5 years.
- Tamoxifen for 2–3 years with early switch to AIs exemestane or letrozole (total 5 years).
- AI for 5-years – letrozole or anastrazole (for large tumours, node positivity or HER2+ disease).
- Tamoxifen for 5 years followed by AI (letrozole) for another 2–3 years (for node positive disease).

The optimal duration of tamoxifen currently appears to be 5 years. Early results of the two randomized studies of extended tamoxifen (aTTom and ATLAS) did not show any significant benefit but an increased risk of endometrial cancer and venous thrombosis with 10 years of tamoxifen.

Early switch to AI, initial AI and extended use of hormones have all shown improvement in DFS with a decrease in distant metastasis, breast recurrence and contralateral tumours.

Mechanisms of action of hormonal agents

Oestrogen stimulates the growth of breast cancer. In premenopausal women 90% of total oestrogen is produced by the ovary which is stimulated by FSH and LH. The remaining oestrogen is produced by peripheral conversion of circulating androgen by the enzyme aromatase which is seen in extraovarian tissues such as subcutaneous fat, liver, muscle, breast and breast cancer cells. In postmenopausal women, ovarian production of oestrogen ceases and extraovarian production from secondary sources continues. Aromatase activity also increases with age.

Hormonal treatment is aimed at decreasing oestrogenic stimulation of breast cancer cells. This is achieved by either preventing the binding of oestrogen to cancer cells (e.g. tamoxifen), or by inhibiting ovarian and extraovarian production of oestrogens (e.g. oophorectomy, GnRH agonists and aromatase inhibitors).

Hormonal agents

Tamoxifen is a non-steroidal antioestrogen which has antagonist activity against breast cancer cells and agonist effect on bone, endometrium and serum lipids. Tamoxifen causes competitive inhibition with oestrogen for oestrogen receptors which results in a G1 block leading to decreased tumour growth. Other mechanisms include induction of apoptosis, and increasing NK cell activity.

The side effects of tamoxifen include hot flushes (50%), vaginal discharge and irregular menses. Tamoxifen increases the risk of endometrial cancer, especially in those above 50 years of age (80 excess cases per 10,000 tamoxifen treated women at 10 years). Other side effects include endometrial polyp and hyperplasia, thromboembolism (1–2%) and retinopathy. The beneficial effects of tamoxifen include increase in bone mineral density and decreased circulating cholesterol and LDL.

Aromatase inhibitors reduce oestrogen levels in postmenopausal women by inhibiting the aromatase enzyme in extraovarian tissue. However these are ineffective in premenopausal women as they increase gonadotropin secretion which leads to reduced feedback of oestrogen on the hypothalamic–pituitary axis, thereby causing increased aromatase activity. There are two groups of AIs:

- Type 1 inhibitor (steroidal analogue–enzyme inactivator) – irreversibly bind to aromatase, e.g. exemestane.
- Type 2 inhibitor – non-steroidal analogue–enzyme inhibitor – reversibly bind to the enzyme, e.g. anastrazole and letrozole.

The usual side effects of AIs are hot flushes, joint pain and muscular stiffness. The long-term risk of osteoporosis is a concern (see p. 61, late effects). All patients need bone mineral density assessment by DEXA scan prior to starting AI. Patients with osteopenia need vitamin D and calcium supplement whereas those with a T-score less than −2.5 SD (osteoporosis) need bisphosphonates. All patients on AI need a 2-yearly DEXA scan.

Adjuvant trastuzumab

In patients with HER2+ disease (immunohistochemical score of 3+ or FISH score >2.0) one year of adjuvant trastuzumab is recommended. Trastuzumab (Herceptin) is a humanized monoclonal antibody again the extracellular domain of HER2. All the six randomized studies have shown improved DFS with addition of trastuzumab to chemotherapy while 4 of the 6 trials showed an overall survival benefit with adjuvant trastuzumab, e.g. HERA study which compared chemotherapy vs. chemotherapy with trastuzumab showed a better 3-year DFS (81% vs. 74%) and OS (92% vs. 90%).

Adjuvant trastuzumab is indicated in patients with >1 cm and/or node positive tumour and who received adjuvant chemotherapy. The role of trastuzumab in <1 cm and node negative disease as well as a single modality is not studied.

A loading dose of 8 mg/kg followed by 17 maintenance doses of 6 mg/kg every three weeks is the recommended schedule. If there are more than 7 days delay treatment needs to be restarted with a loading dose.

Common side effects include hypersensitivity and flu-like symptoms. Cardiotoxicity is a concern (<4% symptomatic or severe cardiac failure). Hence it is not given if the left ventricular ejection fraction is <50%. It is not given concurrently with anthracyclines, but can be given concurrently with taxanes. Cardiac monitoring during treatment is mandatory. A recent study reported no increase in adverse cardiac events in patients receiving trastuzumab with adjuvant radiotherapy.

Locally advanced disease (T3 N1, T1–3 N2–3, T4 N0–3)
(Figure 10.6)

Patients with locally advanced breast cancer are usually treated with neoadjuvant systemic therapy which is aimed at down staging the primary tumour which may facilitate surgery or even avoid the need for mastectomy. Full staging workup is needed in this group of patients.

In older women with receptor positive tumours, initial hormonal treatment can be used. Although studies show that all the AIs result in a higher response than tamoxifen, letrozole is the only licensed drug for neoadjuvant use. Two randomized studies, separately comparing letrozole and anastrazole with tamoxifen, showed that aromatase inhibitors induce a higher rate of regression allowing breast conservation. In the comparative study of 4 months of tamoxifen with letrozole, letrozole has a higher response rate (55%) than tamoxifen (36%). This study also showed that those patients with HER-1 or HER-2+ tumours had a higher response to letrozole (88% vs. 21%). In the second study anastrazole achieved significantly higher breast-conservation rate than tamoxifen (47% vs. 22%, p = 0.03).

Neoadjuvant chemotherapy is the standard treatment for patients with large primary tumours aiming for conservation and for inflammatory breast cancer (see p. 132). Chemotherapy results in a 70–90% response with a 20% pathological complete response. NSABP B-27 showed that an initial anthracycline regime followed by docetaxel results in a better response rate (90.7% vs. 85.5%, p < 0.001) and pathological complete response (64% vs. 40%, p < 0.001). In patients with HER2 positive tumours addition of trastuzumab results in improved pathological response (65% vs. 26%, p = 0.016) and it is advisable to incorporate trastuzumab with the neoadjuvant non-anthracycline chemotherapy. One such approach is to give initial 3–4 courses of anthracycline chemotherapy followed by taxanes with trastuzumab. In breast cancer, type and degree of response to primary systemic treatment predicts disease-free as well as overall survival.

After neoadjuvant chemotherapy, inflammatory breast cancer patients undergo total mastectomy whereas non-inflammatory breast cancer patients undergo mastectomy or conservation if appropriate. If patients had negative SNB prechemotherapy, no axillary surgery is needed. If axillary nodal status is unknown or positive SNB, axillary clearance is needed.

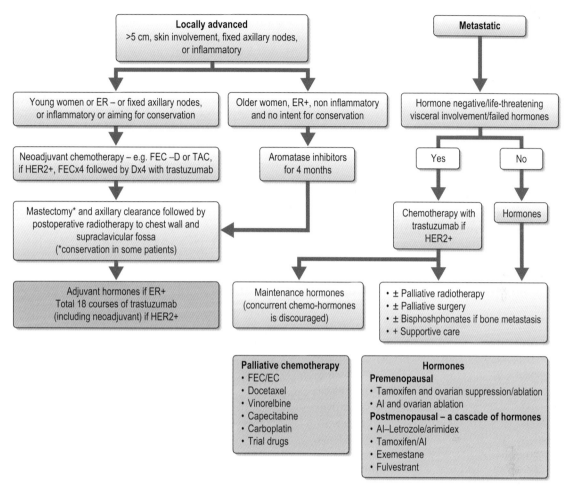

Figure 10.6
Management of locally advanced and metastatic breast cancer.

All patients need postoperative radiotherapy to chest wall or breast (Figure 10.6). Adjuvant systemic treatment depends on hormone receptor and HER2 status.

Metastatic disease (any T, any N, M1) (Figure 10.6)

Approximately 6% patients present with distant metastasis at diagnosis and 40% of patients with early stage disease will eventually develop metastases. The survival of patients with metastatic disease varies from months to years. Bone metastases have the best outcome, followed by lung, liver and brain metastases.

Evaluation includes complete history and examination, blood tests including the tumour marker CA15-3 if available, CT scan chest, abdomen and pelvis, bone scan and receptor status. Imaging of the brain is indicated only if symptomatic.

The aims of treatment are symptom control, improving quality of life and survival. Treatment options include hormones, chemotherapy and biological agents.

Patients with hormone receptor positive disease without life-threatening visceral involvement are treated with hormonal treatment. In premenopausal women who have not previously had tamoxifen or discontinued for >12 months, the standard option is tamoxifen and ovarian ablation or suppression. Otherwise, an AI with ovarian ablation may be considered.

In postmenopausal women studies show that AI have superior results compared with tamoxifen so should be the drug of choice, if not received previously. In one study, letrozole resulted in a significantly longer time to progression (41 vs. 26 weeks, p = 0.0001) and higher response rate (30% vs. 20%, p = 0.0006) compared with tamoxifen in advanced breast cancer. Since data are in more favour of letrozole, it is the agent of choice. There is no definite recommendation for second-line, but the options include tamoxifen, anastrazole, letrozole, exemestane, fulvestrant and megesterol acetate. Unless there is an indication for chemotherapy, various hormonal agents are used as a cascade of treatment until all options are exhausted.

Chemotherapy is used in patients with receptor negative tumours, hormone resistant tumours, and life-threatening progressive disease. Chemotherapy results in a 50% response rate usually lasting less than one year. Based on meta-analysis, anthracyclines result in a greater clinical benefit than a CMF regime and should be considered as first-line treatment if the patient has not previously received an anthracycline. Taxanes are the options after anthracycline failure. Both docetaxel and paclitaxel have proven activity. Other agents used in breast cancer include capecitabine, vinorelbine, gemcitabine, carboplatin, etc. (Box 10.6).

Patients with HER2 positive disease are treated with trastuzumab with or without chemotherapy. In patients who progress on trastuzumab, retrospective data support a change of chemotherapy with continuation of trastuzumab; however, NICE recommends discontinuation if it is systemic progression. Patients with HER2 positive disease have a high risk of brain metastasis. Trastuzumab need not be discontinued on isolated progression/relapse in the brain.

In patients after trastuzumab failure, lapatinib is a treatment option, though currently not yet approved in the UK. It is an inhibitor of HER2 and as well as EGFR (ErbB1) receptor. A randomized study in patients who had been previously treated with trastuzumab showed a significant improvement in time to progression with capecitabine combined with lapatinib compared with capecitabine alone (6.2 months vs. 4.3 months, p = 0.00013).

A very small subset of patients present with bone marrow failure subsequent to extensive bone disease. Modified chemotherapy with low-dose weekly anthracycline or taxanes is the option in these patients (Box 10.6).

In patients with metastatic disease, response to treatment should be evaluated after 3 months of endocrine treatment and after 2–3 cycles of chemotherapy.

Recurrent disease

2–20% patients after conservative surgery and <10% patients after radical surgery will present with loco-regional recurrence within 10 years. 10–70% patients present with metastatic recurrence within 10 years.

Patients presenting with isolated loco-regional recurrence need complete staging prior to potentially curative treatment and 'secondary' adjuvant treatment. Patients with systemic recurrence are treated similarly to those with metastatic disease.

Palliative care

- Bone metastases – treated with pain management as per WHO analgesic ladder (p. 66) and local radiotherapy studies show that 8–10 Gy as a single fraction has similar efficacy to that of prolonged. Women with bone metastases should be given bisphosphonates which help to control pain as well as prevent fractures, need for radiotherapy or orthopaedic surgery and epidoses of hypercalcaemia. Pamidronate, ibandronate, clodronate and zoledronic acid have all been shown to be effective.
- Brain metastasis – management of brain metastases are dealt with in Chapter 16 (p. 278). Patients with HER2+ disease have a high risk of brain metastasis, particularly to the posterior fossa.
- Tumour related symptoms of fungation, discharge and bleeding are treated with either palliative mastectomy or radiotherapy.

- Management of oncological emergencies such as spinal cord compression and hypercalcaemia are discussed in Chapter 23 (p. 328).

Prognostic factors and outcome

Lymph node metastasis is the most important prognostic factor. The number of lymph nodes involved has prognostic implications. Other important prognostic factors include tumour size (affects the risk of nodal involvement, metastasis and survival), grade (affects survival), age (women aged <35 years have twice the risk of local recurrence and 1.6 times higher risk of distant metastasis compared with >35 years), hormone receptor status (patients with ER+ tumours have better survival), lymphatic invasion (presence of which increases local recurrence and systemic recurrence) and HER2+vity (adverse prognosis, more likely to respond to anthracyclines).

Long-term prognosis can be estimated using the Nottingham prognostic index (Figure 10.5) or using online programmes such as adjuvant online (www.adjuvantonline.com).

5-year survival of stage I breast cancer is 85%, stage II 70%, stage III 50% and stage IV 20%.

Screening and prevention

Evidence shows that screening using mammography reduces death from breast cancer by a third. In the UK screening is aimed at those with the greatest proven benefit which includes women aged 50–69 years. The benefit of screening for women aged 40–49 years and >70 years is controversial.

Screening mammography is done every 2 years for the general population and annually for those with a strong family history of breast cancer. In women having screening, the breast cancer prevalence is about 0.5% (i.e. about 1 in 200 women who are screening will be diagnosed to have breast cancer). 10% of women recalled for further assessment with a 'positive' screening mammogram are found to have a breast cancer.

Assessment and prevention of breast cancer in women with family history of breast cancer is given on p. 47.

Special situations

Paget's disease

This is a pre-malignant condition of the nipple and areola occurring in the 5th or 6th decade. Clinically there is erythema, dryness and fissuring of the nipple.

Microscopically it is characterized by Paget's cells located throughout the epidermis. More than 95% of patients with Paget's disease have an associated ductal carcinoma. Fifty percent of patients with Paget's disease have a lump of which more than 90% are invasive carcinoma. Of the other half of patients without a lump, 30% will have invasive carcinoma and 70% have ductal carcinoma-in-situ.

Investigations include breast examination, mammography and biopsy. Prognosis is dependent on the characteristics of associated malignancy.

Conservative surgery followed by radiotherapy is the treatment of choice. The local recurrence with surgery alone is 25–40% from a small series. An EORTC study of complete excision with nipple-areolar complex with postoperative radiotherapy showed a local recurrence of 5.2%. Mastectomy is offered based on patient choice and for multifocal disease. Management of regional nodes and recommendations for systemic treatment are based on the features of underlying malignancy.

Inflammatory breast cancer

Two percent of all breast cancers are inflammatory. Clinically there is ill-defined erythema, tenderness, induration and eczema-like skin changes. This is often misdiagnosed as a breast abscess. Microscopically it is characterized by the presence of cancer cells in dermal lymphatics. All patients need staging investigations with CT of the chest and abdomen and bone scan. Patients without distant metastasis are treated with neoadjuvant chemotherapy followed by mastectomy and axillary clearance and adjuvant radiotherapy. In HER2+ patients, trastuzumab can be added along with neoadjuvant taxanes. Patients receive hormones if ER+.

25% of patients present with metastatic disease when the aim is palliative and the treatment principle is the same as metastatic breast cancer.

Triple negative breast cancer

Triple negative breast cancer lacks the expression of oestrogen, progesterone and HER2 receptors. Up to 15% of breast cancer falls into this category which is associated with a high rate of local and systemic recurrence. These tumours are similar to BRCA-1 associated breast cancer. Currently, these tumours are treated as other breast cancers. Recent understanding of the role of BRCA1 gene pathway dysfunction in these tumours has led to the ongoing research on the role of platinum chemotherapy and poly (ADP-ribose) polymerase (PARP) inhibitors as potential therapeutic strategies. Data show that these tumours are sensitive to platinum-based chemotherapy and hence a number of studies are underway to evaluate various platinum regimes.

Bilateral breast cancer

It occurs in those with a strong family history of breast cancer and those who had breast cancer at an early age. It can be either synchronous (tumours occur simultaneously or within 6 months of initial diagnosis) which occurs in less than 1% or metachronous (tumours diagnosed 6 months or more after initial diagnosis) which has an incidence of 1–2% per year on follow-up. These should be managed as two separate breast cancers.

Male breast cancer

Male breast cancer accounts for 1% of all breast cancers and 0.1% of male cancer deaths. The average age at diagnosis is 10 years later than women. Alterations in testosterone and oestrogen balance may play a role in the aetiology as illustrated by the increased risk in men with undescended testis, or after orchiectomy. Klinefelter's syndrome has 50-fold increase in breast cancer. Other risk factors include obesity, cirrhosis, family history of breast cancer, BRCA1/2 mutations.

90% tumours are invasive of which 80% tumours are infiltrating ductal carcinoma, 5% papillary and 1% lobular. 10% tumours are DCIS. 80% tumours are ER+ and 75% PR+.

Usual presentation is a painless mass (85%) and other features include nipple retraction, ulceration, discharge and pain. Investigations include ultrasound, mammography and histological confirmation.

Primary treatment is total mastectomy with an axillary procedure similar to female breast cancer. Adjuvant radiotherapy indications are similar to female breast cancer. Adjuvant tamoxifen is indicated for ER+ tumours.

Metastatic breast cancer can be treated with hormonal manipulation or chemotherapy. 80% of oestrogen in men is produced peripherally and 20% production is from the testis. Hence, aromatase inhibitors may not be effective. Methods of hormonal manipulation include tamoxifen, orchidectomy, anti-androgens and aminoglutethimide.

Breast cancer during pregnancy

Please see p. 292.

Recent advances

Several biological and target agents are under investigation either as single agents or in combination. A randomized study of bevacizumab (an anti-VEGF) with paclitaxel showed a better response rate (37% vs. 21%, p < 0.001) and progression-free survival (11.8 vs. 5.9 months, p < 0.001) compared with paclitaxel alone. However, overall survival was similar in both groups. An ongoing study (BEATRICE) is evaluating the role of 1 year of bevacizumab along with standard adjuvant chemotherapy in triple negative breast cancer.

Other agents under evaluation include sunitinib (a tyrosine kinase inhibitor), PARP inhibitors, cetuximab (EGFR inhibitor) and ixabepilone (a microtubule inhibitor).

Further reading

Veronesi U, Boyle P, Goldhirsch A, Orecchia R, Viale G. Breast cancer. Lancet. 2005;365:1727–1741.

Benson JR, Jatoi I, Keisch M et al. Early breast cancer. Lancet. 2009;373:1463–1479.

Buchholz TA. Radiation therapy for early-stage breast cancer after breast-conserving surgery. N Engl J Med. 2009;360:63–70.

Pagani O, Senkus E, Wood W et al. International guidelines for management of metastatic breast cancer: can metastatic breast cancer be cured? J Natl Cancer Inst. 2010;102:456–463.

Roy V, Perez EA. Beyond trastuzumab: small molecule tyrosine kinase inhibitors in HER-2-positive breast cancer. Oncologist. 2009;14:1061–1069.

Bosch A, Eroles P, Zaragoza R, Viña JR, Lluch A. Triple-negative breast cancer: molecular features, pathogenesis,

treatment and current lines of research. Cancer Treat Rev. 2010;36:206–215.

Fentiman IS, Fourquet A, Hortobagyi GN. Male breast cancer. Lancet. 2006;367:595–604.

Dawood S, Ueno NT, Cristofanilli M. The medical treatment of inflammatory breast cancer. Semin Oncol. 2008;35: 64–71.

Cancers of the gastrointestinal system

11

TV Ajithkumar and E de Winton

Oesophageal cancer

Epidemiology

Oesophageal cancer is an aggressive cancer with an overall survival rate of less than 10%. There are over 7000 new patients per year in the UK and 16,000 per year in USA. The median age at diagnosis is 69 years. The male to female ratio is 2.5 : 1; but cervical oesophageal cancer is more common in women.

Aetiology

Oesophageal reflux and Barrett's oesophagus are thought to increase the risk of adenocarcinoma. Oesophageal reflux may account for the increased incidence of adenocarcinoma (10% per year) in the Western world.

Box 11.1 shows risk factors for oesophageal cancer. A diet rich in fruit and vegetables has been shown to reduce the relative risk.

Anatomy

The oesophagus extends from the cricopharyngeal sphincter to the gastro-oesophageal junction (GOJ) and is 25 cm in length. Figure 11.1 shows the anatomic sections of the oesophagus. The majority of tumours (85%) arise in the middle and lower third of oesophagus and 15% arise in the upper third.

Pathogenesis and pathology

Oesophageal cancer is thought to be the end result of a multi-step process of carcinogenesis. Adenocarcinoma arising from Barrett's oesophagus is thought to undergo a stepwise progression with associated genetic changes.

The common malignant tumours are adenocarcinoma, squamous cell carcinoma (SCC) or undifferentiated carcinoma. Most adenocarcinomas occur at or immediately above the GOJ which are classified (Siewert Classification) as follows:

- Type I – distal oesophageal cancer which may infiltrate GOJ.
- Type II – straddles the GOJ (cancer of the cardia; also called junctional cancer).
- Type III – subcardial cancer which may infiltrate OGJ and distal oesophagus.

Adenocarcinoma – accounts for 65% of oesophageal cancers in the UK and the major aetiological factor is Barrett's oesophagus. The incidence of carcinoma arising in Barrett's oesophagus is 1 per 100 patient-years.

Squamous cell carcinoma (SCC) accounts for 25% of oesophageal cancer. Alcohol and smoking are the major etiological factors. SCC is common in upper and mid third cancers.

Most common sites of metastatic spread are lymph nodes (70%), lung (20%), liver (35%), bone (9%) and adrenal glands (2%).

Clinical features

Most patients present with progressive dysphagia and difficulty in swallowing liquids indicate an advanced stage. 50% patients experience painful swallowing and other presentations include reflux, regurgitation and vomiting following eating, rapid weight loss. Local invasion of cancer leads to pain, and nerve compression leading to Horner's syndrome, recurrent laryngeal nerve palsy and a raised hemi-diaphragm.

© 2011, Elsevier Ltd
DOI: 10.1016/B978-0-7234-3458-0.00016-6

Box 11.1: Risk factors for oesophageal cancer

- Gastro-oesophageal reflux (achalasia – SCC, hiatus hernia and obesity – adenocarcinoma)
- Barrett's oesophagus (adenocarcinoma)
- Nutritional deficiency (vitamins A, C and riboflavin – SCC)
- Oesophageal injury (SCC)
- Alcohol (SCC)
- Smoking (SCC)
- Fungal toxins (infected cereals)
- Plummer–Vinson syndrome (upper third SCC)
- Tylosis palmaris (50% lifetime risk of SCC)
- History of head and neck cancer (SCC)
- Diet – high fat, low-protein and low calorie (SCC)
- Nitrosamines (both adenocarcinoma and SCC)

Metastatic disease can result in liver capsular pain, bony metastases, ascites or peritoneal deposits. Patients are usually cachectic at this stage.

Evaluation

History: details of symptoms including performance status, weight loss and degree of dysphagia.

Examination: cachexia, anaemia, jaundice, enlarged supraclavicular nodes, chest (for pleural effusion) and abdomen (hepatomegaly, ascites).

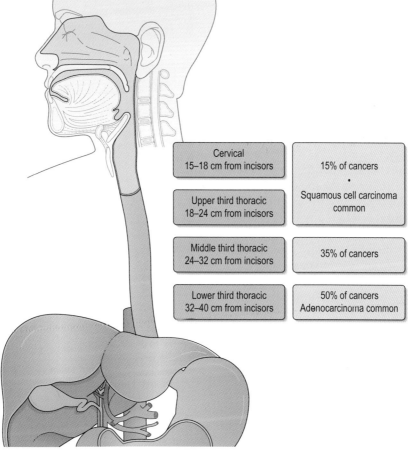

Cervical 15–18 cm from incisors	15% of cancers · Squamous cell carcinoma common
Upper third thoracic 18–24 cm from incisors	
Middle third thoracic 24–32 cm from incisors	35% of cancers
Lower third thoracic 32–40 cm from incisors	50% of cancers Adenocarcinoma common

Figure 11.1
Anatomic section of oesophagus.

Investigations and staging

Investigations are aimed at establishing the extent of disease, obtaining histologic diagnosis and assessing fitness for appropriate treatment:

- Barium swallow is usually the initial investigation of choice which shows the level of obstruction. Malignant strictures appear as asymmetric narrowing with abrupt, shelf-like margins and irregular contours, and may show proximal dilatation (Figure 11.2A).
- Endoscopy allows visual assessment of the tumour and biopsy.
- Endoscopic ultrasound (EUS) helps to assess the depth of invasion through the various layers of oesophagus (>90% accuracy), adjacent structures and neighbouring lymph nodes (70–80% accuracy). The normal oesophagus has five alternating hyperechoic and hypoechoic layers with inner most hyperechoic superficial mucosa. Oesophageal cancers appear as hypoechoic masses that can disrupt this layered pattern (Figure 11.2B, arrow). Malignant lymph node is characterized by more than 1 cm, round, hypoechoic area with distinct margins (Figure 11.2B, arrowhead). EUS guided fine needle aspiration (FNA) of any suspicious lesions, particularly lymph nodes of >5 mm, helps to improve the diagnostic accuracy.
- CT scan of the thorax, abdomen and pelvis is routinely done to assess the local extent of the tumour and local and distant staging.
- Positron emission tomography (PET) is useful in detecting distant metastases (sensitivity of 90% and specificity of >90%) and has been increasingly used in oesophageal cancer.
- Laparoscopy is useful in lower third oesophageal and gastro-oesophageal junction tumours prior to major surgical procedure. This helps to visualize and biopsy small peritoneal metastases, which may not have been detected on CT or PET. Up to 20% patients are up-staged after this procedure and major surgery can be avoided.
- Bronchoscopy is useful as a preoperative procedure in upper and middle third oesophageal cancer to rule out bronchial invasion.
- Tissue diagnosis is obtained via endoscopic biopsy.

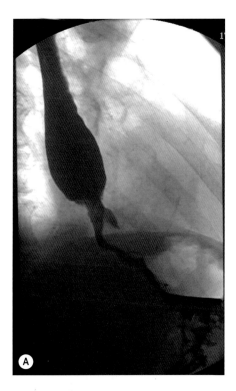

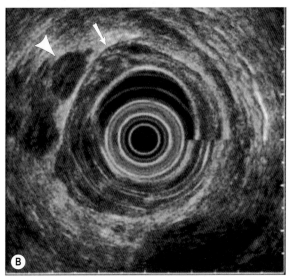

Figure 11.2
Barium swallow (A) and EUS (B) in oesophageal cancer. (Weinstein WM, Hawkey CJ, Bosch J. Clinical Gastroenterology and hepatology, 1st edition, Page 183, fig 32.7 (Mosby, 2005).)

Box 11.2: Staging of oesophageal cancer

Stage I
- T1 N0 M0   Invasion of lamina propria or submucosa

Stage IIa
- T2 N0 M0   Invasion of the muscularis mucosa
- T3 N0 M0   Invasion of the adventitia

Stage IIb
- T1–2 N1 M0   Regional nodal involvement

Stage III
- T3 N1 M0
- T4 N0–1 M0   Invasion of adjacent structures

Stage IVa
- Any T any N M1a

Stage IVb
- Any T any N M1b

  Tumours of upper third cancer
- M1a: Metastasis in cervical lymph nodes
- M1b: Other distant metastasis

  Tumours of middle third cancer
- M1a: Not applicable
- M1b: Non regional lymph node or other distant metastasis

  Tumours of lower third cancer
- M1a: Metastasis in coeliac lymph nodes
- M1b: Other distant metastasis

- Other investigations – include full blood count, biochemistry and coagulation profile. Patients considered for surgery need pulmonary function tests, arterial blood gases, ECG and an exercise test.

Staging

Staging determines prognosis and guides treatment. TNM staging is given in Box 11.2.

Management of oesophageal cancer (Figure 11.3)

Localized disease

This group consists of patients with stages I–III oesophageal cancer as well as a subgroup of operable stage IVa (involving pleura, pericardium and diaphragm). However, only one-third of patients present with localized disease. The majority of these are stage II or III disease and less than half of these patients are curable. Assess-ment of fitness for suitable treatment is an essential component of the decision. A number of treatment options are available depending on the stage, location of tumour, and fitness to undergo treatment, which include:

- Endoscopic mucosal resection (EMR) – for superficial cancer limited to the mucosa.
- Radical surgery alone (T1N0M0 tumours located >5 cm from the cricopharyngeal junction and fit for surgery).
- Radical chemoradiotherapy (tumours within 5 cm from the cricopharyngeal junction, unresectable/medically unfit patients with T1–T3N0–1M0 tumours and selected T4N0–1M0).
- Preoperative chemotherapy followed by radical surgery (operable and medically fit patients with T1–T4N0–N1M0 cancer located >5 cm from the cricopharyngeal junction).
- Radical chemoradiotherapy followed by surgery (only in those with residual disease after radical chemoradiotherapy and fit for surgery).
- Radical radiotherapy (not suitable for surgery and chemotherapy).
- Palliative treatment or best supportive care (PS >2).

Radical surgery

Surgery is the best single modality treatment compared with radiotherapy alone. The best outcome from specialist centres is 5-year survival of approximately 35% with a postoperative mortality of less than 5%.

Type of surgery depends on the site of tumour, histology and the extent of lymphadenectomy required. The surgery involves subtotal oesophagectomy with the upper part of the stomach and anastomosis of the cervical oesophagus and gastroplasty. 60–70% of patients have involved lymph nodes at the time of surgery and hence need dissection of abdominal and mediastinal nodes in middle and lower third cancers (a minimum of 15 nodes should be removed).

The common procedures are as follows:

- Upper third oesophageal cancer: three-phase approach with complete removal of the tumour and mediastinal and supraclavicular lymphadenectomy.

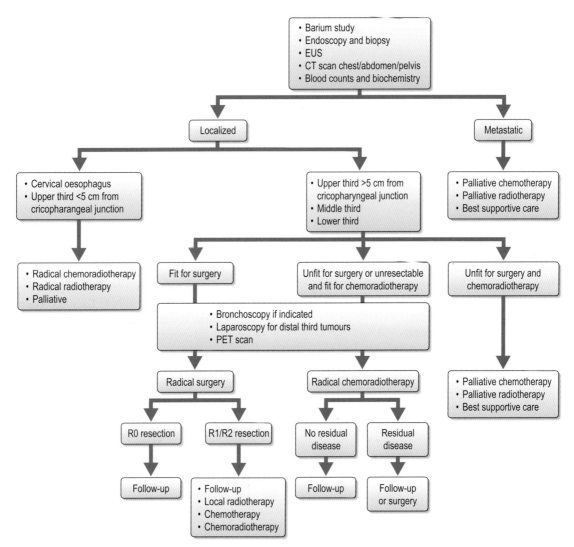

Figure 11.3
Management of oesophageal cancer.

- Middle and lower third cancers: two stage Ivor–Lewis approach. The first stage consists of laparotomy and mobilization of the stomach, followed by right thoracotomy to remove the tumour and to form an oesophagogastric anastomosis.

Minimally invasive surgical approaches are evolving.

Radical radiotherapy (Box 11.3)

Radical radiotherapy is the treatment of choice in patients with localized disease who are medically unfit for surgery and in whom chemother-apy is contraindicated. The best results are an overall 5-year survival of less than 10%.

Radical chemoradiotherapy (CRT)

Radiotherapy is given in combination with chemotherapy which is proven to be superior to radical radiotherapy alone. Chemotherapy improves local control by radiation sensitization and helps to minimize distant metastatic relapses. This approach results in an overall 3-year survival of 30%. The commonly used combination is cisplatin with 5-fluorouracil with radiotherapy at a dose of 50 Gy in 2 Gy per fraction (Box 11.3). However, locoregional recurrence remains the

Box 11.3: Radiotherapy for oesophageal cancer

Position – supine (with arms above head for middle and lower third, and arms by side for upper third)

Localization – CT planning with information from EUS

Target volume

Radical chemoradiotherapy
- GTV – tumour with enlarged nodes
- CTV:
  - Superio-inferior
    - Tumours above carina (cervical and upper-third) – GTV + 2 cm and bilateral supraclavicular nodes
    - Middle third – GTV + 2 cm margin
    - Lower third – GTV + 2 cm margin and coeliac axis basin nodes and gastrohepatic ligament (lesser curve, paracardial and left gastric nodes)
  - Lateral and anterior – GTV + 1 cm
  - Posterior – GTV + 0.5–1 cm
- PTV – CTV + 1 cm
- 2 phase treatment – phase I CTV = GTV + 3–5 cm superio-inferior margin and 1.5–2 cm axial margin and phase II CTV as GTV with 2 cm margin superoinferiorly and 1.5–2 cm axially

Radical radiotherapy

PTV – 5 cm superior inferior margin for phase I and 2.5–3 cm for phase II and 2.5 cm axial margin

Palliative radiotherapy

PTV – tumour and node + 3 cm margin

Dose

Indication	Single phase	2 phase
Radical chemoradiotherapy	50–50.4 Gy in 25–28 fractions	Phase I – 30 Gy in 15 Phase II – 20 Gy in 10
Radical radiotherapy	55 Gy in 20 or 66 Gy in 33 fractions	Phase I – 33 Gy in 12 and phase II – 22 Gy in 8 Phase I – 36 Gy in 18 and Phase II 30 Gy in 15
Preoperative chemoradiotherapy	45 Gy in 25 fractions	
Palliative	30 Gy in 10 fractions or 20 Gy in 5 fractions	

Normal tissue tolerance
- Lung V20 (volume receiving 20 Gy) <25%
- Heart V30 <40%
- Spinal cord total dose below 45 Gy

Care during radiotherapy
- Weekly blood test
- Keep Hb >12 gm%
- Avoid significant weight loss (consider PEG/RIG feeding)

major cause for overall failure with 50% of patients developing locoregional disease. Attempts to increase the radiotherapy dose to improve local control has resulted in increased treatment-related deaths without improvement in local control or survival. Studies comparing CRT with CRT followed by surgery showed similar overall survival, but with high treatment-related mortality with surgery.

Preoperative chemotherapy followed by surgery

A meta-analysis showed that preoperative chemotherapy followed by surgery improved 2-year survival by 7% compared with surgery alone (HR 0.90; CI 0.81–1.00). The largest study (MRC OE02) of 802 patients which compared surgery alone with two cycles of 3-weekly preoperative cisplatin (80 mg/m^2 on day 1 as 4 hour infusion) and 5-fluorouracil (1 g/m²/day continuous infusion for 4 days) followed by surgery showed that chemotherapy improves overall survival from 34% to 43% at 2-years (p = 0.004). Hence, this is the standard treatment option in most UK centres.

Preoperative CRT followed by surgery

A meta-analysis showed that preoperative CRT followed by surgery improved 2-year survival by 13% compared with surgery alone (HR 0.81 95% CI 0.70–0.93; p = 0.002). However, this benefit was only seen with concurrent chemoradiotherapy rather than sequential and treatment-related mortality was increased with preoperative CRT (p = 0.053). Due to concerns about morbidity and mortality, it is not practised in the UK.

Advanced and recurrent disease (Figures 11.3 and 11.4)

Two-thirds of oesophageal cancer patients present with advanced disease and a significant number of patients who had initial radical treatment will relapse. The treatment is essentially palliative, aimed to improve symptoms, quality of life and possibly to extend life. Pre-treatment performance status is important in deciding potentially toxic treatment.

Systemic treatment

Chemotherapy for advanced oesophageal cancer improves survival when compared to best supportive care alone. In the UK, the combination of epirubicin, cisplatin and 5FU (ECF) has been used as the standard regime (Box 11.4). A randomized

study (REAL-2) to explore the role of oxaliplatin instead of cisplatin and capecitabine instead of 5-FU (EOX regime) showed that toxicity of 5FU and capecitabine were similar; oxaliplatin resulted in increased neuropathy and diarrhoea but reduced renal toxicity, thromboembolism, alopecia and neutropenia when compared with cisplatin. Patients receiving EOX survived longer than ECF (38% vs. 47% at 1-year; p = 0.02).

Palliative treatment of dysphagia

Dysphagia is the predominant symptom which needs palliation. The various methods to relieve dysphagia are:

- Endoscopic dilatation – results in immediate but short lived (2–4 weeks) improvement and

---

Box 11.4: Chemotherapy for oesophageal cancer

Preoperative chemotherapy
- Cisplatin 80 mg/m² on day 1 and 5-FU 1 gm/m²/day continuous infusion for 96 hours. Cycles repeated every 3 weeks for 2 cycles.

Chemoradiotherapy
- Cisplatin 60–80 mg/m² repeated 3 weekly for 4 cycles with 5-fluorouracil 250 mg/m²/day initially reducing to 200 mg/m²/day during radiotherapy.

Palliative
ECF regime
- Epirubicin 50 mg/m² day1, cisplatin 60 mg/m²/day1 and 5-FU 200 mg/m²/day; cycle repeated 3-weekly

ECX regime
- Epirubicin 50 mg/m² day1, cisplatin 60 mg/m²/day1 and capecitabine 625 mg/m² orally twice daily ; cycle repeated 3-weekly

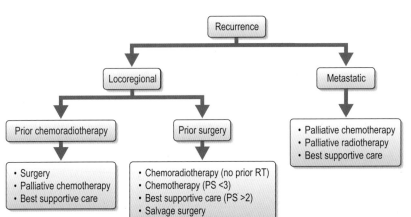

Figure 11.4
Management of recurrence.

hence useful only for those with limited life expectancy.

- Stent – immediate and prolonged improvement. There are two types of stents: uncovered and covered (has risk of migration).
- Local therapies – laser, ethanol injection and photodynamic therapy. Response is short lived.
- Radiotherapy – is delivered by external beam radiotherapy or brachytherapy. Radiotherapy will not result in immediate relief of dysphagia and may cause initial deterioration.
- Palliation of other symptoms follows the principles that of any other cancer (p. 66).

Prognosis and survival

Stage, particularly depth of invasion of the oesophageal wall, is an important prognostic factor. Other prognostic factors include age, performance status and weight loss (>10% in 3 months). Grade and histologic subtypes have no prognostic importance.

The overall 5-year survival of oesophageal cancer is <10%. Less than a third of patients are suitable for surgical resection. Around 80% of patients with stage I disease are alive at 5 years whereas only 15% of stage IIa/III patients are alive at 5 years. The median survival of patients treated with palliative intent is 4 months.

Follow-up

All patients are followed up after curative treatment. The follow-up involves history and clinical examination, 4-monthly for one year, 6-monthly for two years and yearly thereafter. Investigations are done as clinically indicated.

Ongoing studies and new agents

New chemotherapy regimes and drugs are being tested to improve the efficacy of CRT. UK SCOPE 1 trial is testing the addition of cetuximab (an EGFR inhibitor) to standard CRT.

MRC OE05 study is comparing ECF chemotherapy followed by resection versus ECX chemotherapy followed by resection in patients with resectable adenocarcinoma of the oesophagus.

Along with various attempts to improve the loco-regional control of oesophageal cancer, studies are ongoing to assess the benefit of various biological agents. Gefinitib (500 mg daily), a tyrosine kinase inhibitor which acts by blocking epithelial growth factor receptor (EGFR), has been shown to have some benefit in patients with advanced oesophageal cancer (50% 6-month survival). Bortezomib, a proteasome inhibitor, is also being studied along with chemotherapy. Another agent under investigation is a monoclonal antibody, panitumumab (REAL 3 study).

Screening and surveillance

The role of screening is not fully established. In the UK, high-risk patients (tylosis and Plummer–Vinson syndrome) are regularly screened with endoscopy. Routine surveillance of chronic reflux (absolute individual risk of less than 1 in 1000 per annum) is not justified. Patients with Barrett's oesophagus with mild dysplasia are treated with acid suppression therapy followed by a repeat endoscopy and multiple biopsies at 8–12 weeks. If this remains stable, six-monthly repeat biopsy is recommended. Patients with high-grade dysplasia have a 30–40% risk of having invasive adenocarcinoma and hence full staging is undertaken with a view to oesophagectomy.

Small cell carcinoma of oesophagus

This accounts for 0.5–2.4% of oesophageal cancers. The usual presentation is dysphagia (86%) of 1–3 months' duration and presents in patients in their late 50s. Treatment is similar to small cell lung cancer with chemoradiotherapy. There are some reports suggesting that addition of surgical resection may improve long-term survival. The reported median survival ranges from 12–18 months.

Gastric cancer

Epidemiology

Gastric cancer is the second commonest cause of cancer death in the world. There are approximately 8200 new patients per year in the UK and over 26,000 per year in USA. Although the overall incidence has decreased significantly, there has been an exponential rise in tumours of the proximal stomach and cardia. The median age at diagnosis in men is 70 years and in women 74 years. It is common in men (male to female ratio 2.3 : 1).

Only 20% of patients present with localized disease and the overall 5-year survival is 15–20%.

Aetiology

The aetiology of gastric cancer is multifactorial. The following factors increase the risk:

- Diet: low consumption of fruits and vegetables and high intake of salts, nitrates and smoked or pickled foods increases the risk.
- Smoking.
- *Helicobacter pylori* – associated with gastric lymphoma and adenocarcoma (2.8-fold increase).
- Blood group A (20% increased risk for infiltrative type).
- Gastric resection, chronic atrophic gastritis and pernicious anaemia.
- Family history of gastric cancer (2–3-fold increase).
- Genetic syndromes: hereditary non-polyposis colorectal cancer, familial adenomatous polyposis, and Peutz–Jeghers syndrome.

High intake of fruits and vegetables (high in vitamin C and E, and antioxidants) and regular use of aspirin and non-steroidal anti-inflammatory drugs (NSAIDs) are associated with a reduced risk of gastric cancer.

Pathology

Gastric cancer arises through a multistage and multifactorial process. The intestinal type of gastric cancer evolves through the stages of metaplasia to dysplasia to carcinoma. However details of evolution of diffuse type of gastric cancer is not known.

- Adenocarcinoma accounts for 95% of gastric cancers. Histologically these are divided into intestinal or diffuse type. The intestinal subtype usually arises in distal stomach in older patients and the diffuse subtype is common in younger patients. The variant diffuse subtype which extensively infiltrates the stomach wall is known as linitis plastica.
- Primary lymphomas (MALT) are increasing.
- Gastrointestinal stromal tumours (GIST) (p. 261).
- Other tumours include small cell carcinoma, carcinoid and squamous cell carcinoma.

Clinical features

Most patients present with advanced disease. Presenting features are often nonspecific and typically include weight loss, persistent abdominal pain, nausea, anorexia, and early satiety. Dysphagia can occur with GOJ or proximal gastric tumours, whilst distal tumours can produce gastric outflow obstruction. 10–20% patients have haematemesis. Paraneoplastic features include dermatomyositis, acanthosis nigricans, diffuse seborrhoeic keratoses (sign of Leser–Trelat), circinate erythemas and microangiopathic haemolytic anaemia.

Evaluation

- History – detailed history including performance status, recent weight loss and family history.
- Clinical examination:
  - General: anaemia, jaundice, cachexia, enlarged left supraclavicular lymph node (Virchow's node).
  - Abdomen: epigastric mass, hepatomegaly, periumbilical nodule (Sister Mary Joseph nodule), mass on anterior rectal wall on per rectal examination (Blumer's shelf) and ovarian masses (Kruckenberg's tumour).

Investigations and staging

Evaluation of patients helps to establish histological diagnosis, to assess the extent of disease (stage) and assess fitness to undergo appropriate treatment.

Initial assessment

Flexible oesophagogastroduodenoscopy (OGD) is the diagnostic procedure of choice which permits direct visualization of tumour and biopsy of any suspicious lesions. However, the diagnosis of the diffuse-type gastric cancer can be difficult endoscopically as the overlying mucosa may appear normal.

Double contrast barium studies (Figure 11.5) complement endoscopy.

Further assessment

Once histological diagnosis is made, staging investigations are necessary to determine the treatment options.

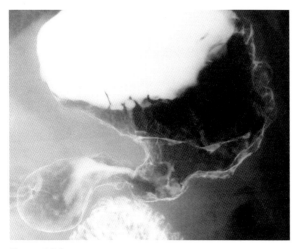

Figure 11.5
Barium study shows a large circumferential lesion in the body of the stomach (with permission).

- CT scan of chest, abdomen and pelvis should be undertaken to establish loco-regional (sensitivity of 65–80%) and metastatic staging. High resolution dynamic two-phase multi-slice CT with contrast and water (600–800 ml) to distend the stomach has improved the diagnostic accuracy. The drawbacks of CT scan are that it is not very accurate for staging early cancer and up to 30% of peritoneal metastases will not be detectable.
- Endoscopic ultrasound (EUS) is useful in predicting depth of tumour invasion and helps to guide FNA of suspicious perigastric lymph nodes. The stomach is seen as five layers of alternating bright (hyperechoic) and dark (hypoechoic) bands.
- Laparoscopy – laparoscopy allows direct visualization of the liver surface, peritoneum and local lymph nodes. Laproscopy alters CT staging by up to 40% (up or down-staging) and is recommended in all patients with gastric cancer and GOJ cancer with a gastric component. Biopsy should be taken from all suspicious lesions. Intraoperative ultrasound may further increase the yield of liver metastasis and is useful in assessing lymph nodes. Cytology of peritoneal washings may be undertaken, but its sensitivity is limited by contamination with mesothelial cells.
- PET scan may be useful for establishing metastatic disease and to predict response to neoadjuvant treatment, particularly for intestinal type cancer.

Preoperative evaluation

Includes full blood count, biochemistry, coagulation profile, arterial blood gas, pulmonary function tests and ECG. All patients should undergo nutritional screening prior to surgery. A body mass index of <18.5, body weight <90% predicted, >20% weight loss and a low albumin predict an increased risk of perioperative complications.

Staging

Box 11.5 shows the pathological staging of gastric cancer. Sixteen nodal stations defined by the Japanese Research Society for Gastric Cancer help to define the extent of lymph node dissection in gastric cancer (Figure 11.6 and see below).

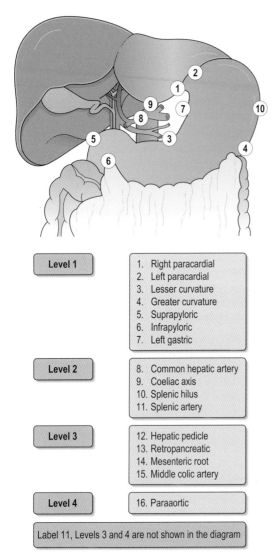

Level 1	1. Right paracardial 2. Left paracardial 3. Lesser curvature 4. Greater curvature 5. Suprapyloric 6. Infrapyloric 7. Left gastric
Level 2	8. Common hepatic artery 9. Coeliac axis 10. Splenic hilus 11. Splenic artery
Level 3	12. Hepatic pedicle 13. Retropancreatic 14. Mesenteric root 15. Middle colic artery
Level 4	16. Paraaortic

Label 11, Levels 3 and 4 are not shown in the diagram

Figure 11.6
Upper abdominal nodal stations.

Management of gastric cancer (Figure 11.7)

All patients should be assessed in a multidisciplinary setting. Assessment of the performance status and co-morbidities should be done.

Early gastric cancer (EGC)

By definition the tumour is limited to the gastric mucosa or submucosa (T1) irrespective of nodal involvement. There is a 10–20% risk of lymph node involvement, depending on the size of the tumour, histologic subtype and presence of submucosal invasion. With treatment the 5-year survival is >90%, whereas if untreated up to two-thirds progress to advanced cancer over 5 years. The treatment options include:

- Endoscopic mucosal resection (EMR) – is appropriate for small well-differentiated polypoidal or raised lesions.
- Gastric resection with lymphadenectomy.

Resectable gastric cancer

All patients should undergo laparoscopy with or without peritoneal washings for malignancy cells prior to open laparotomy to assess the extent of disease and resectability. Surgery is feasible only in less than half of the newly diagnosed patients and only 13–50% patients are cured with surgery.

Surgery

Surgery is aimed at complete removal of the tumour and lymph nodes. When performing gastric resection a 5 cm free margin is required for infiltrative tumours whereas 2 cm may be sufficient for expanding tumours. The pylorus seems to act as a barrier to extension of cancer and hence 2–3 cm surgical margin for pylorus may be necessary.

The extent of gastric resection depends on the size and location of the primary tumour (Figure 11.8).

- Subtotal gastrectomy – for an early or well circumscribed T2 cancer, >2 cm away from GOJ. A 5 cm margin is needed for more infiltrative lesions.
- Total gastrectomy – for tumour located <5 cm from GOJ or the tumour is diffuse with submucosal infiltration.
- Distal gastrectomy – is the option for distal gastric tumours which can be completely excised.

Lymphadenectomy with recovery of a minimum of 14, and an optimal of 25 lymph nodes is recommended. Based on the extent of lymphadenectomy, dissection is categorized as:

- D0 – gastric resection with incomplete dissection of level 1 nodes.
- D1 – gastric resection with complete dissection of level 1 nodes.
- D2 – gastric resection with complete dissection of level 1&2 nodes.

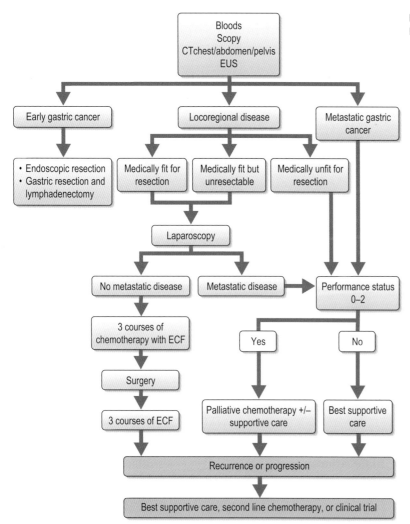

Figure 11.7
Management of gastric cancer.

- D3 – gastric resection with complete dissection of levels 1–3 nodes.
- D4 – gastric resection with complete dissection of level 1–4 nodes.

The current UK practice is to perform D2 lymphadenectomy without pancreatico-splenectomy. Laparoscopic gastrectomy and laparoscopy assisted D2 dissection are shown to be promising.

Adjuvant chemotherapy
Meta-analyses showed improved survival benefit with adjuvant chemotherapy (one study reported HR 0.85–95%; CI: 0.80–0.90); but there was no standard chemotherapy regime. Adjuvant chemotherapy is hence not offered except in a clinical trial.

Adjuvant chemoradiotherapy
A randomized trial showed better 3-year survival with post-operative chemoradiation (50% vs. 41%; p = 0.005) compared with surgery alone. However, it is not an accepted standard treatment in the UK and Europe because of the drawbacks of the study such as only 10% patients had D2 dissection, significant radiotherapy error in 30% patients and 30% patients did not complete chemoradiotherapy due to toxicity.

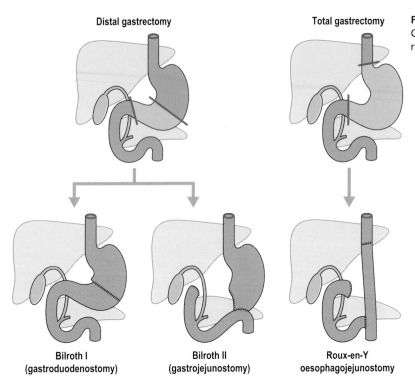

Figure 11.8
Gastric resections and reconstructions.

Distal gastrectomy

Total gastrectomy

Bilroth I
(gastroduodenostomy)

Bilroth II
(gastrojejunostomy)

Roux-en-Y
oesophagojejunostomy

Perioperative treatment

A randomized study (UK MRC MAGIC) showed that three cycles of pre- and postoperative chemotherapy with epirubicin, cisplatin and continuous infusion 5 fluorouracil (ECF) significantly improved 5-year survival (36% vs. 23%; p = 0.009) compared with surgery alone in resectable gastric and lower oesophageal cancers (Box 11.6). This is the standard of care in most of the UK and parts of the Europe (Box 11.6).

Unresectable gastric cancer

The median survival of patients with unresectable non-metastatic cancer is 6 months without treatment. Treatment is aimed at improving the symptoms and quality of life and possible extension of life. The various palliative measures include:

- Bleeding – endoscopic laser photocoagulation or argon plasma coagulation is effective in controlling bleeding. If these measures fail, palliative resection may be considered.
- Obstruction – tumours of the proximal stomach may present with dysphagia whereas distal stomach tumours present with gastric

outlet obstruction. Endoscopic stent placement offers effective palliative. However, 15–40% with develop recurrent symptoms. An alternative option is palliative bypass.
- Radiotherapy – is effective in controlling bleeding or obstruction in patients who are unsuitable candidates for other interventions. Radiotherapy is effective in controlling pain.

Box 11.6: Treatment regimes in gastric cancer

**Perioperative chemotherapy and surgery
(UK MRC MAGIC trial)**

- ECF chemotherapy: Epirubicin 50 mg/m² IV day 1, cisplatin 60 mg/m² IV day 1 and 5-fluorouracil 200 mg/m²/day continuous IV infusion for 21 days. Cycle repeated 3-weekly. Total 3 cycles preoperatively.
- Surgery 3–6 weeks after chemotherapy
- Postoperative chemotherapy – 3 cycles of ECF started 6–12 weeks after surgery

Metastatic or unresectable cancer
ECF regime (see above)
ECX regime
- Epirubicin 50 mg/m² day 1, cisplatin 60 mg/m²/day 1 and capecitabine 625 mg/m² orally twice daily; cycle repeated 3-weekly

Systemic treatment of unresectable gastric cancer

Patients with unresectable and/or disseminated gastric cancer should be considered for a clinical trial, and those with good performance status (0–2) may be offered systemic therapy. Randomized trials suggest that chemotherapy may improve survival compared with best supportive care (9–11 months vs. 3–4 months HR 0.39) and quality of life. A meta-analysis showed that combination chemotherapy improves survival by 6 months and the best survivals are achieved by three-drug regimens containing 5-FU, anthracycline and cisplatin. The standard regime used in the UK is ECF (Box 11.6). A recent study (REAL 2) showed that ECF is comparable to EOX. This regimen has the advantage of avoiding the need for continuous infusion of 5-FU.

Other active agents include taxanes, and irinotecan.

Follow-up

There is no evidence that regular intensive follow-up improves outcome and hence symptom driven follow-up is recommended.

Management of recurrence

The role of second-line chemotherapy is not well-established. The commonly used agents include taxanes, irinotecan and oxalipatin. In the majority of patients management is essentially palliative aiming at best supportive care.

Prognosis

Important prognostic factors in resectable gastric cancer include depth of invasion, number of lymph nodes involved and positive resection margins. Estimated 5-year survival by stage is:

- Stage I: 70%.
- Stage II: 40%.
- Stage III: 20%.
- Stage IV: less than 5%.

Newer agents

Monoclonal antibodies and various agents targeting pathways of cellular proliferation are being evaluated. However data are still limited to early phase studies. Examples of molecules under study are bevacizumab (anti-VEGF), cetixumab (anti-EGFR) etc.

Screening

Routine screening is not recommended for gastric cancer. Role of screening of asymptomatic individuals for gastric cancer from countries with high incidence such as Japan shows inconsistent results of benefit.

Gastric stump cancer

By definition this is the cancer developing in the gastric remnant at least 5 years after surgery for benign peptic ulcer disease. Patients after distal gastric resection have a 4–7 fold increase in gastric cancer attributed mainly to gastroduodenal reflux. Treatment is complete removal of gastric remnants with a D2 lymphadenectomy. The pattern of lymph node metastases in these cancers may differ from primary gastric cancer and the prognosis is the same as primary gastric cancer.

Cancers of the liver

Introduction

Cancers of the liver can be primary (5%) or secondary (95%). The most common primary liver cancer is hepatocellular carcinoma (HCC) which accounts for 90% of primary liver cancers. There are more than 3000 new patients diagnosed in the UK. Males are more commonly affected (male: female ratio is 5:3). Median age of diagnosis is 64 years.

Aetiology

The risk factors include:

- Chronic liver disease – 80–90% HCC arising in patients with cirrhosis.
- Hepatitis infection – hepatitis B and C viruses account for 75% cases of HCC. HCV accounts for the recent rising trend.
- Alcohol accounts for 10% of cancers in Asia and 20% in Europe and USA.
- Non-alcoholic fatty liver disease (NAFLD) – associated with obesity and type 2 diabetes. 5% patients progress to cirrhosis and have an increased risk of HCC.
- Aflatoxin.
- Metabolic disorders – haemochromatosis, alpha-1-antitrypsin deficiency, and Wilson's disease.

Pathology

HCC is the most common primary liver tumour and is multiple in >50% cases. They spread locally and invade blood vessels. Commonly metastasize to lungs. The other histologic types include cholangiocarcinoma, sarcomas and lymphoma.

Clinical features

Commonest presentation is an incidental mass on USS in cirrhotic patients. Other presentations include abdominal pain, weight loss, anorexia, fever, ascites, jaundice, and paraneoplastic syndromes (hypercalcaemia and hypoglycaemia). Spontaneous bleeding of HCC can occur in 5–15% patients who present with abdominal pain, haemorrhagic ascites or even shock.

Diagnosis and staging

In a patient with pre-existing cirrhosis, a mass of ≥2 cm has >95% of chance of being malignant. Serum AFP of ≥400 µg/l is diagnostic.

Imaging

Contrast enhanced CT scan and MRI scan are useful in establishing the diagnosis. Both tests have 80% accuracy. The characteristic feature of HCC is a specific vascular profile – an intense contrast intake during the early arterial phase followed by contrast washout during delayed/portal venous phase.

Tissue diagnosis

In patients with cirrhosis, >2 cm nodule with characteristic dynamic profile on one imaging, biopsy confirmation is unnecessary. In patients with a 1–2 cm nodule, if a characteristic vascular profile is seen in two imaging techniques, biopsy confirmation is needed. Lesions of >1 cm with non-specific vascular pattern need biopsy. However, biopsy can be delayed or avoided depending on the timing of definite treatment. Biopsy has the risk of tumour seeding. Nodules of <1 cm in size needs close follow-up.

Staging

There are two methods of staging: TNM and Okuda staging. Barcelona Clinic Liver Cancer group incorporate Okuda staging (Box 11.7) for staging classification and treatment recommendation.

Box 11.7: Okuda staging of hepatocellular carcinoma

Criteria	Positive	Negative
Tumor size*	>50 percent	<50 percent
Ascites	Clinically detectable	Clinically absent
Albumin	<3 mg/dL	>3 mg/dL
Bilirubin	>3 mg/dL	<3 mg/dL

Stage	
I	No positive
II	One or two positives
III	Three or four positives

Prognosis of untreated patients
- Stage I: 8.3 months
- Stage II: 2 months
- Stage III: 0.7 months

*Largest cross-sectional area of tumour to largest cross-sectional area of the liver.

Management (Figure 11.9)

Treatment of HCC depends on tumour stage, liver function (Child–Pugh grading; Box 11.8), and performance status.

Stage O and stage A

Treated radically and treatment options include:

- Resection.
- Transplantation.
- Percutaneous tumour ablation.

Resection

Surgical resection is the treatment choice in HCC in non-cirrhotic patients. These tumours generally tend to be solitary and large. The 5-year survival is 50% with less than 1% mortality.

Resection is the appropriate treatment for only a subset of cirrhotic patients with HCC. Absence of portal hypertension and normal bilirubin are key factors in selecting the best candidates for resection. Hence the eligibility criteria include:

- Single tumour
- No jaundice
- No portal hypertension
- No extra-hepatic disease

With appropriate selection of patients a 5-year survival of 70% can be achieved with less than 5% operative mortality. There is no role for any adjuvant treatment after resection.

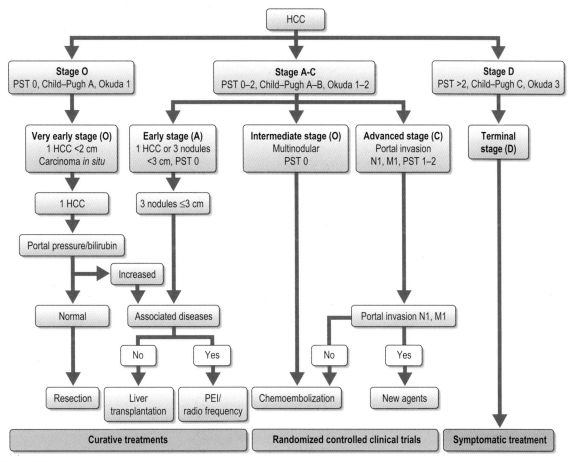

Figure 11.9
Staging classification and treatment of hepatocellular carcinoma (Llovet JM, Burroughs A, Bruix J. LANCET 2003;362;1907–1917, fig 5, with permission). PST – performance status test, PEI – percutaneous ethanol injection.

Box 11.8: Child–Pugh grading of severity of liver disease

Criteria	Score 1	2	3
Hepatic encephalopathy (grade)	None	1–2	3–4
Total bilirubin (mg/dl)	<2	2–3	>3
Ascites	Absent	Mild	Moderate or severe
Serum albumin (g/dl)	>3.5	2.8–3.5	<2.8
Prothrombin time (second prolonged) or INR	<4 or 1.7	4–6 or 1.7–2.3	>6 or >2.3

Child–Pugh Grade A = 5–6 points.
Grade B = 7–9 points.
Grade C = 10–15 points.

Liver transplantation

Liver transplantation is a treatment option for HCC in cirrhotic patients. Indications for liver transplantation (only 10% are eligible) include (Milan criteria):

- Solitary HCC <5 cm.
- Up to three HCC all <3 cm.

In these highly selected patients the reported 5-year survival is >70%. Liver transplantation is not an acceptable option for HCC in non-cirrhotic patients because of the need for intense immunosuppression.

Percutaneous ablation

Percutaneous ablation is a treatment option for patients with stage 0 & A disease who are not suitable for resection or transplantation and those who are waiting for transplantation. Ablation is achieved either by:

- Chemical injection (ethanol, acetic acid and boiling saline).
- Thermal ablation (radiofrequency, laser and cryotherapy).

Percutaneous ethanol injection (PEI) and radiofrequency ablation (RFA) are equally effective for tumours of <2 cm whereas RAF is more effective for larger tumours.

Stage B & C

Treatment is palliative and options include:

- Transarterial chemoembolization (TACE) and transarterial embolization (TAE).
- Systemic treatment.
- Chemotherapy.
- Biological agents, e.g. sorafenib.

Chemotherapy results in low response rate and has no impact on survival. Sorafenib, a multi-kinase inhibitor, has been shown to prolong survival in patients with advanced HCC with good liver function compared with controls (10.7 vs. 7.9 months)

Stage D

Treatment is essentially symptomatic and supportive.

Management of recurrence

After surgical resection 70% of cases recur at 5 years. Some of these recurrences are true recurrences (intrahepatic metastases) and some are de novo tumours (30–40%). True recurrences typically occur within 2 years after resection, and are usually associated with vascular invasion, satellite nodules and poorly differentiated tumours. De novo tumours usually occur late.

The treatment options include re-resection (possible in 10–20%), salvage transplantation or palliative treatment.

Prognosis

Prognosis depends on cancer and cirrhosis. 50–60% patients die of cirrhosis, 30% with hepatic failure and 10% with gastrointestinal bleeding.

- Stage 0 & A after radical treatment – 5-year survival 50–75%.
- Stage B – median survival 16 months without treatment and with TACE 3-year survival is 50%.
- Stage C – median survival 6 months without treatment and with palliative treatment <10% survive for 3 years.
- Stage D – 1 year survival <10%.

Screening

Surveillance is offered to patients with cirrhosis and the two most common tests used for screening are serum alpha-foetoprotein (AFP) and ultrasonography.

Tumours of the biliary tract

Tumours of the biliary tract can occur at any point between the sphincter of Oddi and the gallbladder.

Carcinoma of the gallbladder

Introduction

Carcinoma of the gallbladder is the most common malignant lesion of the biliary tract. It is more common in females with a 4:1 female:male ratio.

Gallstones are considered one of the important risk factors, although the majority of patients with gallstones never do not develop cancer. 65–90% of patients have associated gallstones. Other reported risk factors include 'porcelain' gallbladder, gallbladder polyps of >10 mm diameter, and anomalous pancreaticobiliary duct junction (APBDI).

Pathology

90% of patients with gallbladder cancer have associated dysplasia and carcinoma-in-situ, suggesting a multi-step carcinogenesis. 90% tumours are adenocarcinoma and the remainder are squamous cell carcinoma. Spread of tumour is by local invasion (including liver segments IV and V), through lymphatics and venous blood (to liver).

Clinical presentation

The usual presentation is an incidental finding at cholecystectomy. Other clinical features are that of gallstone disease and unremitting jaundice in some patients.

Investigations and staging

Initial assessment is by ultrasound which may show a complex mass filling the lumen with localized thickening of gallbladder wall. There may be associated liver metastasis, ascites and dilated bile ducts.

- CT – useful in local staging, it can establish infiltration into adjacent tissues and vessels and nodal or distant metastases.
- MRI is useful in identifying invasion of the hepatoduodenal ligament and portal vein encasement, both features suggestive of an unresectable tumour.
- ERCP is not useful in diagnosing gallbladder cancer but can be useful in identifying growth in adjacent intrahepatic ducts or in the common bile duct.

Staging

Staging is given in Box 11.9.

Treatment

Patients with resectable cancer

Surgery is the only curative treatment and no more than 10–30% patients are eligible for surgery. Surgical resection is contraindicated in:

- Multiple liver metastases
- Ascites
- Multiple peritoneal metastases

Box 11.9: Staging of gallbladder cancer

Stage I
- T1N0M0 – tumour invades lamina propria or muscle layer
- T2N0M0 – tumour invades perimuscular connective tissue; no extension beyond serosa or into liver

Stage II
- T3N0M0 – perforates serosa and invades liver or adjacent organ
- T1–3N1M0 – regional lymph node metastasis

Stage III
- T4 any NM0 – invades main portal vein or hepatic artery or multiple extrahepatic organs

Stage IV
- Any T any N M1 – distant metastasis

- Extensive involvement of hepatoduodenal ligament
- Encasement or occlusion of major vessels
- Poor performance status

The surgical options include:

- Simple cholecystectomy
- Radical cholecystectomy (for tumours invading perimuscular connective tissue and beyond – ≥T2) (Figure 11.10)
- Radical cholecystectomy with liver resection – the extent of liver resection is controversial.
- Radical cholecystectomy with extensive node dissection – the role of node dissection is controversial. Para-aortic node dissection does not improve survival.
- Radical cholecystectomy with resection of the bile duct or pancreaticoduodenectomy.

Adjuvant treatment

There is no proven role for adjuvant treatment. A small retrospective study suggests that in patients with completely resected gallbladder cancer adjuvant radiotherapy with 5-fluorouracil chemotherapy may improve survival (5-year survival rate of 64% compared with 33% of historical control).

Patients with unresectable and metastatic cancer

Treatment in this group of patients is essentially palliative. Jaundice is treated with stent placement or biliary bypass.

Palliative chemotherapy

5-fluorouracil is the most extensively studied regime. 5-fluorouracil based combination chemotherapy yields a response rate of 10–38%. Combination of gemcitabine and cisplatin gives a higher response of 61%.

Prognosis

5-year survival of gallbladder cancer is <5%. Stage at diagnosis is the most important determinant of prognosis. Median survival of early stage disease is 7–19 months whereas that of metastatic disease is 2 months.

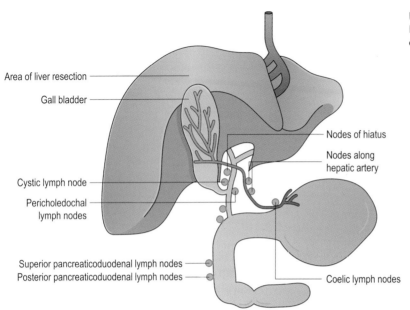

Figure 11.10
Extent of dissection in radical cholecystectomy.

Area of liver resection

Gall bladder

Nodes of hiatus

Nodes along hepatic artery

Cystic lymph node

Pericholedochal lymph nodes

Superior pancreaticoduodenal lymph nodes
Posterior pancreaticoduodenal lymph nodes

Coelic lymph nodes

Carcinoma of the bile ducts

Introduction

Cholangiocarcinoma (CCA), which comprises tumours arising from intrahepatic, perihilar and distal extrahepatic bile ducts, accounts for 3% of all gastrointestinal cancers. There is a slight male preponderance. Peak incidence occurs around 65–70 years.

Aetiology

Risk factors include:

- Primary sclerosing cholangitis (PSC; life time risk 5–20%) – occurs at an earlier age (30–50 years) and tends to present as a diffuse, multicentric tumour.
- Liver fluke infestation (*Opisthorchis viverrini*, *Clonorchis sinensis*) – 8–10% cases. These are endemic in Japan and Southeast Asia.
- Chronic typhoid carriers (6-fold increased risk).
- Chronic intraductal gallstones (10% risk).
- Choledochal cysts (life time risk 3–15%) – average age for development of CCA is 34 years. Higher risk on those with anomalous pancreatico-biliary ductal junction and mutations in p53 and Smad-4 tumour suppressor genes and K-ras oncogene.

- Thorotrast (a radiological agent which is no longer used).
- Smoking increases the risk in patients with PSC.

Pathology

CCA can arise anywhere in the biliary tree. 90% of tumours are adenocarcinoma whereas tumours arising from choledochal cysts and or gallstones may be adenosquamous or squamous carcinomas.

Clinical features

The presentation of CCA depends on the anatomical location. 10% tumours arise from intrahepatic ducts, 50–60% from hilar (called Klatskin tumours) and 20–30% from the distal common bile duct. Intrahepatic tumours present as a mass lesion detected by abdominal imaging or with non-specific symptoms, whereas hilar or extrahepatic tumours present with jaundice (>90%), pruritus, weight loss and abdominal pain. Patients presenting with a triad of cholestasis, abdominal pain and weight loss should be evaluated for cancer.

Diagnosis of malignancy in patients with PSC is challenging. The new development of jaundice and a dominant bile duct stricture in an individual with previously stable PSC should raise the suspicion of malignancy.

Diagnosis and staging

Blood tests include raised markers of biliary obstruction. CA19.9 of >100 U/mL has a sensitivity of 89% and a specificity of 86%.

Imaging

- USS is used as a first line test in patients presenting with abnormal liver function tests, jaundice or abdominal pain. USS can differentiate obstructive from non-obstructive jaundice, detect a mass lesion in intra-hepatic CCA, and confirm ascites in patients with advanced disease. Further imaging is always needed to evaluate and stage the disease.
- CT of the chest, abdomen and pelvis is useful in locoregional and metastatic staging.
- MR cholangiography (MRCP) and endoscopic retrograde cholangiopancreatography (ERCP) are useful in accurate local staging.
- MRI is particularly useful for hilar CCA.
- Cholangiography assesses biliary drainage and can be used to obtain a biopsy.

Tissue diagnosis

Patients with resectable tumours do not need preoperative diagnosis whereas tissue diagnosis is needed for unresectable or metastatic disease. Tissue diagnosis can be obtained by biliary cytology, endoscopic ultrasound or CT guided biopsy depending on the location of tumour.

Laparoscopy and laparoscopic ultrasound are useful in identifying patients with superficial liver or peritoneal metastases and thus laparotomy can be avoided.

Staging

The Bismuth and Corlette classification of proximal bile duct cancers are shown in Figure 11.11.

Treatment

Resectable tumour

The aim of surgery in resectable disease is R0 resection which involves resection of tumour with regional nodes and extended liver resection. Criteria which exclude resectability include:

- Distant metastases
- Encasement of coeliac trunk
- Portal vein occlusion with collaterals

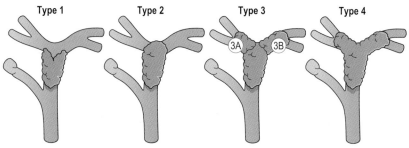

Figure 11.11
Classification and treatment of biliary tumours.

Type 1 – proximal to the bifurcation
Type 2 – involving hepatic duct confluence but not hepatic duct
Type 3 – extending to the right (type 3A) or left (type 3B) hepatic ducts
Type 4 – extends into both the right and left hepatic ducts or with multi-focal duct involvement

---

Treatment
- Types I and II: en bloc resection of the extrahepatic bile ducts and gall bladder, regional lymphadenectomy, and Roux-en-Y hepaticojejunostomy
- Type III: as above plus right or left hepatectomy
- Type IV: as above plus extended right or left hepatectomy
- Distal cholangiocarcinomas are managed by pancreatoduodenectomy as with ampullary or pancreatic head cancers
- The intrahepatic variant of cholangiocarcinoma is treated by resection of the involved segments or lobe

- Lymph node metastasis (N2 nodes).
- Poor clinical status and co-morbidities.

Type of primary surgery depends on location of tumour (Figure 11.11).

Adjuvant treatment

There is no proven role for adjuvant treatment after R0 resection.

Liver transplantation

Neoadjuvant chemoradiotherapy followed by liver transplantation may be an appropriate treatment for a subgroup of patients with unresectable localized disease with no lymph node and vascular involvement. The reported 5-year survival is 82% from USA.

Management of unresectable tumours

Management of unresectable tumours is essentially palliative and supportive. Jaundice is managed with stent or biliary bypass. Other evolving treatments include photodynamic therapy, high intensity focused ultrasound (HIFU), radiofrequency ablation, palliative radiotherapy and drug coated stents.

Palliative chemotherapy with gemcitabine alone or in combination with platinum agents or capecitabine may be considered for fit patients. The reported response rate is 15–40% with median survival of 4–16 months. A recent randomized phase III study (ABC-02) has shown that a combination of cisplatin and gemcitabine yields a better median overall survival compared with gemcitabine alone (11.7 months vs. 8.1 months $p < 0.001$).

New agents

Growth factor receptors HER-1 and HER-2 are overexpressed in biliary tract cancers. New agents studied include erlotinib (EGFR-1 inhibitor) and lapatinib (EGFR-1/HER-2 dual inhibitor) (p. 370).

Prognosis

CCA has a poor 5-year survival of <5%. The majority (75%) of patients die within 1 year. Surgery is the only curative treatment and outcome depends on completeness of surgical resection. R0 resection has a 5-year survival of 20–40%, R1 has 5–10% and R2 has 0%. The median survival after palliative chemotherapy is 4–16 months.

Pancreatic cancer

Introduction

Approximately 7400 new cases are diagnosed in the UK and 37,000 new cases in USA every year. The peak incidence is in the 65–75 year age group with 60% of patients being older than 65 years of age. The male:female ratio is 1.25:1. Only 10–15% patients present with early stage disease amenable to curative surgery, and 4% survive more than 5 years.

Aetiology

Exact aetiology is unknown and the suggested risk factors include:

- Cigarette smoking – increases the risk by two fold and accounts for 30% of cases.
- Increasing age – more than 50% pancreatic cancers occurring in individuals aged 70 years or older.
- Chronic pancreatitis – increases risk by 15–25%.
- Late onset diabetes mellitus.
- Hereditary pancreatitis – autosomal dominant condition, mutation of PRSS1 gene and results in a 70-fold increase.
- Cancer family syndromes – account for 10% of cases. Common syndromes associated with pancreatic cancer include Peutz–Jeghers, familial atypical multiple mole melanoma, familial adenomatous polyposis and Li–Fraumeni syndrome.

Pathology

Ductal adenocarcinoma develops through an adenoma–carcinoma sequence of epithelial pre-neoplastic lesions called pancreatic intra-epithelial neoplasia (PanIN).

Ductal adenocarcinoma is the most common malignant tumour of the pancreas. There are several variants such as undifferentiated (anaplastic), adenosquamous, signet ring cell carcinoma, and mucinous non-cystic. 65% tumours are located within the head, 15% in the body, 10% in the tail and 10% are multifocal.

Clinical features

Tumours of the head of the pancreas tend to present with obstructive jaundice or acute pancreatitis, but the onset is usually insidious. Tumours of the body and tail tend to present even later and are associated with a worse prognosis. Other presenting features include fatigue, back pain, weight loss, late onset diabetes mellitus, steatorrhoea and duodenal obstruction.

Signs
- General examination – anaemia, jaundice, cachexia, enlarged left supraclavicular node (Troisier's sign).
- Abdominal examination – abdominal mass, ascites, hepatomegaly, umbilical nodule.

Diagnosis and staging
Initial investigations include abdominal ultrasound and CT scan.

- Abdominal ultrasound – is the initial evaluation which can detect biliary and pancreatic duct dilatations, tumours >2 cm and liver metastases.
- CT scan of the chest, abdomen and pelvis is helpful in local (Figure 11.12A) and distant staging. It can also help to determine the resectability of a tumour with 80–90% accuracy.

Further investigations include:

- Magnetic resonance cholangio-pancreatography (MRCP) – useful in assessing cystic tumours.
- Endoluminal ultrasonography (EUS) – useful in detecting small tumours and biopsy of small lesions.
- Endoscopic retrograde cholangiopancreatography (ERCP) – rarely used in the diagnosis except to insert biliary stent to relieve obstructive jaundice and obtain biopsy (Figure 11.12B).
- Percutaneous transhepatic cholangiography (PTC) useful to relieve jaundice when ERCP has failed or not possible.

Tissue diagnosis
Tissue diagnosis is usually obtained by EUS with fine needle aspiration (FNA). The technique has a sensitivity of >90% and specificity of almost 100%. Percutaneous fine needle aspiration (FNA) biopsy is less sensitive (69%) and carries a risk of intraperitoneal seeding (16%).

Blood tests
- FBC, biochemistry and clotting profile.
- Serum CA19.9 is the commonly used tumour marker which has a sensitivity of 70–90%

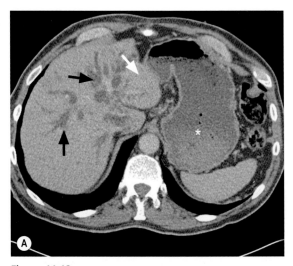 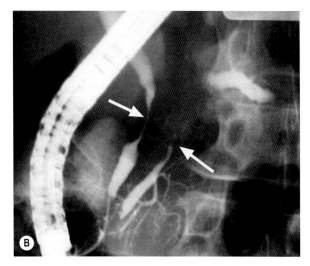

Figure 11.12
CT scan and ERCP in pancreatic cancer. Carcinoma pancreas (white arrow) leading biliary obstruction (black arrow) and duodenal obstruction with gastric dilatation (white asterix) (A) and ERCP shows strictures of common bile duct and pancreatic duct ('double duct sign') (B).

and specificity of 90%. It is useful to assess response and identify tumour recurrence. A level of <200 u/ml suggests longer survival.

Further tests prior to surgery

Laparoscopy with laparoscopic ultrasound alters the management of 15% of patients already assessed as resectable by CT. Selective laparoscopy based on the serum level of CA19-9 and large tumour, is a more efficient strategy, reducing the proportion of patients undergoing laparoscopic ultrasound from 100% to around 45% while increasing the yield from 15% to 25%.

Staging

Staging is shown in Box 11.10.

Management of pancreatic cancer

Treatment of resectable cancer

Surgery

Patients with good performance status and resectable tumours are treated with radical resection. Criteria for resectability are given in Box 11.11. Though the aim of surgery is a complete microscopic resection (R0), 30–60% of resections result in microscopic residual disease (R1).

Patients with jaundice may be considered for pre-operative biliary drainage. The type of surgery depends on location of the tumour:

- Tumours of head of the pancreas – pancreaticoduodenectomy (classic Whipple) or pylorus preserving pancreatoduodenectomy (pp Whipple) are considered curative. A meta-analysis showed that both procedures carry equal morbidities and survival. There is no survival advantage for extended radical lymphadenectomy in pancreatic cancer.
- Tumours of the body and tail of pancreas – left pancreatectomy which includes splenectomy and en bloc removal of the hilar lymph nodes.

The postoperative morbidity of radical surgery is around 40% and the mortality is <5%.

Neoadjuvant therapy

Neoadjuvant treatment using a combination of external beam radiotherapy with 5-FU or Gemcitabine based chemotherapy may improve resectability in a borderline resectable tumour. Several studies report a resection rate of 60% and negative resection margin of 90%. However, this is not routinely practised in the UK.

Postoperative treatment

- Adjuvant chemotherapy – a meta-analysis showed that adjuvant chemotherapy improves 5 year survival (19% vs. 12%) and median survival (19 months vs. 13.5 months) compared with no chemotherapy. The recently reported ESPAC-3 study comparing gemcitabine and 5-FU/FA in patients who had R0/

Box 11.10: Staging of pancreatic cancer

Stage 0
TisN0M0   Carcinoma-in-situ

Stage IA
T1N0M0   Tumour limited to the pancreas, ≤2 cm in diameter

Stage IB
T2N0M0   Tumour limited to the pancreas, >2 cm in diameter

Stage IIA
T3N0M0   Tumour beyond pancreas, but without involvement of coeliac axis or superior mesenteric artery

Stage IIB
T1–3N1M0   Regional lymph node metastasis

Stage III
T4 any NM0   Tumour involving coeliac axis or superior mesenteric artery

Stage IV
Any T any N M1   Distant metastasis

Box 11.11: Criteria for resectable pancreatic cancer

- No coeliac, hepatic or superior mesenteric artery involvement
- A patent superior mesenteric-portal venous confluence
- Portal venous involvement of not more than 2 cm in length or more than 50% circumference
- No liver, peritoneal or other distant metastases
- Absence of portal hypertension and cirrhosis
- No severe co-morbidity to exclude surgery

R1 resection showed no difference in survival (median survival of 23.0 months with 5-FU/FA and 23.6 months with gemcitabine).

- Adjuvant chemoradiotherapy – a meta-analysis showed that chemo-radiotherapy did not improve survival compared with no treatment (median survival 15.8 months vs. 15.2 months).
- Adjuvant chemoradiotherapy and chemotherapy – RTOG 9704 trial reported no statistically significant survival benefit with gemcitabine to adjuvant 5-FU based chemoradiotherapy.

Unresectable and metastatic cancer

70% of patients will present with unresectable disease and treatment of these patients is essentially palliative. Treatment options include:

- Palliative chemotherapy (for locally advanced and metastatic cancer).
- Palliative chemoradiotherapy (locally advanced cancer).
- Symptom control (poor performance status).

Palliative chemotherapy – single agent response rate is seldom more than 10%. A meta-analysis showed that chemotherapy improves survival compared to best supportive care (HR 0.64; 95% CI, 0.42–0.98). Single agent 5-FU results in a median survival of 5–6 months. Single agent gemcitabine has a better median survival (5.7 vs. 4.4 months, p = 0.0025), 1-year survival (18% vs. 2%) and relatively mild toxicity compared with 5-FU. Hence the current drug of choice is gemcitabine.

A recent meta-analysis has confirmed that gemcitabine combination chemotherapy improves survival compared with gemcitabine alone (HR = 0.91; 95% CI, 0.85–0.97). Capecitabine and platinum are the commonly used drugs with gemcitabine.

Palliative chemoradiotherapy – the role of external beam radiotherapy given concurrent with 5-FU or gemcitabine is not clear. However, a meta-analysis showed that chemoradiotherapy increases survival compared with radiotherapy alone (HR 0.69, 95% CI 0.51–0.94). There was no survival difference between chemotherapy alone and chemoradiotherapy followed by chemotherapy.

Symptom control

- Pain control – measures include analgesics, celiac plexus block or unilateral thoracoscopic splanchnicectomy.
- Obstructive jaundice – managed with biliary stent or surgical bypass. Plastic stents are used for patients with metastatic disease and tumours of >3 cm diameter whereas self-expanding metal stents are used for patients with good performance status and locally advanced disease of <3 cm.
- Duodenal obstruction – treated with endoscopically placed stents or bypass surgery.

New agents

Early studies combining gemcitabine with EGFR inhibitor erlotinib has shown some activity but the exact role of EGFR inhibitors is still evolving.

Prognosis and outcome

The most important prognostic factors are resectability and performance status. Median survival following surgical resection ranges from 11–20 months. Without active treatment, metastatic pancreatic cancer has a median survival of 3–6 months and 6–10 months for locally advanced disease, which increases to around 11–15 months with surgical resection. Five-year survival ranges from 7–25%. Radical resection alone gives a 5-year survival rate of around 10%.

Pancreatic endocrine tumours

Pancreatic endocrine tumours arise from the islet cells of the pancreas and the main types are insulinoma, gastrinoma, glucagonoma and VIPoma. The mean age at presentation is 47 years. Genetics syndromes of MEN1, Von Hippel–Lindau, neurofibromatosis type 1 and tuberous sclerosis are associated with an increased risk of pancreatic endocrine tumours.

Clinical presentation is either due to tumour mass or from excessive peptide secretion.

- Insulinomas present with features of hypoglycaemia associated with fasting or vigorous exercise, and rapidly relieved by eating a snack or drinking a liquid rich in glucose. Diagnosis is based on a very low blood sugar (<2 mmol/l) and a high level of insulin and C-peptide (indicative of endogenous insulin).

- Gastrinoma presents with refractory multiple peptic ulcers and diarrhoea. It is diagnosed by high gastrin levels (>100 pg/ml, or >200 pg/ml after secretin stimulation).
- Glucagonoma presents with features of hyperglycaemia, stomatitis, weight loss, diarrhoea and psychiatric disturbances. Necrolytic migratory erythema of the skin is a characteristic feature. Diagnosis is by high plasma glucagon levels.
- Vasoactive intestinal polypeptide tumour (VIPoma) causes watery diarrhoea and hypokalaemia. Diagnosis is by high plasma levels of vasoactive intestinal polypeptide.

Staging investigations of pancreatic endocrine tumours include CT scan, MRI scan, EUS, ^{111}In-octreotide and selective portal/splenic venous sampling and intraoperative ultrasound.

Surgical resection is the treatment of choice which may be indicated even in metastatic disease. 5-year survival following surgical resection is 50–95%.

Cystic tumours of pancreas

These constitute around 15% of all pancreatic cystic masses. The common types are:

- Serous cystic neoplasms predominantly affect women, are found mostly in the head of the pancreas and represent 30% of cystic neoplasms. Conservative approach with regular imaging is the management.
- Mucinous cystic neoplasms are also common in women affecting the body and tail of the pancreas, and represent 40% of primary cystic neoplasms. These are treated with resection to avoid malignant transformation.
- Intraductal papillary mucinous neoplasms (IPMNs) commonly affect men and constitute 30% of pancreatic cysts. IPMNs arising from main duct should be resected whereas those from branch duct may be managed with regular follow-up imaging.

Carcinoid tumours

Carcinoid tumours are neuroendocrine neoplasms arising from enterochromaffin cells. These can be functioning or non-functioning. The mean age at presentation is 49 years and women are more commonly affected.

The clinical presentation of a carcinoid tumour can be a non-specific abdominal symptom, although carcinoid syndrome can occur in 25% of cases. CT is the diagnostic image of choice. Surgery is the treatment of choice for resectable tumours. However, 70–80% patients present with advanced disease. Treatment options for advanced disease include:

- Symptom control using octreotide or a long acting version.
- Radioisotope treatment using ^{131}I-MIBG or ^{111}In/90Y octreotide in patients with positive scans.
- Palliative chemotherapy – streptozosin plus 5-FU/dacarbazine and doxorubicin plus 5-FU.

The overall five-year survival rate is 30–40% and the median survival of patients with metastatic disease is approximately 7 months.

Malignant tumours of the small intestine

Small intestinal malignancies constitute 2–3% of all malignant GI cancers. The ileum is the most frequent site of tumours and is more common in males.

Aetiology

The risk factors include:

- Familial adenomatous polyposis (FAP) – small intestinal adenocarcinoma is one of the common causes of death in patients with FAP after colectomy.
- Crohn's disease (adenocarcinoma).
- Coeliac disease (adenocarcinoma and lymphoma) – type of lymphoma in coeliac disease is enteropathy associated T cell variant.
- Tropical sprue (lymphoma).
- MEN type-1 (gastrin producing tumour of duodenum and jejunum).

Pathology

Tumours of small intestine can be of epithelial, mesenchymal or lymphoid origin. The following are the common types of cancers occurring in the small intestine:

- Adenocarcinomas (45%) – occur in ampulla of Vater in the duodenum and jejunum.

- Carcinoids or neuroendocrine tumours (30%) – common in terminal ileum.
- Sarcomas (10%) – common in ileum, majority of tumours are GIST (p. 261).
- Lymphomas (15%) – B cell NHL is the most common.
- Metastatic cancers – are commoner than primary and usual primaries are GI tract, breast, uterus, ovary and melanoma.

Clinical features

Clinical presentation depends on the type of cancer, site and size. The majority of patients with small intestinal malignancies present with advanced disease. Nonspecific symptoms include abdominal pain, anaemia, nausea, bleeding, and weight loss. Patients can also present as a surgical emergency with perforation or intussusception. Duodenal tumours can present with obstruction as well as jaundice. Metastatic liver carcinoid can present with carcinoid syndrome. Lymphoma may present with pain, weight loss and features of malabsorption. GIST commonly presents with anaemia, sometimes with an abdominal mass.

Investigations

The initial investigations depend on the presenting symptoms.

Imaging

- Plain X-rays – useful in suspected obstruction.
- Abdominal ultrasound – useful to detect liver metastasis, ascites and biliary dilatation.
- CT scan of chest, abdomen and pelvis can delineate primary tumour and disease extent. Different histological types exhibit different features, e.g. lymphoma appears as diffuse segmental thickening of the small intestine and GIST as a well circumscribed mass.
- Small bowel follow-through.
- Endoscopic ultrasound (EUS).
- Small bowel endoscopy.
- ^{111}In-octreotide scan – in carcinoid to rule out metastatic disease.

Tissue biopsy

Biopsy confirmation is essential prior to definitive treatment. Tissue diagnosis can be obtained by endoscopic, CT guided or laparoscopic methods or by laparotomy.

Staging

Adenocarcinoma is staged similar to colonic cancer (p. 163). Lymphomas are staged using the Ann Arbor staging (p. 299).

Management

Small intestinal adenocarcinoma

In patients with localized adenocarcinoma, resection of visible disease and regional lymph nodes is done. In advanced disease, surgery may help with palliation of symptoms.

Chemotherapy regime is same as that of colonic cancer (p. 165). A small study reports a response rate of 50% and a median survival of 20 months with a combination of oxaliplatin with capecitabine.

Small intestinal lymphoma

Stage I and II B-cell NHL are treated surgically with or without chemotherapy, whereas III–IV disease is treated with primary chemotherapy with or without surgical debulking. Chemotherapy regimens are similar to NHL (p. 305).

GIST

Managed similar to GIST occurring elsewhere (p. 261).

Prognosis

Prognosis depends on the type of cancer and stage. Adenocarcinoma usually presents with advanced disease and the reported 5-year survival is 30%. Duodenal tumours have a better prognosis with 5-year survival of 50%.

Lymphomas have a 10-year survival of 60%. The prognosis of small bowel GIST depends on their size and mitotic rate (see p. 262 for NIH prognostic index).

Colorectal cancer

Epidemiology

Colorectal cancer (CRC) is the third commonest cancer in the UK after breast and lung. Over 36,000 new cases per year are diagnosed in the UK and 105,500 per year in the USA.

Over 80% of cases occur in people over 60 and is rare below the age of 40 (except in hereditary forms). The male:female incidence ratio is 1.2 : 1.0. In the UK, the lifetime risk is 1 in 18 for men and 1 in 20 for women. Two-thirds of primaries are in the colon and one third in the rectum. Left-sided cancers are more common than right (sigmoid and rectal cancers account for over half).

Aetiology

The majority of colon cancers are sporadic and not associated with known hereditary genetic mutations. Hereditary bowel cancer is characterized by early age at diagnosis, right-sided cancers, synchronous/metachronous colorectal tumours or other characteristic tumours in same individuals or families (see below). Up to 25% of patients with CRC give a positive family history, suggesting involvement of genetic factors.

- Genetic (p. 50):
  - Familial adenomatous polyposis (FAP) accounts for 1% of all cases of CRC.
  - Hereditary non polyposis colorectal cancer (HNPCC) accounts for about 5% of all CRC cases.
- Familial – those with an affected first-degree relative are at increased risk of developing CRC (relative risk 2.25).
- Inflammatory bowel disease – increases the risk. In ulcerative colitis the cumulative risk of developing CRC is estimated to be 8% at 20 years and 18% at 30 years.
- Diet and supplements – high intake of red meat, calorie and high body mass index increase the risk whereas high vegetable intake and high-fibre diet are protective.

- Drugs – females on hormone replacement therapy and those using regular aspirin are at low risk of developing CRC.
- Lifestyle – long-term smokers are at high risk of adenomas and CRC mortality. Regular physical activity reduces the risk of CRC, particularly in men.

Pathogenesis and pathology

Almost all colorectal cancers are adenocarcinomas and arise in adenomatous polyps through a multi-step process (Figure 11.13). Most adenocarcinomas are moderate to well differentiated with typical morphology. About 80% of primary colorectal adenocarcinomas and 70% of metastases will be CK7– CK20+. Rare histologic types include squamous cell carcinoma, small cell carcinoma, adenosquamous carcinoma and medullary carcinoma.

Presentation

About 85% of patients with bowel cancer have these symptoms at the time of diagnosis. Approximately one-third presents with altered bowel habit or obstructive symptoms (usually left sided tumours as the distal bowel is narrower and faecal content more solid) and one-third with iron deficiency anaemia (usually right-sided tumours). For rectal cancers other symptoms include faecal incontinence, passage of mucus and tenesmus. Up to 30% present with acute colonic obstruction. More advanced tumours may cause weight loss,

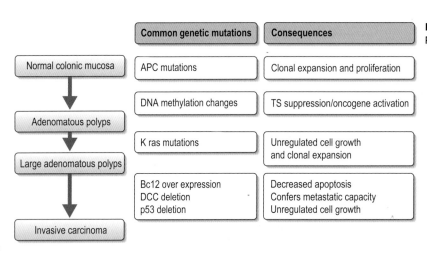

Figure 11.13
Pathogenesis of colorectal cancer.

nausea and anorexia, and abdominal pain and distension from ascites or hepatomegaly.

Investigations and staging

Initial investigations include double contrast barium enema (DCBE), sigmoidoscopy (allows visualization up to splenic flexure at 60 cm) and colonoscopy (Figure 11.14A & B). The whole colon should be imaged as approximately 5% of patients have synchronous cancers and up to 40% have synchronous adenomas. CT colonography is an alternative DCBE (Figure 11.14C). Endoscopy also allows biopsy confirmation.

Those patients presenting with suspected intestinal obstruction should have cross-sectional imaging preoperatively unless there are signs of peritonitis when emergency surgery will take precedence.

Further investigations

- Blood – full blood count, liver function tests, U&E and serum carcinoembryonic antigen (CEA). The majority of patients will have an elevated CEA preoperatively, and this can be used to detect early recurrence in patients who may be appropriate for further curative surgery. It is also useful in monitoring response to treatment in recurrent and metastatic disease. It is less likely to be elevated in poorly differentiated carcinomas.
- All patients with confirmed CRC need CT scan of the chest, abdomen and pelvis for staging.
- Patients with rectal cancer need locoregional staging with pelvic MRI (Figure 11.15); including T2W image MRI helps to define the extent of the tumour and to identify mesorectal margin invasion by tumour which helps to decide need for neoadjuvant treatment.
- If MRI suggests a small (<3 cm) early T1 lesion endorectal ultrasound is useful to access feasibility of local excision and exclude tumour penetration into the muscle of the bowel wall (T2 disease) with an accuracy of 87%.
- PET scan is not routinely used in CRC but may be useful in the context of a rising

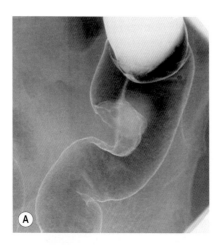
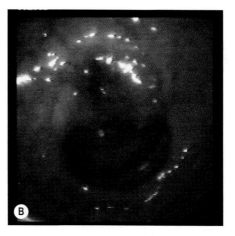
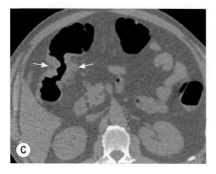

Figure 11.14
Double contrast barium enema shows a polypoid cancer with an irregular indrawn base (A), colonoscopy showing T1 high rectal cancer (B) and CT colonography showing an annular carcinoma (C). Parts A and C from Adam A, et al: Grainger & Allison's Diagnostic radiology, 5th Edition, Volume 1, 2009 (Elsevier), with permission.

CEA or clinical suspicion of metastatic disease or local recurrence, where CT is negative or equivocal and confirmation of relapse would alter management. PET scan may also have a role in potentially resectable metastatic disease such as lung to rule out extensive metastasis.

- In patients with resectable or potentially resectable liver metastasis, MRI of the liver is done to exclude more extensive disease prior to perioperative chemotherapy (Figure 11.16).

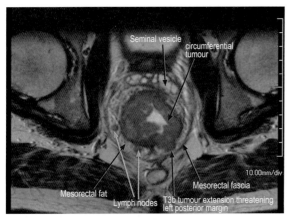

Figure 11.15
T2W MRI of mid rectal cancer shows threatened mesorectal margin.

Staging

Figure 11.17 shows TNM and Dukes' staging which are postoperative staging. After radical resections, 12 or more nodes should be examined as this correlates with prognosis for Dukes' B cancers. Pathology reports should also inform about presence or absence of tumour perforation, extramural vascular invasion, radial margins, lymph nodes (number examined and involved) and assessment of completeness of resection.

Management of colon cancer (Figure 11.18)

Stage I (Dukes' A)
- Surgery

Stage II (Dukes' B)
- Surgery
- Consider adjuvant chemotherapy in patients with PS0-2 if:
  - high risk factors (vascular invasion, peritoneal involvement or T4 tumours, perforation, poorly differentiated adenocarcinoma and surgical margins with tumour cells).
  - or young age (<70 years).

Stage III (Dukes' C)
- Surgery.
- Consider adjuvant chemotherapy in all patients with PS 0–2.

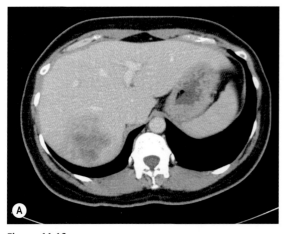
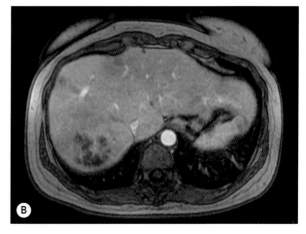

Figure 11.16
CT scan of liver in portal venous phase shows resectable liver metastases (A) and MRI liver with hepatocyte specific contrast reveals more extensive metastases (B).

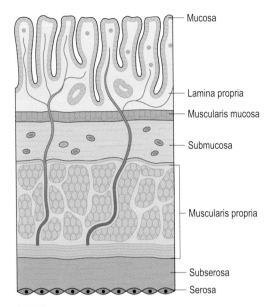

Mesorectal tissue/mesorectal
membrane in rectum

Tis – confined to mucosa or lamina propria
      (no significant metastatic potential)
T1 – invades submucosa
T2 – invades muscularis propria
T3 – invades subserosa/pericolic/mesorectal tissue
T4 – invades other organs or tumour on serosal surface

Stage group	TNM stage	Dukes stage	% Patients
O	Tis N0 M0	–	
I	T1-2 N0 M0	A	11
IIA	T3 N0 M0	B	34
IIB	T4 N0 M0		
IIIA	T1-2 N1 M0	C1 or 2	26
IIIB	T3-4 N1 M0		
IIIC	T1-4 N2 M0		
IV	T1-4 N1-2 M1	D	29

N1 = 1–3 lymph nodes (LN) contain metastatic carcinoma,
N2 = ≥4 LN contain metastatic carcinoma,
C1 = apical LN negative,
C2 = apical LN positive

Figure 11.17
Staging for colorectal cancer.

Stage IV

- Consider radical surgery with perioperative chemotherapy if resectable liver +/− lung metastases.

- Palliative chemotherapy
- Palliative radiotherapy
- Other palliative treatments
- Active symptom control

Surgery

Surgery is curative and several studies have shown equal survival with better cosmesis and shorter hospital stays for laparoscopic versus open surgery for colectomies. Emergency surgery has higher perioperative mortality than that of elective surgery. Hence emergency stenting may be useful to temporarily decompress an obstructed lesion prior to definitive surgery.

Adjuvant chemotherapy

Table 11.1 shows current recommendations for adjuvant chemotherapy. There is no benefit of adjuvant chemotherapy in Dukes' A disease. In stage III (Dukes' C) disease, 5-fluorouracil/folinic acid (5FU/FA) chemotherapy gives an absolute survival benefit of between 8–13%, with 6 months chemotherapy as effective as 1 year. In stage II disease, chemotherapy results in a similar proportional reduction (approximately 33%) in recurrence, but absolute benefits are less because of lower mortality rates (QUASAR 1 showed an absolute increase in 5-year OS of 3.6% for patients less than 70 years). Patients with stage II disease with adverse features have a higher disease-related mortality rate (with >1 risk factor this approaches that of Dukes' C cancers) and hence absolute benefits of adjuvant chemotherapy are greater.

Capecitabine has been shown to have equal efficiency with favourable toxicity profiles compared to bolus 5FU in patients with stage III disease. This is now standard of care for high risk Dukes' B cancers and those patients with Dukes' C not fit for combination chemotherapy. In patients with stage II and III CRC, addition of oxaliplatin to 5FU/FA improved 3-year DFS by 5% over infusional 5FU/FA alone at the cost of increased neurotoxicity. Absolute benefit was greater for stage III vs. stage II disease (6.9% vs. 2.7%). Hence oxaliplatin in combination with 5FU/FA is a treatment option for stage III colon cancer.

Ideally chemotherapy should begin within six weeks of surgery dependent on wound healing and patient recovery. The benefit of adjuvant

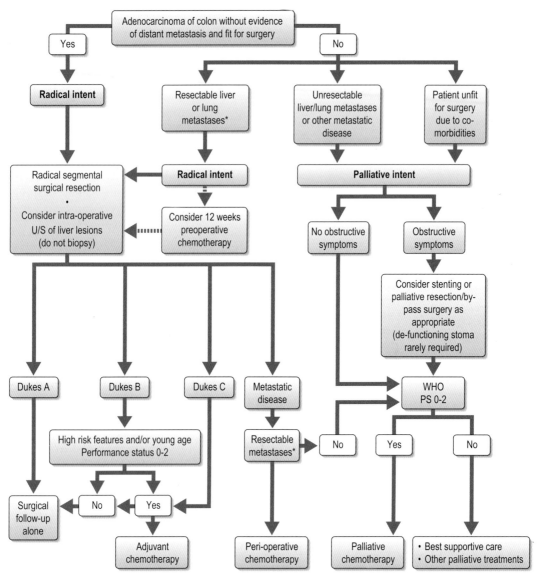

* <4 lung resectable metastases following cardiothoracic surgical review and/or liver metastases resectable or potentially resectable with downstaging Ox/MdG chemotherapy following liver surgeons review (requires >30% of liver intact post surgery. Note that age, number, size and proximity of metastases to major vessels are not exclusions to this) Patients WHO PS 0-1

Figure 11.18
Management of colon cancer.

treatment starting beyond 3 months of surgery is uncertain.

Management of isolated lung or liver metastases

Liver or lung metastasectomy should be considered in fit patients following radical resection of their primary disease (Figure 11.16). However, resection is feasible only in 10% of patients with metastatic disease. Preoperative chemotherapy, in selected patients whose liver metastases are initially extensive for surgery, can enable curative resection in about 30%. A maximum of 12 weeks treatment is recommended prior to surgery as

Table 11.1: Chemotherapy regimens for colorectal cancer

Regimen	Drugs	Doses	Schedule	Indications	PS
Modified Roswell Park	5FU Folinic acid	500 mg/m² 20 mg/m²	IV B weekly 6/8 IV B weekly 6/8	Adjuvant patients <70 years Dukes' B (equivalent efficacy to Mayo Clinic regimen with less mucositis)	0–2
Capecitabine	Capecitabine	1250 mg/m²	po bd 14 d 3 weekly	Adjuvant Dukes' B (high risk) Adjuvant Dukes' C First line palliative	0–2
Modified de Gramont (MdG)	Folinic acid 5FU	350 mg 400 mg/m² 2800 mg/m²	IV 2 h d1 IV B d1 IVI 46 h d1–3	First line palliative (capecitabine not tolerated or severe renal impairment)	0–2
Oxaliplatin modified de Gramont	Folinic acid Oxaliplatin 5FU	350 mg 85 mg/m² 400 mg/m² 2400 mg/m²	IV 2 h d1 IV 2 h d1 IV B d1 IVI 46 h d1–3	Adjuvant Dukes' C First or second line palliative Perioperative resectable liver metastases	0–1
Irinotecan modified de Gramont	Folinic acid Irinotecan 5FU	350 mg 180 mg/m² 400 mg/m² 2400 mg/m²	IV 2 h d1 IV 90 min h d1 IV B d1 IVI 46 h 1–3	First or second line palliative	0–1
Irinotecan	Irinotecan	350 mg/m²	IV 90 min d1	Second line palliative	0–1
Concurrent RT schedules	Capecitabine 5FU Folinic acid	825 mg/m² 350 mg/m² 20 mg/m²	po bd 5 weeks IV B d1–5 weeks 1+5 IV B d1–5 weeks 1+5	Neoadjuvant locally advanced rectal cancer	0–1

both oxaliplatin and irinotecan are associated with liver parenchyma damage and the risks increase with higher cumulative chemotherapy doses.

A recently published trial has shown a 9% increase in 3-year PFS (42% vs. 33%) for patients undergoing surgery with perioperative oxaliplatin/modified de Gramont (Ox/MdG) chemotherapy (12 weeks pre- and 12 weeks post-resection) in patients with four or less resectable liver metastases without increased postoperative mortality.

In patients who underwent combined liver and lung metastasectomy the reported 5-year survival is around 30% whereas that of lung metastasectomy is around 50%. Patients who relapse with isolated liver disease after a previous resection of liver metastases, may be considered for re-resection depending on hepatic reserve and PS.

Management of rectal cancer (Figure 11.19)

Traditionally rectal cancers are defined as tumour arising <15 cm from the anal verge (<12 cm in USA). With the advent of MRI imaging, rectal cancers are defined as those arising below the peritoneal reflection.

Stage I
- Surgery TME AR or APR
- Local excision for T1 tumours of mid or lower rectum
- Short course pre-op RT for T2 low rectal cancers requiring APR

Stage II
- Surgery TME AR or APR
- Short course preoperative RT for T3 low rectal cancers requiring APR

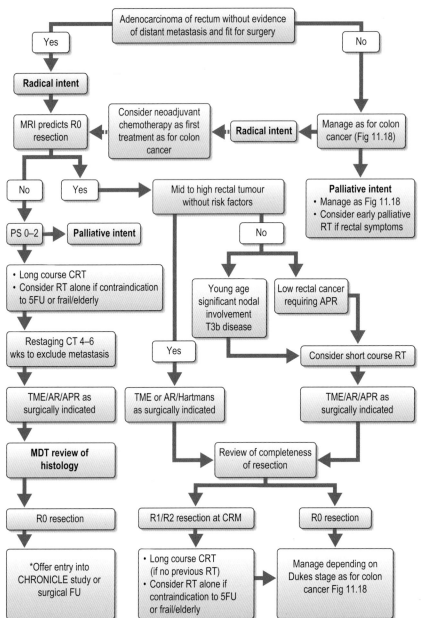

Figure 11.19
Management of rectal cancer.

* In patients not receiving concurrent neoadjuvant fluropyrimidine chemotherapy manage as for colon cancer according to Dukes stage

- Long course preoperative CRT if MRI predicts involved or threatened (<1 mm from tumour) circumferential resection margin (CRM).
- Consider adjuvant chemotherapy as for colon cancer in patients who did not have preoperative CRT.

Stage III
- Surgery TME AR or APR
- Long course preoperative CRT if MRI predicts involved or threatened CRM (from tumour or nodes)
- Short course preoperative RT for T1–3 N1–2 low rectal cancers requiring APR

- Consider short course preoperative RT in patients with rectal cancer at any level if multiple risk factors for recurrence (young age, involved nodes, EMVI, bulky tumour).
- Consider adjuvant chemotherapy as for colon cancer in patients who did not have preoperative CRT.

Stage IV
- As for colon cancer.

Surgery

Local recurrence is a significant risk in rectal cancer, with rates historically as high as 40% with surgery alone. Approximately 25% of patients fail with locoregional disease alone which is rarely curable and often associated with distressing symptoms. In recent years strategies have focused on reducing local recurrence rates in rectal cancer. The most important factor in this is R0 resection, i.e. no tumour cells at the circumferential excision margin which reduces the rate of local recurrence by 90% and mortality rate by 66% of that if margins are involved.

Total mesorectal excision (TME), involves careful dissection with the resection plane outside the mesorectum. It has led to significant improvements in local recurrent rates, survival and decreased morbidity such as impotence in men. It should be standard for all rectal cancer surgery, with either anterior resection (AR) for mid to high tumours or abdominoperineal resection (APR) for low rectal tumours if clearance <1 mm or there is sphincter involvement or poor anal tone. Since laparoscopic surgery results in higher rates of CRM involvement and sexual and urinary complications compared with open resection, open TME surgery remains the gold standard.

Though there are no randomized studies, local excision is an option for T1 tumours in the absence of risk factors for relapse (nodes, high grade, vascular invasion, >3 cm). Transanal excision is the commonly used technique.

Radiotherapy (Table 11.2)

Data show that preoperative radiotherapy is more effective (relative reduction in recurrence rates 57% vs. 37%), less toxic and requires lower dose than post operative treatment (biologically effective dose >30 Gy vs. >35 Gy).

Preoperative short course radiotherapy has been shown to reduce the risk of local recurrence (LR) by >50% in resectable locally advanced rectal cancer (Swedish study 5-year LR 27% with surgery alone vs. 12% surgery and radiotherapy). With TME surgery this advantage persist and there is much lower LR rates (Dutch study 2-year LR 8.2% TME alone vs. 2.4% TME with radiotherapy). Side effects of radiotherapy are increase in early (wound complications) and late (bowel, anorectal and sexual function) morbidity.

The accuracy of preoperative MRI staging in rectal cancer has led to a more selective approach to the use of RT in the UK with short course treatment being offered to those patients with predicted R0 resections but significant risk factors for relapse (Figure 11.19). Early reports from the MRC CR07 study show reduced LR rates (4.7% vs. 11.1%) for all stages and sites of rectal cancer with preoperative short course RT compared to selective postoperative RT if CRM was positive, and an improved 3-year DFS of 4.6%.

Downstaging of locally advanced disease

In patients where MRI identifies risk of CRM involvement preoperative long course chemoradiotherapy (LCCRT) is used to downstage tumours enabling R0 resection in up to 80%. Concurrent chemotherapy improves pathological complete response rates and reduces LR over RT alone at the cost of increased acute toxicity.

Adjuvant chemotherapy in rectal cancer

There is no proven benefit for postoperative adjuvant 5FU chemotherapy after preoperative bolus 5FU CRT schedule, regardless of stage. In patients who haven't had preoperative CRT the benefit of adjuvant chemotherapy is thought to be similar to that in colon cancer, although the number of rectal cancer patients in adjuvant chemotherapy studies is small.

Local recurrence of rectal cancer

In selected cases exenteration (if not involving pelvic side walls or sacrum) may be curative. In these cases metastatic disease should be excluded

Table 11.2: Radiotherapy for rectal cancer

Indication	Technique	Target volume	Dose and timing
Low rectal cancer requiring APR (T2–3N0, T1–3N1–2)	Simulator 2D Patient prone Anal marker 3 or 4 field	PTV borders Sup – L5/S1 Inf – anal marker/3 cm below disease (spare anal canal for mid-high tumours) Lat – 1 cm outside bony pelvis Post – post sacrum Ant – mid femoral head/2 cm ant sacral promontory	25 Gy/5# over 1 week Preoperative Surgery within 7 days
MRI predicted Involved or threatened CRM	CT planned 3D conformal Patient prone 3 or 4 field	PTV = CTV (GTV and mesorectum) + 3 cm margin sup/inf/lat 2 cm ant Post to sacrum	45 Gy/25# over 5 weeks With chemotherapy Preoperative Surgery 6–8 weeks
R1 or R2 resection	Simulator 2D Patient prone Anal marker 3 or 4 field	Field borders Sup – L5/S1 Inf – anal marker/3 cm below disease Lat – 1 cm outside bony pelvis Post – post sacrum Ant – mid femoral head/3 cm ant to rectum	50.4 Gy/28# over 5½ weeks with chemotherapy Postoperative
Unresectable or recurrent disease	Simulator A + P field	Field borders To cover gross disease and pelvic nodes as above Consider 2 cm on gross disease if poor PS	30 Gy/10# or 27 Gy/6# over 2 weeks

by PET before committing patients to such morbid surgery. If preoperative CRT is previously not given, it should be used to decrease the risk of further recurrence. Re-irradiation is not a standard practice but may be considered in selected cases.

Palliation of colorectal cancer

Unresectable locally advanced or recurrent disease and stage IV disease (excluding limited liver and or lung metastases) is treated with palliative intent.

Endoluminal procedures

Expanding metal stent can be placed endoscopically in upper rectal and left or right-sided colonic lesions (technically difficult to place through tumours involving the flexures). It relieves obstructive symptoms in 90% of patients for more than a year (10% migration rate is 10% and 10% re-obstruction rate) and avoids the need for a stoma. Endoscopic laser ablation is

useful to control bleeding in colonic and previously irradiated rectal cancers.

Radiotherapy

For unresectable rectal cancer radiotherapy can offer symptom control, particularly for bleeding, tenesmus and pain.

Palliative chemotherapy

Chemotherapy given early, rather than after development of severe symptoms, is associated with better outcomes without adverse effects on quality of life.

Fluropyrimidines improve median survival by approximately 4 months over best supportive care alone (10 vs. 6 months). The infusional regimen Modified de Gramont (MdG) and oral capecitabine have a response rate of approximately 30% and favourable toxicity profiles in comparison to other 5FU/FA regimes. The addition of either irinotecan or oxaliplatin to MdG or capecitabine as first line treatment increases response rates to 50–60% and median survival to 14–16 months at the cost of increased toxicities. The addition of second line treatment prolongs median survival to more than 20 months.

Targeted systemic therapy

Bevacuzimab (anti-VEGF) as first line in combination with irinotecan/5FU increased median survival by 4.7 months (20.3 m vs. 15.6 m), and with oxaliplatin/5FU increased 18 month survival by 10% (63% vs. 53%), compared to respective chemotherapy alone. The common side effects of bevacuzimab include hypertension, proteinuria, gastrointestinal perforation, intra-abdominal infections, impaired wound healing, and increased arterial thromboembolic events. Treatment should not be given within 28 days of major surgery.

Cetuximab and panitumumab are anti-EGFR antibodies. Cetuximab in combination with irinotecan/5FU (CRYSTAL study) increased response rate (RR) (39% vs. 47%) and improved progression free survival (PFS) (8 m vs. 8.9 m). In combination with oxaliplatin/5FU, it increased RR (36% vs. 46%) but did not improve PFS. The most common toxicities of cetuximab are skin reaction and diarrhoea.

The K-ras gene is emerging as both a predictive and prognostic factor for response to targeted anti-EGFR antibodies. Improved response rate and RR and PFS are associated with wild type K-ras. Mutated K-ras appears to be associated with lack of response and worse survival compared to wild type K-ras, with some evidence that anti-EGFR antibodies are actually detrimental compared to chemotherapy alone.

Palliation of liver metastases

Percutaneous radio-frequency ablation (RFA) can be useful to palliate inoperable or recurrent liver metastasis in selected patients (achieves a median survival of up to 36 months). However, lesions >4–5 cm, superficial lesions and those close to vessels are not effectively treated by RFA.

Follow-up

Eighty percent of recurrences from CRC occur within the first 2 years and 90% within 3 years. 5- and 7-year survivals equate to cure for colon and rectal cancer respectively with <5% relapsing after this. Aims of follow-up following radical treatment are to detect recurrent disease at a potentially curable stage and surveillance for metachronous polyps or bowel cancers. Optimum follow up strategy is uncertain and varies widely.

Routine surveillance of the bowel

Patients who do not have their entire colon imaged at diagnosis should have colonoscopy within 6 months of treatment to exclude synchronous polyps or cancers. For patients who have had complete bowel imaging at staging, initial colonoscopy 1–3 years following treatment is recommended, followed by 5-yearly (more frequently in patients with ≥5 polyps) colonoscopy in polyp free patients with a life expectancy of ≥15 years.

Routine surveillance for distant disease

Studies suggest that intensive follow-up is associated with significantly improved 5-year OS (HR 0.81) in Dukes' B and C patients. A significant proportion recurs with asymptomatic liver metastasis and with active surveillance up to 20% patients are candidates for curative surgery. Hence following radical treatment for Dukes' B or C cancer, patients fit for further active treatment are followed up as follows:

- 6-monthly CEA for 2 years followed by yearly until 5 years.
- CT liver (and pelvis in rectal cancer) at 12 and 18–24 months.
- CT if rising CEA with PET if CT fails to identify relapse.

Screening

General population

A meta-analysis has shown that screening by faecal occult blood (FOB) reduces the risk of death from CRC by 16% overall, and by 23% (RR 0.77) in those who are actually screened. The NHS Bowel Cancer Screening Programme (BCSP) for people aged 60–69 offers 2-yearly FOB tests and colonoscopy to those with abnormal results. Those >70 can request screening.

High-risk populations (p. 50)

Prognosis and outcome

Stage is the most important prognostic factor. Stage-wise 5-year survival rates are >90% for stage I (Dukes' A), 70–85% for stage II (Dukes' B) without risk factors, 40–60% for stage II with risk factors and stage III (Dukes' C) and 5% for stage IV disease. Median survival of inoperable metastatic disease is 6 months with best supportive care alone, 18–20 months with chemotherapy and over 2 years with targeted agents.

Anal cancer

Squamous cell cancers (SCC) of the anal canal are uncommon. The peak incidence occurs in the seventh decade. There is a slight predominance of females of 2–3:1 for cancers of the anal canal. Risk factors include genital infection with human papillomavirus (HPV, most frequently type 16), chronic immunosuppression in transplant and HIV positive patients, and smoking (2–5 fold increase).

Pathogenesis and pathology

The anal canal is 3–4 cm long and extends to the palpable upper border of the anal sphincter. Perianal cancers by definition occur within 5 cm of the anal verge with no extension into the canal.

Anal cancer may arise in anal intraepithelial neoplasia (AIN), which can progress from low to high grade and is found in areas adjacent to squamous cell carcinoma.

Ninety percent of anal cancers are squamous cell, histological subtypes which include large cell keratinizing, basaloid, and transitional (large cell non-keratinizing). Collectively they are referred to as cloacogenic or epidermoid cancers. All have a similar natural history, response to treatment, and prognosis.

Approximately 5–10% tumours are adenocarcinoma of the anal glands and are managed as low rectal cancers. Other histologic types are melanoma, basal cell and small cell carcinoma.

Presentation

Anal carcinoma presents with discomfort, itching and bleeding in 50%. Symptoms are often dismissed as haemorrhoids. Any patient over the age of 60 should be examined to exclude carcinoma as should those with a mass, enlarged inguinal nodes, pain or persistent symptoms. Faecal incontinence and vaginal fistula are late symptoms of locally advanced disease. Distant metastases are rare at presentation.

Investigations and staging

Initial assessment includes digital rectal examination, examination under anaesthesia (EUA) and biopsy. Transanal US is useful in assessing depth of invasion and perirectal nodes. CT or MRI is useful to assess pelvic nodal metastases. Up to 50% of palpable or radiologically suspicious inguinal nodes are not involved and hence a fine needle aspiration (FNA) of clinically suspicious nodes, with excision biopsy if FNA is non-diagnostic, is recommended. Distant metastasis is seen in <5% at diagnosis and staging includes CT chest and abdomen. Apart from routine blood tests, patients with risk factors should be tested for HIV.

TNM staging is given in Table 11.3.

Management

The treatment options for localized tumours are:

- Local excision (selected stage I patients)
- Concurrent chemoradiotherapy (CRT) (stage I–III)
- Radical surgery (T3 or 4 causing sphincter destruction and salvage after CRT)

Table 11.3: Staging for anal cancer

Stage group	TNM stage	% patients
I	T1 (tumour ≤2 cm) N0	12
II	T2 (tumour 2–5 cm) N0 T3 (tumour >5 cm) N0	55
IIIA	T1–3 N1 (perirectal nodes) T4 (tumour invading adjacent organ) N0	30
IIIB	T4N1 Any T N2 (unilateral internal iliac or inguinal nodes) Any T N3 (perirectal and inguinal or bilateral internal iliac +/– inguinal nodes)	
IV	M1 (extra pelvic metastases)	<5

NB Invasion of rectum, subcutaneous tissue, skin or sphincter muscles is not T4

Treatment options for patients with stage IV disease are palliative chemotherapy, palliative radiotherapy and active symptom control.

Local excision

Local excision with curative intent is an option for selected patients with stage I disease not invading the sphincter muscles. The 5-year overall survival with local excision alone is approximately 70%. However CRT gives better chance of overall disease control and should therefore be considered for all patients who are fit for this approach, even if local excision has been performed as first line treatment.

Chemoradiation (CRT)

There are no RCTs of surgery versus CRT; but CRT offers sphincter preservation for the majority of patients. Chemoradiation using concurrent mitomycin C (MMC) and 5 FU is the standard of care for all stages of locoregional disease (Box 11.12). The UKCCCR ACT I and an EORTC study confirmed the benefit of CRT over RT

> ### Box 11.12: CRT for anal cancer
>
> #### Radiotherapy
> **Phase I**
> Patient prone with anal marker (canal tumours) and palpable disease wired (margin tumours and inguinal nodes)
>
> Ant and post fields
>
> *Borders*
> Superior = 2 cm above bottom of SI joints
> Inferior = 3 cm below anal margin or most inferior extent of disease
> Lateral = lateral to femoral heads
> Dose 30.6 Gy in 17 fractions of 1.8 Gy
>
> **Phase II**
> Field borders are a 3 cm margin on GTV in all planes.
> N0 canal tumours = 3 field (posterior, right and left lateral)
> N0 margin tumours = direct field
> N+ tumours = anterior and posterior fields
> Dose 19.8 Gy in 11 fractions of 1.8 Gy
>
> #### Chemotherapy
> Week 1 mitomycin C 12 mg/m^2 d1 and 5FU 1000 mg/m^2/d d1–4
> Week 5 5FU 1000 mg/m^2/d d1–4
>
> RT fields and doses are as per ACT II protocol. Chemotherapy schedule is as per ACT I study

---

alone in terms of reduction in locoregional failure, improvement in colostomy free and disease specific survival. Acute toxicities are increased by concurrent treatment, without significant increase in late morbidity.

Radiation dose and technique

The dose of radiation concurrent with chemotherapy required to treat anal cancer is debatable.

There is evidence to suggest doses as low as 30 Gy in combination with chemotherapy are sufficient for microscopic disease and 45 Gy adequate to treat non bulky gross disease. This underlies current UK practice. Since the median potential doubling time of anal cancer is 4 days (similar to that of cervix cancer), local control rate is likely to be decreased by prolonging overall treatment time.

The failure rate in untreated clinically normal inguinal nodes is up to 25%. This has led to the practice of elective nodal irradiation which reduces the risk to <5% without significant morbidity.

The role of cisplatin

Cisplatin in combination with 5 FU is under investigation as neoadjuvant, concurrent and adjuvant treatment in anal cancer. The current UK–ACT II is comparing two CRT schedules (standard MMC/5FU versus cisplatin/5FU) and adjuvant chemotherapy with two cycles of cisplatin/5FU versus no further treatment.

HIV positive patients

Prior to the advent of highly active antiretroviral therapy (HAART), tolerance of CRT in patients with HIV and CD4 counts <200 at doses of RT >30 Gy was poor, with excessive toxicities. The majority of patients can now be treated with standard doses (p. 297).

Radical surgery

Patients with confirmed local relapse following CRT who are fit to consider salvage surgery should be restaged with CT chest and abdomen to exclude metastatic disease as well as MRI pelvis to stage regional disease. Approximately 50% can be cured by a salvage surgical resection, but local recurrence rates approach 50% even in patients undergoing complete resections. Inguinal node dissection similarly is reserved for patients with residual or recurrent inguinal metastases after CRT. It carries a high risk of postoperative wound complications and chronic lymphoedema.

Other occasional indications for surgery include a contraindication to primary CRT, incontinence due to sphincter damage or a vaginal fistula and late toxicity from CRT.

Metastatic disease

Distant metastases develop in up to 15% of patients and the most effective chemotherapy is a combination of 5-FU with cisplatin. Response rates in metastatic disease are approximately 55% but rarely complete and their duration usually only a few months.

Follow-up

Follow-up is to diagnose local recurrence at an early stage so that salvage surgery may be offered. Anal cancers regress slowly over several months following CRT and therefore early random biopsy is not helpful. Local recurrences usually appear within three years and distant metastases within five years after CRT. Follow-up therefore commonly comprises rectal and inguinal node examination at regular intervals – initially 6-weekly if there is continuing treatment response, but possible residual disease, until resolution. Then 2, 3 and 4-monthly for the first 3 years followed by 6-monthly review to 5 years. The development of a hard-edged ulcer after previous healing, an enlarging mass, or increasing pain at the site of the primary tumour site are suggestive of recurrence and should be confirmed by biopsy.

Serious late toxicity including ulceration, radionecrosis and stenosis causing loss of anorectal function and requiring colostomy occurs in 5–12% and is related to radiation dose. Perineal fibrosis, rectal urgency and diarrhoea, and dyspareunia are relatively common.

Prognosis and survival

Size of the primary tumour, in the absence of metastases, is the most useful predictor of

Table 11.4: Survival and local control with CRT by T stage

T stage	5-year OS %	5-year local control %
T1	80	90–100
T2	70	75
T3/4	45–55	55

survival. Overall 5-year survivals are in the region of 75%. A lesion size of 4 cm represents the threshold for local control, with up to 95% of tumours ≤4 cm achieving complete pathological response to CRT (Table 11.4).

Spread to the regional nodes is an adverse factor for survival, with 5-year survivals up to 20% lower than in node-negative patients. If inguinal nodes are not invading skin or deep structures, control rates with CRT alone are approximately 80%. Perianal lesions have a more favourable prognosis than those of the anal canal, due to the decreased risk of nodal metastases.

Median survival of patients with distant metastases remains 9–12 months.

Further reading

Mariette C, Piessen G, Triboulet JP. Therapeutic strategies in oesophageal carcinoma: role of surgery and other modalities. Lancet Oncol. 2007;8:545–553.

Hartgrink HH, Jansen EP, van Grieken NC, van de Velde CJ. Gastric cancer. Lancet. 2009;374:477–490.

Rampone B, Schiavone B, Martino A, Viviano C, Confuorto G. Current management strategy of hepatocellular carcinoma. World J Gastroenterol. 2009;15:3210–3216.

Eckel F, Jelic S; ESMO Guidelines Working Group. Biliary cancer: ESMO clinical recommendation for diagnosis, treatment and follow-up. Ann Oncol. 2009;20 Suppl 4:46–48.

Hidalgo M. Pancreatic cancer. N Engl J Med. 2010;362: 1605–1617.

Cunningham D, Atkin W, Lenz HJ et al. Colorectal cancer. Lancet. 2010;375:1030–1047.

Uronis HE, Bendell JC. Anal cancer: an overview. Oncologist. 2007;12:524–534.

Cancers of the genitourinary system

12

M Beresford

Cancer of the kidney

Introduction

Renal cell carcinoma (RCC) accounts for 2–3% of all cancers, with 6600 new diagnoses and 3600 deaths per year in the UK. There has been an increasing incidence over the past 10–15 years, at least in part due to more incidental tumours being found with the increased use of cross-sectional imaging. Peak age at presentation is between 65–75 years, with very few cases in the under 40 age-group. The male to female ratio is 3:2.

Aetiology

Risk factors for renal carcinoma are as follows:

- Smoking – smokers are more likely to develop RCC than non-smokers and the effect seems to be dose-dependent, with heavy smokers having a relative risk of 2.0.
- Occupational exposure – risk ratios of 1.3 to 1.6 have been observed in individuals exposed to petroleum, hydrocarbon, steel, asbestos, cadmium or dry cleaning products.
- Analgesic nephropathy – there is an increased risk of RCC in patients who develop nephropathy associated with the use of phenacetin-containing analgesics.
- Obesity – obesity increases the risk of developing RCC, with a linear relationship between body weight and risk (odds ratios of up to 4.8). Excessive consumption of red meat and dairy products might increase risk, but there appears to be no relationship with alcohol or caffeine intake.

- Acquired cystic kidney disease – in dialysis patients.
- Genetic factors – Von Hippel–Lindau disease is a familial disorder characterized by the development of multiple tumours including bilateral renal cell carcinomas, retinal/central nervous system haemangioblastomas and phaeochromocytomas. Hereditary papillary renal cell carcinoma (HPRC) is a condition in which patients are at risk of developing multiple, bilateral type 1 papillary renal carcinomas and involves mutation in the c-met oncogene.

Pathology

In adults, 85% of malignant lesions arising from the kidney are renal cell carcinoma, with most of the remainder being metastases from other primary tumours. Other rarer cancers include clear cell sarcoma, lymphoma, oncocytoma and adult form of Wilms' tumour.

- Renal cell carcinomas (RCCs) – most RCCs are well-differentiated and usually arise within the upper pole. The majority are of clear cell origin although they often contain several different cell types, including granular cells and spindle cells (the poor prognosis sarcomatoid variant).
- Transitional cell carcinomas – are relatively uncommon, accounting for 5% of malignancies in the kidney, and are sometimes a result of analgesic nephropathy. They arise in the renal pelvis and often affect multiple sites of the urothelial mucosa with 50% having a history of bladder tumours. Transitional cell carcinomas of the renal pelvis are usually

© 2011, Elsevier Ltd
DOI: 10.1016/B978-0-7234-3458-0.00017-8

discovered late, although occasionally present earlier with obstructive symptoms. Due to the proximity to the renal vein, they tend to spread early, typically with metastases to lung and bone. 5-year survival varies from 10–70% depending on tumour grade.

- Squamous cell carcinomas – these are rare and usually associated with chronically infected staghorn renal calculi. Presentation tends to be late, with locally extensive disease.

Presentation

Renal tumours often remain asymptomatic and unnoticed until large. The classical triad (also known as 'too late' triad) of presenting symptoms (loin pain, haematuria and flank mass) occurs in less than 10% of patients. Up to 20% of patients have a history of fever at presentation, and a third report weight loss and cachexia. 30% have metastatic disease at presentation and a further 25% have locally advanced disease. Typical sites of metastases include lungs (75%), lymph nodes/soft tissue (36%), bone (20%) and liver (18%). Patients may also demonstrate a number of paraneoplastic manifestations such as polycythaemia, hypercalcaemia etc.

Investigations and staging

Initial investigations include urinalysis for protein, blood and cytology. Blood tests should include full blood count, urea and electrolytes, liver function, clotting and calcium levels.

Imaging

CT scan: CT scan appearance (Figure 12.1) is important in determining the appropriate surgical procedure – laparoscopic, partial or radical nephrectomy. Size is important in diagnosis – benign cortical adenomas can look like malignancies but tend to be less than 3 cm in diameter.

Other investigations: for small tumours, a chest X-ray is sufficient for staging if the CT scan does not include the chest. Ultrasound and colour flow Doppler are useful in assessing renal vein and inferior vena caval invasion. A bone scan should be considered if there are symptoms or a raised alkaline phosphatase.

If there are concerns about renal reserve from imaging or renal function blood tests, then more formal assessment of renal function is appropriate.

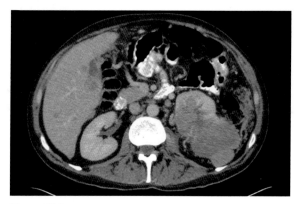

Figure 12.1
CT scan showing an irregular mass lesion arising from the left kidney.

Staging

Stage (Table 12.1) determines the prognosis and treatment of renal tumours.

Management

Surgery of the primary tumour

Curative

The definitive treatment for renal cancer is surgical resection. Radical nephrectomy is performed by an anterior approach and en bloc removal of the kidney, adrenal and perirenal fat. The adrenal gland is rarely involved in T1 or T2 tumours and can be left behind. If tumour invades the renal vein, this can be ligated distal to the tumour thrombus and even partial vena caval resection may be undertaken if necessary.

Regional lymphadenectomy is sometimes performed during the radical procedure, but its role in prolonging survival is debatable.

Recent improvements in surgical techniques have enabled laparoscopic partial or total nephrectomies as a less invasive technique for removing kidneys with small volume tumours. Nephron-sparing surgery should be considered particularly for patients with poor renal reserve or non-functioning contralateral kidneys.

Palliative

Nephrectomy should also be considered as a palliative procedure in patients with metastatic disease. Although very rarely (<1%) this may result in regression of metastases ('abscopal effect'), it is not the main reason for considering surgery. It is aimed mainly at reducing symptoms

Table 12.1: Staging of tumours of the renal parenchyma

Stage			
I	T1 N0 M0	7 cm or less in size, confined to kidney T1a ≤4 cm T1b >4 cm ≤7 cm	
II	T2 N0 M0	>7 cm in size, confined to kidney	
III	T1/2 N1 M0	Confined to kidney, metastases in a single regional node	
	T3 N0/1 M0	T3a	Invades adrenal gland or perinephric tissues but not beyond Gerota fascia
		T3b	Extends into renal vein(s) or vena cava below diaphragm
		T3c	Extends into vena cava above diaphragm
IV	T4 N0–2 M0	T4	Invades beyond Gerota fascia
	T1–4 N2 M0	N2	Metastases in >1 regional node
	T1–4 N0–2 M1	M1	Distant metastases

such as pain, haematuria and hypercalcaemia. Removal of the tumour bulk may also improve the efficacy of any subsequent systemic treatment – trials have shown that patients with metastatic disease who are treated with interferon have improved survival if they undergo palliative nephrectomy prior to the immunotherapy.

Adjuvant therapy

Adjuvant therapy with interferon-α following nephrectomy has been investigated and does not appear to confer any survival advantage. More complicated and toxic regimes using combinations of interferon, interleukin-2 and 5-fluorouracil (known as the Atzpodien regimen) have not proved any better and in fact may be detrimental.

Metastatic disease

Interferon-alpha

Interferon alpha is a cytokine with anticancer and antiviral activity. Response rates in metastatic RCC are reported as 10–15% with a 2% complete response rate (although there are also occasional reports of spontaneous remissions off treatment) and a stable disease rate of approximately 25%. A Cochrane review showed a 3-month survival benefit with interferon compared with no interferon. Interferon may be better in 'good' prognosis metastatic disease, based on the number of disease sites, performance status and diagnosis to metastases interval.

The optimal regimen of interferon is not yet known. Typical dose schedules are of 9–12 mega-units subcutaneously three times per week, often starting at a lower dose to assess tolerability. Treatment is discontinued at disease progression or after 6–9 months, whichever comes first. Blood counts and liver function should be monitored during treatment.

Interferon has significant side effects (Box 12.1) that impact on quality of life. These effects are dose dependent, but the majority tend to stop quickly on discontinuation of treatment. Common side effects include fatigue, flu-like symptoms, diarrhoea, nausea and vomiting, anorexia, bone marrow suppression and rash at injection site.

Interleukin 2

Interleukin works by stimulating cytotoxic T-cells. It can be given subcutaneously, by high-dose bolus intravenous injection or by continuous infusion (all give similar results). It has been used instead of or in combination with interferon, and seems to result in improved response rates (of 15–20%), but with no improvement in overall survival and significantly worse toxicity than interferon.

Medroxyprogesterone-acetate

The response rate is only 5–7%. Trials comparing progestins and interferon therapy show a survival benefit of approximately 2.5 months in favour of the interferon.

Chemotherapy

Response rates with chemotherapy are less than 10%. A few cases of sarcomatoid variants of RCC have responded to sarcoma chemotherapy regimes such as doxorubicin and ifosfamide.

Novel agents

Various new targeted therapies have shown positive results in the treatment of metastatic renal cell carcinoma and are generally better tolerated than interferon-α and interleukin-2. Studies are now concentrated on the use of these agents in the adjuvant setting and their sequencing in metastatic disease.

Sorafenib and sunitinib are oral multiple kinase inhibitors affecting VEGF, PDGF and c-KIT tyrosine kinases among others (p. 370). They have both antiproliferative and antiangiogenic activity. A phase III trial of sorafenib versus placebo in metastatic RCC patients on second-line systemic therapy showed an improvement of progression-free survival (5.5 months versus 2.8 months respectively).

In the first line setting sunitinib has shown a median progression-free survival of 11 months in comparison with 5.1 months with interferon-α ($p < 0.000001$) and the median overall survival was 26.4 months with sunitinib and 21.8 months with interferon ($p = 0.51$). Sunitinib is the recommended treatment in the UK for patients with performance status 0–1. The dosage is 50 mg once daily for 4 weeks with a 2-week rest period (6-week cycle). Dose may be decreased in steps of 12.5 mg according to tolerance, but there is evidence that efficacy is related to dose-intensity. Adverse events include rash, diarrhoea, hand–foot skin reaction, fatigue, thrombocytopaenia and hypertension. These are usually easily managed and rarely result in permanent discontinuation of therapy.

Temsirolimus inhibits activity of mTOR, which features downstream in the cell signalling pathway and is thought to be a point into which other critical pathways feed. It is an intravenous agent which appears to improve progression-free survival when compared with interferon in metastatic RCC and has shown particular benefit in poor prognosis patients. Everolimus, an oral mTOR inhibitor, has proven benefit in the second-line setting on progression after previous tyrosine kinase inhibitor treatment.

Bevacizumab is a monoclonal antibody which inhibits VEGF. In conjunction with interferon it has been shown to double progression-free survival in previously untreated metastatic RCC when compared with interferon alone.

Radiotherapy

Radiotherapy can be used to control bleeding and pain from primary tumour sites and to treat symptoms associated with bone and central nervous system metastases.

Surgical management of metastases

Resection of metastases from RCC should be considered, particularly for pulmonary lesions, where excellent results can be achieved. Consideration of surgical management should not be confined to solitary metastases, although the best survival figures are seen after complete resection of solitary lesions, with 5-year survival rates of up to 50% compared with 20% following complete resection of multiple lesions. A longer interval between primary tumour and development of metastases correlates with a longer disease-specific survival. Resection of cerebral metastases has also shown favourable results, particularly when there is a long interval from resection of the primary.

Prognostic factors and survival

Survival remains limited for patients with RCC, however in selected patients with metastatic disease, long-term survival is recognized. Characteristics associated with a better prognosis include stage I disease, absence of invasion into the collecting system and predominance of clear cell pattern.

The Memorial Sloan–Kettering prognostic stratification is often used for metastatic disease. Five major prognostic factors are identified: poor performance status (KPS <70), raised lactate dehydrogenase (>1.5× normal), raised serum calcium, low haemoglobin and no nephrectomy. Patients are categorized into three risk groups based on the number of these prognostic factors present: 0 = favourable risk, 1–2 = intermediate risk, 3–5 = poor risk. 3-year survival rates for these risk groups are reported as 31%, 7% and 0% respectively.

Stage-wise 5-year survival for renal cell carcinoma is 66% for stage I, 64% for stage II, 42% for stage III and 11% for stage IV.

Cancers of the urinary bladder and renal pelvis

Introduction

Bladder cancer accounts for 4% of all malignancies, with over 10,000 new diagnoses and almost 5000 deaths each year in the UK. Worldwide it is the 9th most common cancer, but is more common in North America and Western Europe, where it is the 4th most common cancer in males and 8th most common in females. The worldwide male to female ratio is 10:3. Bladder cancer is rare in the under 50 age group, and most common in over 70-year-olds.

Aetiology

Risk factors for bladder tumours include the following:

- Smoking (2–5 fold increased risk).
- Infections – especially schistosomiasis which increases the risk of squamous cell carcinoma.
- Occupational/chemical (aniline dyes, aromatic amines, printing industry, rubber industry, firelighter manufacturers, tar manufacturing, sewage workers, pest control, benzidine, cyclophosphamide, 2-naphthyline, xenylamine, phenacetin).
- Bladder calculi (chronic cystitis).
- Chronic indwelling catheters.
- Previous radiotherapy (risk of sarcoma).

Pathology

In Western countries, over 90% of bladder tumours are predominantly transitional cell carcinoma (TCC), often with elements of squamous, adenocarcinoma or sarcomatous differentiation. 80% are papillary and 20% flat in appearance and the most likely areas affected are the posterior and lateral bladder walls. Flat tumours tend to be of higher grade and more aggressive. Less common histological types are squamous cell carcinoma, adenocarcinoma and very rarely small cell carcinoma.

Tumours often present initially as low grade and superficial, but tend to be multiple and recurrent. With each recurrence there is a tendency to progression in cytologic atypia. The whole of the uroepithelial tract is at risk of transitional cell carcinoma with tumours occurring in the ureters and renal pelvis as well as the urinary bladder.

Carcinoma-in-situ manifests as severely dysplastic cells through all layers of the epithelium. It carries a poor prognosis and often has an invasive component. At least 30% of grade III carcinoma-in-situ will become invasive.

Presentation

The most common presentation is with painless haematuria. A patient presenting with macroscopic haematuria has a 25% chance of having a bladder tumour (5% if microscopic haematuria). Other symptoms include frequency, urgency, dysuria and loin pain due to ureteric obstruction. Occasionally patients present with symptoms caused by metastases such as bone pain, fractures or shortness of breath.

Lymph node involvement is strongly related to tumour grade. Less than 10% of grade 1 tumours have nodal involvement, compared with 80% of grade 3. Metastatic spread is predominantly to the lungs and bones.

Investigations and staging

Investigations

Initial investigations include urine cytology, intravenous urogram (IVU) and cystoscopy. Cystoscopy should include bimanual examination, complete inspection of the urethra and bladder, biopsies of all suspicious areas, transurethral resection of visible tumour and a detailed diagram of the findings to assist in comparison at follow-up procedures.

Once a bladder tumour is confirmed further investigations should be considered, including blood tests (renal function, full blood count, liver function and calcium level), chest X-ray, histology review and for muscle-invasive tumours, CT or MRI scan of the abdomen and pelvis (Figure 12.2). MRI is better for showing early invasion of adjacent organs and extravesical spread. A bone scan is only necessary if indicated by symptoms or a raised alkaline phosphatase. Chest X-ray or CT chest is useful to rule out metastatic disease (Figure 12.3).

Staging

The staging of bladder tumours is shown in Table 12.2.

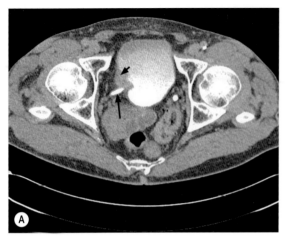 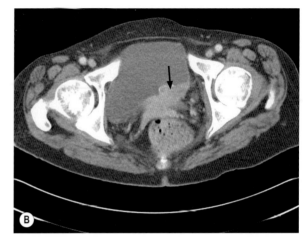

Figure 12.2
CT scan of bladder tumour: tumour shown as filling defect in the right side of base of bladder (short arrow) with contrast filled ureter (long arrow) entering the bladder through the tumour (A). Scan shows an irregular mass arising from base of the bladder (B).

> **Box 12.1: Indication for radical cystectomy**
>
> - Severe/persistent carcinoma-in-situ
> - Muscle invasion
> - Multiple recurrences of T1 disease despite intravesical treatment
> - T1 G3
> - Squamous cell carcinoma and adenocarcinoma
> - Unreliable patient (surveillance is not realistic)

Management

The management of bladder tumours is dependent upon the degree of invasion into the bladder wall and the histological grade of the cancer. Superficial, non-muscle invasive tumours are generally treated by transurethral resection, with intravesical chemotherapy or immunotherapy for multiple or recurrent tumours. Localized muscle invasive disease is treated by primary cystectomy or radiotherapy to the bladder and perivesical tissues. Figure 12.4 shows the management of bladder tumours by tumour stage. Indications for radical cystectomy are shown in Box 12.1.

Intravesical therapy

Intravesical therapy reduces short-term recurrence rates following transurethral resection. The options are chemotherapy with agents such as mitomycin, or immunotherapy with BCG. The incidence of chemical cystitis is approximately 40% with chemotherapy but 90% with BCG, so the latter is often reserved for resistant disease.

Intravesical chemotherapy

Mitomycin reduces recurrence rate following first cystoscopy from 25% to 12%. It is administered as a single dose within 6 hours of transurethral resection or weekly for 6–8 weeks. It should be left in contact with the bladder for 1–2 hours. Response rates are reported as 65%, with a 35% complete response. Side effects include cystitis, reduced bladder capacity, palmer desquamation and a rash.

Intravesical immunotherapy

Intravesical BCG results in a response rate of 75%, with a mean time to recurrence of 2 years. It has been shown to reduce cystectomy rate in CIS patients. Side effects include cystitis, fever, haematuria and prostatitis.

Following resection, BCG treatment should be withheld for a month to allow the mucosa to heal. A 6-week induction course (81 mg of BCG in 50 ml of normal saline) of weekly treatments is followed by cystoscopy. If there is a response a second 6-week course is initiated. If there is progression, cystectomy should be considered.

Trials of maintenance therapy have shown variable benefits using a schedule following the initial 6-week course with three consecutive weekly treatments every 6 months for 3 years

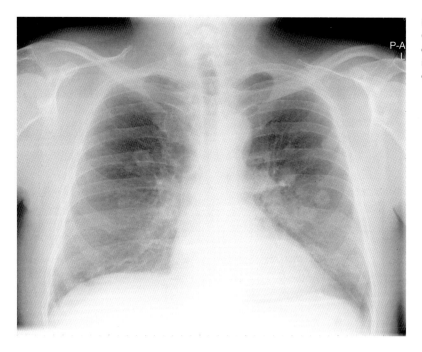

Figure 12.3
Chest X-ray of a patient with cannonball lung metastases from metastatic transitional cell carcinoma of the bladder.

Table 12.2: Staging of tumours of the bladder

Stage		
I	T1 N0	Invades sub-epithelial connective tissue T1a – deep lamina propria T1b – muscularis propria
II	T2 N0	Invades muscle T2a – inner half of muscle (superficial) T2b – outer half of muscle (deep)
III	T3 N0	Perivesical tissue invasion T3a – microscopic T3b – macroscopic
	T4a N0	T4a – invades prostate, uterus, vagina
IV	T4b N0	T4b – invades pelvic or abdominal wall
	T1–4 N1–3	N1 – single regional node ≤2 cm N2 – 2–5 cm single node or multiple nodes ≤5 cm N3 – >5 cm node
	M1	Distant metastases

(but less than a fifth of patients can tolerate this schedule).

Muscle invasive disease

If disease is localized, the aim is for cure with bladder preservation if possible. In disease confined to the bladder, radical cystectomy is curative in 60–70%. Radical external beam radiotherapy might allow preservation of bladder function, but reported cure rates are lower at 50% (although no direct comparisons between surgery and radiotherapy exist). If there is spread beyond bladder (T3 disease), radical treatment is curative in <30% of patients and half of patients will develop distant metastases within 1–2 years.

Radical cystectomy

Radical cystectomy involves excision of the bladder, perivesical fat and the attached peritoneum. In men the prostate and seminal vesicles are removed. In women the uterus, urethra, adnexa, ovaries and a cuff of vagina are resected. Reconstructions tend to be more difficult in women. The role of lymphadenectomy has been controversial, but is now generally accepted as standard. If the urethra is left in-situ, there is a 5–10% risk of urethral recurrence.

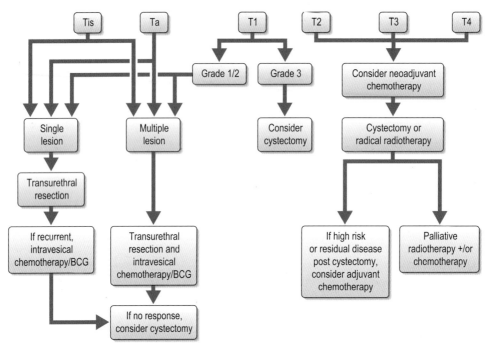

Figure 12.4
Management of transitional all bladder carcinoma by T stage.

Techniques for urinary diversion:

1. Ileal conduit (stoma)
2. Continent diversions
   - Mainz II (if no urethra, insert ureters into rectum – increased risk of bowel cancer and lifelong diarrhoea).
   - Mitrofanoff diversion (ureters implanted into a small bowel reservoir and use a native tube (e.g. fallopian or appendix) to link reservoir to skin; self-catheterization is required).
   - If the urethra is preserved (i.e. no CIS, high tumour) the ureters can be diverted into a reservoir of small bowel which empties via the urethra – no voiding sensation so need bladder training.

Side effects of radical cystectomy include up to 3% mortality, impotence in men (70–100%), dyspareunia in women, uterocutaneous fistulas, infection and small bowel fistulas (30%).

Radical radiotherapy
The aim of radical radiotherapy is cure with bladder preservation. The decision between radical cystectomy and radiotherapy should be made at a multidisciplinary meeting and with involvement of the patient. Randomized studies have shown radiotherapy to have higher rates of local recurrence, but similar overall survival with close follow-up and salvage cystectomy on relapse. Approximately a third of patients treated with radiotherapy will remain cystectomy-free.

There is no survival advantage from nodal irradiation and no evidence of any benefit of adjuvant pelvic radiotherapy following cystectomy.

Poor prognostic factors for radiotherapy include ureteric obstruction, incomplete transurethral resection, sessile (worse than papillary) tumour and persistence/recurrence at first cystoscopy.

Radical radiotherapy is contraindicated in those who had previous pelvic radiotherapy, history of inflammatory bowel disease or small bowel adhesions, extensive CIS, poor bladder function and multiple transurethral resections or multiple intravesical chemotherapy installations (due to reduced bladder function which may worsen with radiotherapy).

Radical radiotherapy is typically CT-planned with a target volume including a 1.5–2 cm margin around the empty bladder, prostatic urethra and tumour extension. This margin is to allow for considerable bladder movement. The rectum and femoral heads should be identified as organs at risk. Treatment is usually delivered via a 3-field plan (anterior and two laterals) to a dose of 55 Gy in 20 fractions over 4 weeks or 64 Gy in 32 fractions over 6.5 weeks using 6–10 MV photons.

Complications of radiotherapy include radiation cystitis (<5%), radiation proctitis (<5%), bowel obstruction (<3%) and erectile dysfunction (60%).

There is interest in partial bladder irradiation (or whole bladder with a second phase tumour boost to a smaller volume) with the intention of reducing toxicity whilst maintaining an effective dose to the tumour.

Palliative radiotherapy

For node positive or locally advanced disease, palliative radiotherapy can be beneficial, particularly for patients with haematuria or pelvic pain. Palliative fields are planned conventionally, sometimes with use of a cystogram to localize the bladder at simulation. Typical dose schedules include 30 Gy in 10 fractions over 2 weeks, 21 Gy in three fractions over 1 week or, in particularly frail patients, a single fraction of 8–10 Gy. Improved symptoms are observed in approximately half of patients, but a similar proportion suffers acute side effects.

Chemotherapy

Chemotherapy in bladder cancer has been primarily used in the palliative and metastatic settings, but there is good evidence to support the use of neoadjuvant chemotherapy prior to cystectomy. However, the platinum-based regimes are toxic and emetogenic, and many patients with invasive bladder cancer are frail with poor renal function so tolerate the chemotherapy poorly.

Chemotherapy in metastatic disease

Response rates of 40–70% have been observed with combinations such as CMV (cisplatin, methotrexate, vinblastine) and MVAC (methotrexate, vinblastine, adriamycin, cisplatin). Newer combinations such as gemcitabine and cisplatin have similar response rates and survival

---

Box 12.2: Chemotherapy regimes in bladder cancer

Gem/Cis:	Gemcitabine – 1 g/m^2 Day 1, 8, 15 Cisplatin* 70 mg/m^2 Day 1
	Repeat every 28 days (or 21 days omitting day 15 gemcitabine)
CMV:	Cisplatin* 100 mg/m^2 Day 2 only (70 mg/m^2 if palliative) Methotrexate 30 mg/m^2 Day 1 and 8 Vinblastine 4 mg/m^2 Day 1 and 8
	Repeat every 21 days
MVAC:	Methotrexate 30 mg/m^2 Day 2, 15, 22 Vinblastine 3 mg/m^2 Day 2, 15, 22 Adriamycin 30 mg/m^2 Day 2 Cisplatin* 70 mg/m^2 Day 2
	Repeat every 28 days

*For patients with poor renal function (creatinine clearance of 30–60 ml/min), consider replacing cisplatin with carboplatin (AUC 4–5).

---

outcomes, with less toxicity (Box 12.2). Single agent platinum regimes are less effective (response rates of 30%).

Neoadjuvant chemotherapy

A meta-analysis of neoadjuvant trials in muscle invasive bladder cancer has revealed a 5% absolute benefit in overall survival for patients treated with cisplatin-based combination chemotherapy. This benefit was seen irrespective of the type of local treatment (surgery or radiotherapy) and applied across all patient groups. There may also be a role for neoadjuvant chemotherapy in bladder preservation, with responding patients being treated with radiotherapy and non-responding patients going on to cystectomy. This is currently being investigated in randomized trials.

Adjuvant chemotherapy

There is conflicting evidence on benefit and a Cochrane review did not recommend this as routine treatment. Studies of immediate versus delayed chemotherapy in high risk (node positive or T3/4) patients post-cystectomy have failed to recruit sufficient numbers.

Concurrent chemo-radiotherapy

There is no definite evidence that concurrent cisplatin with radiotherapy is better than radiotherapy alone. Concurrent 5-fluorouracil and mitomycin-C is being investigated as a less toxic regime to combine with radiotherapy.

Management of carcinomas of the renal pelvis and ureter

The staging of tumours of the renal pelvis and ureter is given in Table 12.3. Renal pelvic and upper urothelial transitional carcinomas are treated by radical resection of the kidney and ureter. Nephron-sparing procedures can be undertaken in small, localized tumours if there are concerns about function of the remaining kidney. Adjuvant radiotherapy confers no survival advantage following complete resection, but may be considered in patients with positive margins or residual local disease. Doses are limited by surrounding structures, but typically 45–50.4 Gy in 25–28 fractions can be delivered. There is some evidence to suggest that the addition of concurrent cisplatin chemotherapy to radiotherapy improves overall and disease-free survival in T3/4 and/or node-positive disease following surgical resection. The majority of relapses are distant, so systemic adjuvant therapy using platinum-containing chemotherapy regimes should be considered, although there is little published data as to the benefits of this approach. The current evidence for adjuvant chemotherapy is stronger for node positive disease than for locally advanced but node negative disease.

Metastatic disease is treated with similar platinum-based chemotherapy regimes to those used in metastatic bladder cancer.

Management of small cell carcinoma of the bladder

Small cell bladder cancer accounts for less than 1% of bladder cancers and commonly presents at an advanced stage. In localized disease patients should be treated with neoadjuvant platinum-based chemotherapy prior to surgery or radiotherapy. Responses to chemotherapy are seen in metastatic disease, but median survival is less than 12 months. Most published data relates to the use of neuroendocrine regimes such as carboplatin/cisplatin with etoposide.

Survival

5-year survival rates for bladder cancer are as follows:

Stage	5-year survival
Ta, T1, CIS	70–95%
T2	50–80%
T3a	40–70%
T3b	20–50%
T4	10%

Survival with metastatic disease is poor despite reasonable response rates to chemotherapy, with <10% 2-year survival.

Cancer of the prostate

Introduction

Prostate cancer accounts for 12% of all cancers (23% of cancer in men), with 32,000 new diagnoses and 10,000 deaths each year in the UK. There has been a large increase in incidence over the past 10–15 years due to increased detection through PSA screening and surgery for benign prostatic disease. The majority of cases occur in the over 70 age-group and the disease is rare in the under 50s. As yet there is no evidence that PSA screening reduces mortality rates from prostate cancer.

Table 12.3: Staging of tumours of the renal pelvis and ureter

Stage		
I	T1 N0 M0	Tumour invades subepithelial connective tissue
II	T2 N0 M0	Tumour invades muscularis
III	T3 N0 M0	Tumour invades peripelvic (or periureteric) fat or renal parenchyma
IV	T4	T4 Invades adjacent organs or perinephric fat
	or N1–3	N1 Metastases in single node ≤2 cm
		N2 Metastases in single node >2 cm but ≤5 cm or multiple nodes
		N3 Metastases in single node >5 cm
	or M1	M1 Distant mets

Aetiology

The exact aetiology is not known and there are various suggested risk factors such as a high fat diet, anabolic steroids, oestrogen exposure and genetic. A hereditary prostate cancer gene on chromosome 1p has been identified. Mutation of the androgen receptor domain may be associated with high grade disease, extraprostatic extension and distant metastases. Mutation of the vitamin D receptor gene may also play a role. There is a link with BRCA genes as well.

Pathology

The vast majority of prostate tumours are adenocarcinomas. Malignant areas are frequently multifocal and most often involve the posterolateral part of the gland. 70% arise in the peripheral zone of the prostate. Rare variations include mucinous, small cell, squamous cell, adenoid cystic and endometrioid carcinoma (the latter is characterized by a normal PSA and lack of hormone response). Transitional cell carcinoma of the prostatic urethra may occur and there are rare reports of secondary spread from other tumours such as melanoma and lung cancer.

The Gleason grading system, an important prognostic factor, describes the degree of differentiation of the malignant cells (Box 12.3). Each tumour is graded twice, each out of five to give a total score out of 10 – the first grade relates to the most commonly observed pattern (primary pattern) and the second to the next most common pattern.

Presentation

The majority of prostate cancers are initially detected following a raised serum prostate specific antigen (PSA) level and approximately half of patients are completely asymptomatic. The PSA blood test may have been taken as part of investigations into non-specific lower urinary tract symptoms of bladder outflow obstruction such as hesitancy, frequency, nocturia and terminal dribbling, or increasingly as part of a well-man screening programme. In symptomatic patients who require a transurethral resection of the prostate (TURP) for presumed benign prostatic hypertrophy, it is not uncommon to discover cancer cells in the prostatic chippings.

Box 12.3: Gleason grading

1. Well differentiated; uniform gland pattern
2. Well differentiated; glands variable
3. Moderately differentiated; papillary/cribriform features or well-spaced acini
4. Poorly differentiated; cords, sheets, fused cells
5. Very poorly differentiated; minimal gland formation and necrosis

Box 12.4: Roach formulae

Risk of lymph node involvement (%):	2/3 PSA + 10 (Gleason-6)
Risk of seminal vesicle involvement (%):	PSA + 10 (Gleason-6)
Risk of extracapsular extension (%):	3/2 PSA + 10 (Gleason-3)

Locally advanced cancers can be detected on rectal examination, and occasionally patients may present with symptoms due to local extension such as pain or bleeding. Metastases to bone are common and bone pain or pathological fracture can be presenting features. Other areas of spread include obturator, perivesical and para-aortic lymph nodes and rarely liver, lung or brain metastases.

The strongest predictors of metastasis are a high PSA, high Gleason score (8–10) and age >70 years. The Roach formulae (based on Partin's tables) are commonly used in treatment algorithms to predict the risk of local extension and lymph node spread (Box 12.4).

Investigations and staging

Initial investigations include a PSA blood test and digital rectal examination (DRE). Patients with raised PSA are offered a transrectal biopsy of the prostate to obtain histological diagnosis (usually 8–12 core biopsies of the prostate are obtained, half from each lobe).

If cancer is confirmed, further investigations are determined by the grade, volume of disease and PSA level, but may include a pelvic MRI scan to define extracapsular spread and seminal vesicle or lymph node involvement (generally offered to patients with Gleason 4+3 disease or above, or with PSA >20 ng/ml, in whom radical treatment is being considered) and a bone scan (if PSA

Table 12.4: Staging of prostate cancer

Stage		Description	
I	T1a	Not palpable, confined to prostate	Diagnosed on TURP, <5% of chippings involved, Gleason grade 2–4 only
II	T1a		Diagnosed on TURP, <5% of chippings involved, Gleason grade ≥5
	T1b		Diagnosed on TURP, >5% of chippings involved
	T1c		Diagnosed by needle biopsy in response to a raised PSA
	T2a	Palpable, but confined to prostate	Confined to 1 lobe, <50% involved
	T2b		Confined to 1 lobe, >50% involved
	T2c		Both lobes palpably involved
III	T3a	Breaches prostate capsule	Extension through the prostate capsule
	T3b		Involvement of one or both seminal vesicles
IV	T4	Local invasion	Invasion of other nearby structures
	Any N1		Spread to regional lymph nodes
	Any M1		Distant metastases

>10–15 ng/ml). If there is doubt over lymph node involvement, a laparoscopic retroperitoneal lymph node biopsy might be considered prior to proposed radical treatment.

Table 12.4 shows the staging of prostate cancer.

As well as the absolute PSA level, various other PSA parameters have been developed in an attempt to improve the predictive value of the test for diagnosis and monitoring:

- PSA density (PSA/volume of gland) allows for higher PSA levels in older men with large, hypertrophied glands. A value of 0.1 ng/ml/cc is considered normal (e.g. a PSA of 5 ng/ml with a 50 cc prostate volume).
- Percent-free PSA (fPSA) is the ratio of how much PSA circulates free compared with the total PSA level, including that attached to blood proteins. The percentage of free PSA is lower in men who have prostate cancer than in men who do not and may be useful in determining which patients with intermediate PSA levels should have a prostate biopsy for diagnosis. There is some controversy over where the cut-off should lie, but fPSA levels of <10% are very suspicious.
- PSA kinetics give an indication of the rate of tumour growth, and include the PSA doubling time, expressed in months or years, and the PSA velocity, expressed as ng/ml/year (this is commonly utilized in patients on active surveillance – see below). To get an accurate indication of PSA velocity, at least three measurements should be taken over a period of 18 months.

Note that very poorly differentiated cancers may not secrete PSA and are therefore more difficult to diagnose, predict and monitor.

Management of localized disease

The treatment options for localized disease are:

- Active surveillance (for patients suitable for radical treatment).
- Watchful waiting (for patients not suitable for radical treatment).
- Radical treatment with surgery or radiotherapy or both.

Active surveillance and watchful waiting

Many patients will have slow-growing disease which may have little or no impact on their life-expectancy, and they might therefore be spared the toxicities and inconvenience of radical treatment. Active surveillance implies close monitoring with early curative treatment offered to patients who show signs of progression. There are no absolute criteria for considering active surveillance and the decision should be made with the patient, but typical parameters would be T1–T2b disease, Gleason grade ≤7, PSA ≤15 (with favourable kinetics). A surveillance programme might consist of 3-monthly visits for the first 2 years, followed by 6-monthly visits thereafter, with a DRE and PSA checked at each visit. Repeat transrectal biopsies should be performed at 18 months. Criteria for consideration of radical treatment would be PSA progression (doubling time <2 years), clinical progression or upgrading of the Gleason score on repeat biopsy.

'Watchful waiting' is appropriate where patients deemed unsuitable for radical treatment are treated with palliative endocrine therapy when there is symptomatic progression.

Radical treatment

Radical treatment options for prostate cancer include radical prostatectomy, external beam radiotherapy and brachytherapy (low-dose rate or high-dose rate). Each treatment has its own characteristics and may be suitable for certain types of patients, but reported success rates are similar if patients are chosen appropriately.

Radical prostatectomy

Perineal, retropubic or laparoscopic approaches can be considered. There is a 5–15% risk of urinary dysfunction after surgery. Nerve-sparing techniques have improved morbidity, with approximately 50% impotence rates.

External beam radiotherapy

Conformal CT planning is well established in prostate radiotherapy (Box 12.5 and Figure 12.5). The Medical Research Council RT01 study randomized between 64 Gy and 74 Gy and found a hazard ratio for biochemical progression free survival of 0.67 (CI 0.53–0.85; p = 0.0007) in favour of the escalated group. However this was achieved at the expense of increased late bowel and bladder toxicity. It is not yet known whether there will be any improvements in overall survival.

Newer techniques such as intensity modulated radiotherapy (IMRT) might enable even further increases in the dose administered or further sparing of normal tissues.

Radiobiological studies have suggested a surprisingly low alpha-beta ratio for prostate cancer

---

> **Box 12.5: Radiotherapy for prostate**
> *(see Figure 12.5)*
>
> **Localization**
> CT planning with empty rectum. Target volume defined on planning CT or co-registered CT/MRI
>
> **Target volume**
> *Primary radical treatment*
> CTV = Whole prostate + tumour extension
> Whole seminal vesicles included if risk of involvement ≥15%
> Consider treating pelvic nodes if risk of nodal involvement ≥15%
> Phase I PTV = CTV + 1 cm margin
> Phase II PTV = CTV + 0.5 cm margin
> *Salvage radiotherapy*
> Prostate bed, any surgical clips and residual seminal vesicle with 1 cm margin
>
> **Dose**
> Prostate and seminal vesicle
>   Phase I – 56 Gy in 28 fractions
>   Phase II – 18 Gy in 9 fractions
> Whole pelvis and prostate
>   Phase I (whole pelvis with prostate) – 50 Gy in 25 fractions
>   Phase II (prostate alone) – 18–24 Gy in 9–12 fractions
> Salvage radiotherapy
>   66–70 Gy in 33–35 fractions
>
> **Tolerance**
> - Rectum: 55.5 Gy to no more than 50% of the rectum, 70 Gy to no more than 25% and 74 Gy to no more than 3%.
> - Bladder: Less than 50% of the bladder should receive 67 Gy.

(1.2–1.5 Gy), which implies that hypofractionated courses of radiotherapy with a high dose per fraction might result in improved cancer control for a similar level of side effects. For this reason doses such as 57–60 Gy in 19–20 fractions over 4 weeks are being investigated. These shortened schedules have the additional advantage of sparing resources and being more convenient for patients.

Though the survival benefit of whole pelvic radiotherapy in high risk of pelvic lymph node involvement (≥15% on Roach criteria) remains to be demonstrated, it is commonly practised.

Acute side effects of radiotherapy include dysuria, frequency, diarrhoea, lethargy and erythema. Late effects include proctitis (diarrhoea, rectal bleeding, tenesmus: 30% mild, 5% severe),

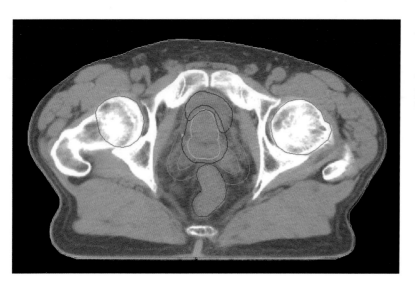

Figure 12.5
Target volumes for radical prostate radiotherapy. Orange line phase I PTV including prostate and seminal vesicle with a 10 mm margin and purple line phase II PTV including only prostate with a 5 mm margin.

impotence (30–40%) and urinary incontinence (1–5%).

Brachytherapy

Low-dose rate (LDR) brachytherapy
Permanent radioactive seeds are implanted directly into the prostate via transperineal needles that are inserted with ultrasound guidance under general or spinal anaesthetic. Approximately 50–100 Iodine-125 or Palladium-103 seeds are implanted to achieve a prescribed dose of 145 Gy. Patients eligible for this treatment are those with a prostate volume of <50 cc, Gleason ≤6, PSA ≤15, T2 or less disease, those haven't had a previous TURP and not at high risk of extracapsular extension or lymph node involvement. Patients should have a transrectal ultrasound volume study to assess suitability for brachytherapy.

Although there is good evidence to confirm the efficacy of brachytherapy in terms of PSA control and biopsy findings, there is as yet no long-term survival data. The procedure has not been directly compared with external beam radiotherapy or radical surgery in randomized studies, but comparative and cohort studies show similar 5-year biochemical recurrence-free and overall survival.

High-dose rate (HDR) brachytherapy
HDR brachytherapy is suitable for intermediate-high risk patients. It is typically given as a boost following a shortened course of external beam radiotherapy but can also be used as monotherapy. Treatment is delivered through catheters implanted with ultrasound guidance into the prostate under general anaesthetic. HDR boost patients are typically treated in two or three fractions, 12 hours apart, necessitating overnight stay with the catheters and template in-situ. Box 12.6 shows some of the HDR boost schedules currently in use.

Role of hormones in curative treatment

Patients undergoing radical radiotherapy are commonly treated with 3 months of neoadjuvant luteinizing hormone releasing hormone (LHRH) analogues. This approach may enable a reduction in the volume of tissue irradiated due to shrinkage of the prostate gland. An EORTC study compared radiotherapy alone versus radiotherapy with immediate androgen suppression started on the first day of radiotherapy and continued for 3 years. 5-year clinical disease free survival was 40% versus 74% and overall survival was 62% versus 78% in favour of the adjuvant endocrine group.

Prolonged adjuvant treatment for 2–3 years should be offered to all patients with high risk disease (Gleason 8–10, clinical T3/4 tumours or lymph node risk >30%). The role in low and intermediate risk patients is being assessed in randomized studies, but these patients are cur-

Box 12.6: High-dose rate brachytherapy boost schedules

External beam dose and fractionation	HDR brachytherapy boost dose and fractionation
35.7 Gy in 13	17 Gy in 2
46 Gy in 23	16.5 Gy in 3
46 Gy in 23	17 Gy in 2
50 Gy in 25	18 Gy in 2
45 Gy in 23	16.5 Gy in 3
46 Gy in 23	23 Gy in 2

Box 12.7: Side effects of LHRH analogues

Hot flushes
Weakness/loss of muscle bulk
Weight gain
Fatigue
Osteoporosis/fracture risk
Loss of libido and erectile function
Mood changes
Poor concentration/memory

rently treated with 3–6 months of LHRH analogues before and during radiotherapy.

It should be noted that LHRH analogues are not without side effects (see Box 12.7) and can add considerably to the morbidity of patients undergoing radiotherapy.

There is no established role for neoadjuvant or adjuvant hormonal manipulation in patients undergoing radical prostatectomy.

Management of locally advanced and metastatic disease

Locally advanced disease

For patients with locally advanced disease radical radiotherapy or surgery may add little or no additional benefit over hormone therapy alone, although there is emerging evidence that radiotherapy does improve biochemical control in patients with PSA levels up to 70 ng/ml. The mainstay of treatment is with LHRH analogues or anti-androgens. Prolonged treatment with LHRH analogues results in significant toxicity due to reduction of testosterone levels (see Box 12.7). Androgen receptor inhibitors, such as bicalutamide, or 5-alpha reductase inhibitors effectively reduce the delivery of testosterone to the prostate without reducing serum testosterone levels and therefore tend to have a better side effect profile, although they can cause significant gynaecomastia. Prophylactic radiotherapy to the breast buds or prophylactic tamoxifen 10–20 mg/day can reduce and sometimes prevent the painful gynaecomastia. Typical radiotherapy doses are 8–10 Gy in a single fraction or 15 Gy in three fractions given on alternate days, using electron radiotherapy delivered to an 8–10 cm circle around each nipple.

Metastatic disease, elderly and those with significant comorbidities

Metastatic disease (Figure 12.6) is generally treated with endocrine therapy, usually LHRH analogues in the first instance, with the addition of an anti-androgen to give maximal androgen blockade on biochemical or clinical progression. The typical duration of response to first line endocrine therapy with LHRH analogues is 18–24 months. There is increasing interest in intermittent LHRH analogue therapy as a way of prolonging the useful lifespan of the drug and of allowing patients to have periods of time off treatment and therefore avoid some of the side effects. Typical schedules are to treat until PSA falls below 4 ng/ml (or <80% of initial value) and restart when PSA rises above 10 ng/ml. Studies have shown no difference in survival when compared with continuous therapy, but significant improvements in quality of life, with patients spending a median of 1 year off treatment.

Third line hormonal therapy with oestrogens can be considered but response duration tends to be short unless response to first and second line treatment has been particularly good.

Elderly patients and those with significant co-morbidities can be treated symptomatically with or without hormones.

Management of relapse after radical treatment

Some authorities advocate postoperative radiotherapy to the prostatic bed in cases with a positive margin at radical prostatectomy, whilst others would wait and offer radiotherapy if the PSA fails to completely suppress or subsequently rises. In these situations, salvage radiotherapy is

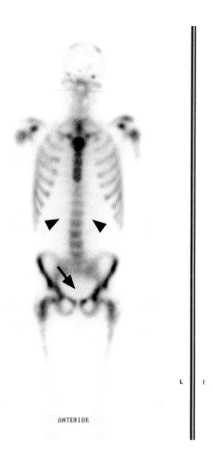
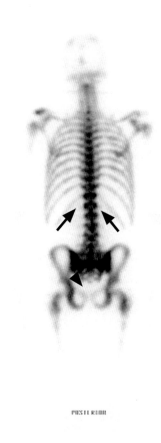

Figure 12.6
Bone scan in metastatic prostate cancer. Note the absence of uptake in the kidneys and bladder (arrows) suggesting that uptake is preferentially by the extensive metastases. This picture is called a 'superscan' which is a contraindication for radioisotope treatment (risk of lethal bone marrow suppression)

most effective if given before the PSA reaches a value of 2 ng/ml (Box 12.5).

Salvage surgery for radiotherapy failures is rarely undertaken due to the complicated nature of the procedure and questionable results. Newer invasive techniques such as cryotherapy and high frequency ultrasound (HiFU) have shown some success in terms of PSA control after radiotherapy failures (and perhaps as primary treatments in place of radiotherapy), but long-term outcomes are awaited.

Role of chemotherapy in prostate cancer

Until recently, chemotherapy has been reserved for advanced metastatic prostate that has become refractory to endocrine treatment (known as hormone refractory prostate cancer, HRPC, or more accurately as castration resistant prostate cancer, CRPC). Docetaxel is now well established in this setting, with studies showing quality of life and overall survival benefits (in the order of 10–12

weeks) when compared with the previous standard regimen of mitoxantrone and prednisolone. Doses of 75 mg/m^2 are administered on a 3-weekly basis for up to 10 cycles. Although low-grade neutropenia is fairly common, the rates of febrile neutropenic sepsis are reassuringly low (<3%) without colony-stimulating factor support.

Chemotherapy agents are now being investigated in earlier stages of prostate cancer, both in metastatic disease prior to the development of CRPC or as an adjuvant to radical prostatectomy for localized disease. There is also interest in second-line chemotherapy after failure of taxanes; there is some evidence for PSA response with satraplatin, an orally active platinum-based drug. Cabazitaxel, a new taxane, has demonstrated a 2.5 month survival benefit in the second-line setting.

Palliative treatment

- Steroids: Low-dose steroids (0.5–2 mg of dexamethasone daily) are effective in some patients in terms of both quality of life improvements and PSA control.

- Bisphosphonates: Zoledronic acid administered intravenously once a month has been shown to reduce the incidence of skeletal events, including fractures or the need for radiotherapy, in men with bone metastases. It is effective at controlling refractory metastatic bone pain.
- Radiotherapy: External beam radiotherapy is very effective in controlling metastatic bone pain and symptoms of primary tumour invasion such as haematuria and pain. Prolonged fractionation regimes have not been shown to be more beneficial than a single fraction of 8 Gy. Radiotherapy is also commonly used in cases of spinal cord or nerve root compression from vertebral metastases (p. 328).
- Radioisotopes: Strontium-89 and Samarium-153 are effective at controlling pain in up to 80% of patients with widespread bone metastases. Radioisotope treatment is particularly useful in patients with diffuse bone pain that cannot easily be targeted with external beam radiotherapy (Figure 12.6). Care must be taken if chemotherapy is to be considered at a later date because of a suppressive effect on the bone marrow.

Prognostic factors and survival

Survival figures from prostate cancer vary widely, depending on histology, stage, PSA level and therapeutic intervention. Patients with localized disease treated with either radiotherapy or radical surgery have 5-year biochemical control rates of 75–85% and 10-year overall survival rates of 60–70%. Patients with metastatic disease can survive for many years, particularly if the tumours are hormone-responsive and if the metastatic spread is confined to the bones.

Cancer of the testes

Introduction

Testicular cancer accounts for 0.7% of all cancers, with fewer than 2000 new diagnoses each year in the UK. There has been an increase in incidence over recent years for reasons unknown. The majority of cases occur in younger men, with around half in men under 35 years of age and 90% in men under 55 years.

Aetiology

Apart from age and race, other risk factors include a previous history of testicular cancer or carcinoma-in-situ. Cryptorchidism (undescended testes at birth) increases the risk by 2–4 fold. There are some reports of increased incidence in men with subfertility and also suggested links with high dietary dairy product intake and a sedentary lifestyle.

Pathology

The majority of testicular malignancies are germ cell tumours (>90%), either seminomas or teratomas. Approximately 20% are of mixed cell type and should be classified as non-seminomatous germ cell tumours (NSGCT). Other types include sex cord tumours, lymphomas and sarcomas.

Intratubular germ cell neoplasia has features similar to carcinoma-in-situ, seen in the contralateral testes in 5% of testicular cancer patients. There is a risk of progression to malignancy of 50% at 5 years. This risk can be prevented with radiotherapy (20 Gy in 10 fractions), which will result in infertility, but avoids the need for a second orchidectomy. It is diagnosed by open or needle biopsies and is more likely in young patients with an atrophic contralateral testis.

Presentation

The majority of testicular tumours (75%) present with a painless, firm swelling of the testis. Occasionally patients present with lower back pain due to intra-abdominal or pelvic lymph node spread, or indeed palpable lymphadenopathy, particularly in the left supraclavicular fossa. Other methods of presentation include infertility, gynaecomastia, secondary hydrocoeles or with symptoms due to secondary spread to other organs such as lung or liver.

Investigations and staging

Preoperative investigations should include testicular ultrasound, chest X-ray and tumour markers including alpha-foetoprotein (AFP), beta-human chorionic gonadotrophin (beta-HCG) and lactate dehydrogenase (LDH). One or more tumour marker is raised in 75% of teratomas and 35% of seminomas. If AFP is raised or beta-hCG is >200, then treat as a non-seminomatous germ cell tumour (NSGCT). Tumour markers should be done preoperatively and repeated a minimum of 7 days after orchiectomy.

Postoperative investigations should include a CT scan of the thorax, abdomen and pelvis for full systemic staging. In case of borderline lymph node size (normal <1 cm), a repeat CT scan after 6 weeks is indicated prior to deciding further management; CT of the brain is indicated if there are multiple lung metastases or beta-HCG levels >10,000 IU/L.

Postoperative tumour markers should be repeated (the half-life of the markers is up to 7 days) and are useful in measuring treatment response and monitoring for recurrence. A bone scan is usually only requested if indicated clinically. Sperm storage should be considered, particularly if chemotherapy is planned.

The staging and risk classification of testicular cancer is shown in Tables 12.5 and 12.6.

Management of testicular cancer

Primary management is a radical inguinal orchidectomy and ligation of the spermatic cord at the internal ring which should be performed within one week after diagnosis. In patients with advanced life-threatening testicular cancer, orchiectomy should not delay chemotherapy. In these situations, if clinical picture and markers are diagnostic, treatment with chemotherapy can be started. Organ sparing surgery may be an option in cases of bilateral testicular cancer.

Postoperative management of seminoma (Figure 12.7)

Stage I disease

Around 80% of patients with seminoma present with stage I disease and survival is >99%. There are two risk factors for recurrence: rete testis invasion and tumour size of >4 cm. 5-year relapse rate is 12% with no risk factors, 16% with one factor and 32% with both factors. Current treatment is active surveillance irrespective of risk factors. If surveillance is not an option the active

Table 12.5: TNM staging of testicular cancer

Stage 0	T1sN0M0 – intracellular germ cell neoplasm
Stage IA	pT1N0M0 – tumour limited to testis and epididymis with no LVI or tunica vaginalis invasion (TVI)
Stage IB	pT2–4N0M0 – pT2 – tumour limited to testis and epididymis with LVI or TVI pT3 – invades spermatic cord pT4 – invades scrotum
Stage IIA	Any T, N1 (≤2 cm regional node) M0
Stage IIB	Any T, N2 (>2–5 cm) M0
Stage IIC	Any T, N3 (>5 cm) M0 node
Stage IIIA/B	Any T, any N, M1A (non-regional nodes and/or lung metastasis)
Stage IIIC	Any T, any N, M1b (other visceral metastasis) Mediastinal primary, any N and any M

Table 12.6: International Germ Cell Consensus Classification prognostic criteria for non-seminomatous tumours

Good prognosis	Intermediate prognosis	Poor prognosis
AFP <1000 ng/ml	AFP 1000–10,000 ng/ml	AFP >10,000 ng/ml
β-HCG <5000 iu/l	HCG 5000–50,000 iu/l	HCG >50,000 iu/l
LDH <1.5 times the upper limit of normal (ULN)	LDH 1.5–10 × ULN	LDH >10 × ULN
Testis or retroperitoneal primary	Testis or retroperitoneal primary	Mediastinal primary site
No non-pulmonary visceral metastases	No non-pulmonary visceral metastases	Non-pulmonary visceral metastases

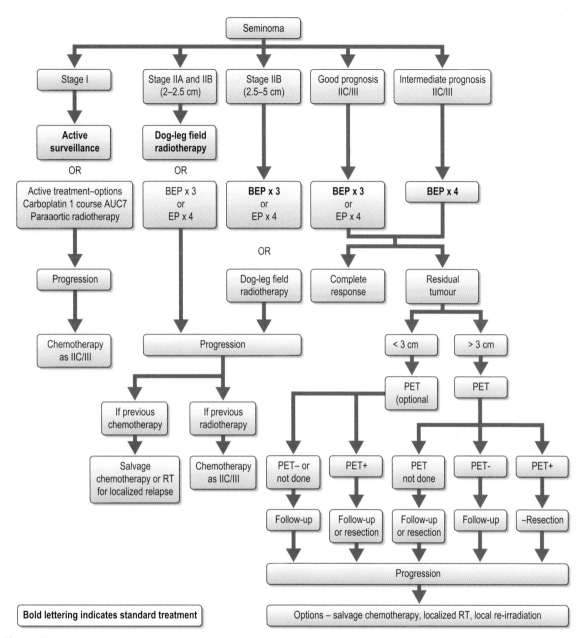

Figure 12.7
Postoperative management of seminoma.

treatment options are a single dose of carboplatin (AUC7) and para-aortic radiotherapy (20 Gy in 10 fractions) (Box 12.9).

Stage II–IV disease
Clinical stage IIA disease should be verified beyond imaging (e.g. needle biopsy) before sys-temic treatment. Standard treatment for stage IA and stage IB with 2–2.5 cm node is radiotherapy to para-aortic and ipsilateral iliac nodes ('dog leg field'). An alternative option is three cycles of PEB chemotherapy (3 or 5-day schedule). Treatment option of stage IIB with 2.5–5 cm node is three courses of PEB (Box 12.8).

Box 12.8: Testicular cancer chemotherapy regime

PEB

3-day schedule

Cisplatin 50 mg/m^2 Days 1–2

Etoposide 165 mg/m^2 Days 1–3

Bleomycin 30 mg on Days 1, 8, 15

5-day schedule

Cisplatin 20 mg/m^2 Days 1–5

Etoposide 100 mg/m^2 Days1–5

Bleomycin 30 mg Days 1, 8, 15

Chemotherapy is repeated 3-weekly independent of leukocyte count but with platelets of >100 × 10^9 on Day 22. Chemotherapy is only delayed if platelet count is not adequate or active infection. Prophylactic G-CSF is used if necessary.

Box 12.9: Radiotherapy in testicular seminoma

Para-aortic strip – field definition (shaded area in Figure 12.8)

- Superior: top of T11 vertebra
- Inferior: bottom of L5 vertebra
- Ipsilateral border (to primary tumour): renal hilum
- Contralateral border (to primary tumour): transverse process of vertebrae

'Dog-leg field – field definition (green line in Figure 12.8)

- Superior: top of T11 vertebra
- Inferior: lower border of ipsilateral acetabulum
- Ipsilateral border (to primary tumour): renal hilum and include iliac nodes
- Contralateral border (to primary tumour): transverse process of vertebrae

Dose

Stage I – 20 Gy in 10 fractions to midplane

Stage II (1–2.5 cm) – 30 Gy in 15 fractions

Stage II (>2.5–5 cm) – 36 Gy in 18 fractions

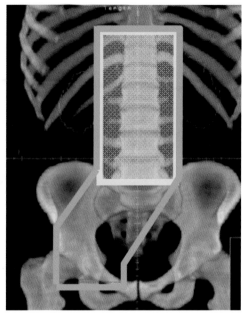

Figure 12.8

Radiotherapy in seminoma. Outline any enlarged lymph nodes on the CT scan and modify the field to ensure that nodes are covered with a 1.5 cm margin.

The treatment of stage IIC/III is three cycles of PEB for good prognosis patients (3 or 5-day schedule) and four cycles for intermediate prognosis patients (5-day schedule). Three cycles of PEB may be substituted by four cycles of PE in cases of increased bleomycin toxicity.

Residual disease and relapse

Management of residual disease is shown in Figure 12.7. In general, patients with >3 cm residual mass need PET scan or frequent follow up or resection.

Patients relapsing after radiotherapy are treated with chemotherapy. Patient who relapse >3 months after initial chemotherapy are platinum sensitive and the standard options are VIP, TIP or VelP. There is no benefit of high dose chemotherapy as second or third line chemotherapy.

Patients who are truly platinum-resistant (relapse during or within 3 months post treatment) have a very poor prognosis (approximately 10% survival) and there is no standard treatment. Gemcitabine/paclitaxel, high dose chemotherapy and surgery if localized disease are the options.

Postoperative management of non-seminomatous germ cell tumours (NSCGTs) (Figure 12.9)

Stage I patients are divided into low (20% relapse rate) and high risk (40–50% relapse) based on absence or presence of vascular invasion. The management is outlined in Figure 12.9. Treatment choice is based on toxicity, tumour burden and patient preference. Active surveillance is intense follow up with frequent clinical examination, tumour marker estimation and scans. Frequency of follow-up depends on risk of relapse.

Management of stage IIA–III disease is outlined in Figure 12.9. It is important that in patients undergoing chemotherapy, dose intensity is maintained (Box 12.8, see also Box 4.3).

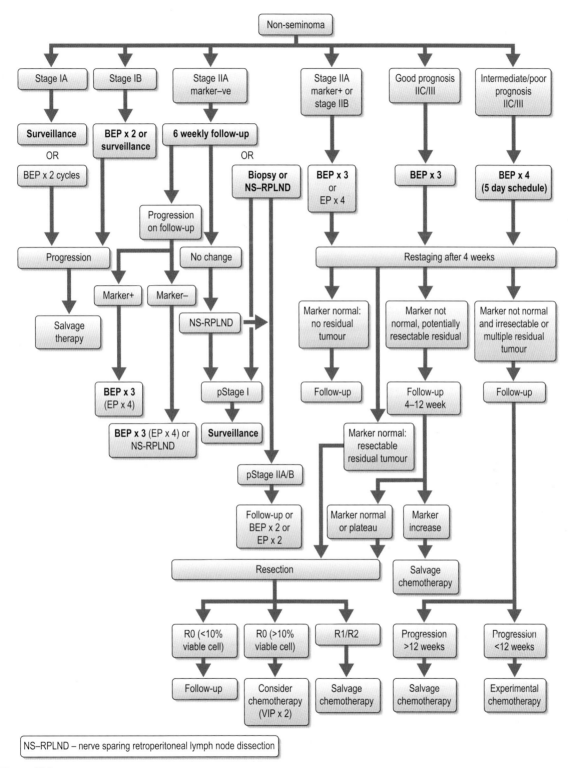

Figure 12.9
Postoperative management of non-seminoma.

Management of residual masses and recurrence

Residual masses >1 cm in size should be resected. Management after resection is based on the extent of resection and proportion of viable tumour cells (Figure 12.9). Chemotherapy for relapse is similar to seminoma.

Management of testicular intraepithelial neoplasia (TIN)

3–5% of patients with testicular cancer have TIN in the contralateral testis with the highest risk if testicular volume <12 ml and age <40 years (34%) and in patients with extragonadal germ cell tumours (≥33%). If untreated, 70% of TIN progress to testicular cancer in 7 years.

Patients should be offered the choice of testicular biopsy or monitoring only (both strategies have excellent survival outcomes). If chemotherapy is given, biopsy should be delayed at least 2 years after treatment. The treatment options in proven TIN include surveillance and active treatment with radiotherapy (20 Gy in 10 fractions) or orchiectomy (in patients with no gonadal tumour, e.g. incidental finding during biopsy for infertility or extragonadal tumour).

Prognostic factors and survival

Seminoma has >90% long-term survival with that of stage I disease at >99%. Stage I non-seminoma has a long-term prognosis of 98–100%. In advanced non-seminoma, survival is 90% for the good prognostic group, 80% for intermediate group and 60% for poor prognostic group.

Follow-up

Follow-up after active treatment involves frequent clinical examination, estimation of tumour markers, chest X-ray and CT-scan up to 5 years. Follow-up beyond 5 years is useful in detecting late toxicities and second cancers.

Cancer of the penis

Introduction

Penile cancers account for less than 1% of all cancers in men, with an annual incidence of 1.5/100,000 in Western Europe. Peak age of occurrence is 60–70 years and they are extremely rare in men under the age of 40.

Aetiology

Risk factors for penile cancer include human papilloma virus (HPV) infection, smoking and previous carcinoma-in-situ. Circumcision is protective.

Pathogenesis and pathology

Pre-malignant conditions include condylomata acuminat, leukoplakia (chronic irritation) and balanitis xerotica obliterans. The following conditions can also progress to cancer:

- Bowen disease (carcinoma-in-situ): solitary, grey plaque with shallow ulceration on the skin of shaft/scrotum. Approximately 10% progress to invasion.
- Erythroplasia of Queryat: single/multiple shiny red plaques on glans/prepuce. Approximately a third progress to invasion.
- Bowenoid papulosis: multiple pigmented plaques (very similar to Bowen's). Rarely becomes malignant.

The vast majority (>90%) of cancers are squamous cell carcinomas (SCC). Verrucous carcinoma is an indolent variant which can present with bulky cauliflower-like lesions. Other rare malignancies of the penis include melanoma, sarcomas (particularly Kaposi's sarcoma), basal cell carcinomas and metastases from bladder, prostate or bowel primary tumours.

Presentation

Penile cancers present as erythematous patches, exophytic growths, nodules or ulcers. There may be associated discharge from the prepuce and/or phimosis. Advanced cases can present with inguino-femoral lymphadenopathy.

Investigations and staging

Diagnosis is made by biopsy of the lesion. Investigations should include a full blood count, urea and electrolytes and liver function. The inguinal, pelvic and abdominal lymph nodes should be assessed with a CT or MRI scan. Clinically enlarged inguinal nodes can be assessed with fine needle aspiration or biopsy. A MRI of the pelvis with an artificial erection may be useful in assessing cavernal invasion (Figure 12.10). A chest X-ray is usually sufficient for distant staging unless there is suspicion of disease else-

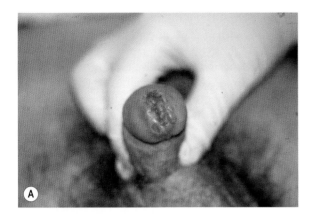

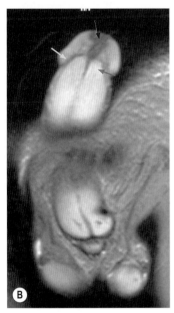

Figure 12.10
Figures show a cancer of the glans penis (A) and an MRI (B) of the pelvis with artificial erection showing a tumour involving the meatus (T3) (red arrow) but without involvement of tunica albuginea (yellow arrow) or corpora cavernosa (green arrow). (Courtesy of Mr. David Ralph, Institute of Urology, London, UK.)

where. It is sensible to photograph the lesion prior to treatment for future reference. The staging of penile cancers is shown in Table 12.7.

Management

Management of the primary tumour

Carcinoma-in-situ

Carcinoma-in-situ can be treated with topical 5-fluorouracil applied twice a day. Patients should be warned to avoid contact with their hands and to abstain from sexual intercourse during the treatment. Alternatively, laser excision can be considered.

Invasive disease

Surgery is the treatment of choice and radiotherapy is an alternative. Amputation with good margins has the best long-term outcome with 90% 5-year survival. Radiotherapy has a 30% long-term failure rate. Circumcision should be performed in all patients, even if treated with radiotherapy.

Surgery

For very small foreskin lesions, circumcision and laser surgery can be curative. For other T1/2 lesions of the glans, a glansectomy or partial amputation may suffice. For larger tumours, particularly if the urethra is involved, total amputation is required.

External beam radiotherapy

If disease is limited to the glans, treatment is with electron-beam radiotherapy with a 2 cm margin around the tumour. Perspex or bolus is placed over the cut-out section to ensure that the skin surface dose is 100%. For more extensive disease, photon irradiation is appropriate. Two lateral fields are applied with the penis placed between two halves of a wax block. The testis and groin are shielded with lead. The conventional dose is 60–64 Gy in 30–32 daily fractions using 4–6 MV photons. If there is residual disease following radiotherapy, surgical excision should be considered as a salvage treatment. Box 12.10 lists the side effects of penile radiotherapy.

Brachytherapy

Patients are circumcised and catheterized before treatment. Brachytherapy is generally only suitable for T1/2N0 tumours of less than 4 cm in size. Two techniques are in use.

- The mould technique employs two Perspex cylinders, the outer of which is loaded with iridium 192 wires. The device is worn for 8–10 hours per day for 1 week, giving a typical dose of 60 Gy.
- The interstitial technique involves insertion of radioactive implants to give 65 Gy to the 85% isodose over 1 week using the Paris system. A 2 mm lead shield is applied to the testes and it is wise to consider stilboestrol

Table 12.7: Staging of penile cancers

Stage		
I	T1 N0	Invasion of sub-epithelial tissue
II	T2 N0	Invasion of corpora or cavernosum
	T1/2 N1	Single superficial inguinal lymph node involvement
III	T3 N0/1	Invasion of urethra/prostate
	T1–3 N2	Multiple or bilateral superficial inguinal nodes
IV	T4 N0–2	Invasion of adjacent structures
	T1–4 N3	Deep inguinal or pelvic nodes involved
	M1	Distant metastases

Box 12.10: Side effects of radiotherapy to the penis

Early	Mucositis
	Oedema of the prepuce
	Local infections
	Dysuria
	Difficulty with micturition
Late	Telangiectasia
	Superficial necrosis
	Urethral meatal stenosis
	Deep fibrosis
	Loss of sexual function

treatment to prevent erections during the week of treatment. Local control rates of up to 90% have been reported for T1 tumours.

Patients who recur after brachytherapy are salvaged with surgery.

Palliative radiotherapy

Palliative treatment with external beam radiotherapy can be considered in unfit patients with locally advanced disease. A typical dosage schedule is 21 Gy in three fractions over a week.

Management of the lymph nodes

Inguinal lymphadenectomy should be considered for patients with enlarged or involved nodes. There is controversy over the need for bilateral dissection, but prophylactic contralateral dissection is appropriate if one side is heavily involved. Prophylactic lymph node dissection in patients without clinically palpable nodes is indicated for patients with T2/3 cancers, when the risk of lymph node involvement is >80%.

In patients with large or fixed nodal disease, preoperative groin radiotherapy (45–50 Gy in 2 Gy daily fractions) or chemotherapy can be considered to downsize the nodes prior to dissection. Radiotherapy is also an option as prophylaxis in clinically node negative patients in place of surgery. Neither surgery nor radiotherapy is curative when there is involvement of the pelvic lymph nodes, and treatment becomes palliative. In these cases it is best to avoid the morbidity of dissecting the groin nodes, but palliative radiotherapy to prevent groin ulceration and leg oedema may be appropriate.

Chemotherapy

There may be a role for primary neoadjuvant chemotherapy in patients with fixed inguinal metastases, approximately 50% of which can be made resectable. Possible chemotherapy regimes include cisplatin and 5-fluorouracil or cisplatin, methotrexate and bleomycin.

Chemotherapy may also be used in fit patients with metastatic disease. There is interest in taxane and platinum combinations.

Prognosis

Nodal status is the major determinant of prognosis. The 5-year disease-free survival rates of patients with N+ and N0 disease are approximately 40% and 80%, respectively.

Further reading

Rini BI, Campbell SC, Escudier B. Renal cell carcinoma. Lancet. 2009;373:1119–1132.

Rini BI. New strategies in kidney cancer: therapeutic advances through understanding the molecular basis of response and resistance. Clin Cancer Res. 2010;16: 1348–1354.

Kaufman DS, Shipley WU, Feldman AS. Bladder cancer. Lancet. 2009;374:239–249.

Damber JE, Aus G. Prostate cancer. Lancet. 2008;371: 1710–1721.

Horwich A, Shipley J, Huddart R. Testicular germ-cell cancer. Lancet. 2006;4;367:754–765.

Pliarchopoulou K, Pectasides D. Late complications of chemotherapy in testicular cancer. Cancer Treat Rev. 2010;36:262–267.

Pagliaro LC, Crook J. Multimodality therapy in penile cancer: when and which treatments? World J Urol. 2009;27:221–225.

Cancers of the female genital system

13

C Parkinson, TV Ajithkumar and HM Hatcher

Epithelial ovarian cancer

Introduction

Epithelial ovarian cancer (EOC) is the sixth most common cancer in women. There are 6,800 new patients per year in the UK and 25,600 per year in the USA. The median age at diagnosis is 61.

Aetiology

Age and family history are the most important risk factors for ovarian cancer. Other risk factors which have been identified are nulliparity, history of infertility, hormone replacement treatment (HRT), early menarche and late menopause, high body mass index (BMI), and endometriosis. Protective factors include multiparity, oral contraceptive use and tubal ligation.

Approximately 5–10% of ovarian cancer are familial, most of which are associated with BRCA1/BRCA2 gene mutations (90%) (p. 48). Women with a BRCA1 mutation have a 40% lifetime risk of ovarian cancer, and those with BRCA2 have an 18% lifetime risk. Women with HNPCC have a 10% lifetime risk of ovarian cancer.

Pathogenesis and pathology

Most EOCs are high grade (G2/3) serous carcinoma (70%) (HGS). p53 mutation is almost universal (97%) in HGS. Downregulation (rather than mutation) of BRCA1 is also thought to be important in the aetiology of non-heriditary HGS. The following are the different types of EOCs:

- Papillary serous tumors (70%) have an appearance resembling the glandular epithe-lium lining the fallopian tube and 70–80% respond to first line chemotherapy.
- Clear cell carcinomas (10%) resemble 'clear cells' of renal cell carcinoma and they have higher rate of recurrence, with a 20–30% response to first line chemotherapy.
- Endometrioid tumours (10%) contain cells resembling the endometrium and 70–80% respond to first line chemotherapy.
- Mucinous tumours (5%) resemble the endocervical epithelium. Mucinous tumours are less chemosensitive to carboplatin and paclitaxel than other histiotypes.
- Mixed carcinomas (5%) have two or more histologic histiotypes comprising at least 10% of the tumour mass.

Within each histiotype, tumours may be classed as benign, malignant, or of low malignant potential (borderline). Low malignant potential tumours are composed of atypical epithelial proliferation without stromal invasion. They present early and have a low likelihood of recurrence, and are therefore treated with surgery alone.

Primary peritoneal carcinoma or papillary serous carcinoma of the peritoneum is histologically indistinguishable from papillary serous ovarian cancer. Primary peritoneal carcinoma is treated identically to serous papillary ovarian cancer and has similar response rates to chemotherapy.

Pattern of spread

The most common pattern of spread is peritoneal. Lymphatic dissemination to the pelvic and para-aortic nodes occurs in advanced disease. Spread through the diaphragm can lead to pleural

DOI: 10.1016/B978-0-7234-3458-0.00018-X

effusion, although some effusions may be reactive. Haematogenous spread to the liver or lung is unusual (2–3%).

Presentation

Overall 95% of patients diagnosed with ovarian cancer are symptomatic. The most common symptoms are abdominal distension (61%), abdominal bloating (57%) or pain (36%), indigestion (31%), pelvic pain (26%), constipation (24%) and urinary incontinence (24%), back pain (23%) and dyspareunia (17%). Half of patients experience constitutional symptoms (anorexia, weight loss or nausea). The median duration of symptoms is 3–6 months.

Signs

Physical findings are rare in patients with early disease. Patients with advanced disease may present with abdominal distension (ascites or tumour), cachexia, bilateral swollen legs (low albumin, or large pelvic masses) signs of pleural effusion which is more often right sided, and pelvic or abdominal mass.

Investigations and staging

All patients with suspected ovarian cancer should have estimation of serum CA-125 and ultrasound scan of the abdomen +/– transvaginal ultrasound scan. The CA-125 is raised in 50% of patients with stage I disease, and in 90% of stage II–IV. Mucinous tumours often have a normal CA-125. Raised CA-125 is not specific to ovarian cancer. Young patients should also have estimation of germ cell tumour markers (AFP, betaHCG, and LDH).

The risk of malignancy index (RMI) scoring system is used to predict whether a pelvic mass is malignant (Box 13.1). Women with an RMI of >200 should be referred to a specialist centre for further management and surgery. An RMI of >200 has a positive predictive value of 87% and a sensitivity of 88% for diagnosing malignant disease.

To assess operability patients should have a CT of the abdomen and pelvis (Figure 13.1), and a CXR. In patients with a pleural effusion, cytological diagnosis is required to determine if the effusion is malignant.

Patients with ascites without a mass on CT, should have cytological and immunohistochemical analysis, in addition to CA-125, CEA and

Box 13.1: Risk of malignancy index (RMI)	
Feature	RMI score
Ultrasound features:	0 = none
multilocular cyst	1 = one abnormality
solid areas	3 = two or more
bilateral lesions	abnormalities
ascites	
intra-abdominal metastases	
Premenopausal	1
Postmenopausal	3
CA-125	U/ml

RMI score = ultrasound score × menopausal score × CA-125 level in U/ml.

CA19-9 (p. 287). The immunohistochemical profile of an ovarian tumour is typically CK 7 positive and CK 20 negative. A serum CA125:CEA ratio >25 is strongly suggestive of an ovarian rather than a GI primary.

Tissue diagnosis

Patients in whom neo-adjuvant chemotherapy is indicated should have a tissue diagnosis prior to surgery, usually by ultrasound or CT guided biopsy.

Preoperative investigations

In addition to imaging and tumour markers, patients should have full blood count and biochemistry for renal and hepatic function. Patients who may require bowel surgery should be referred to the stoma team for discussion pre-operatively.

Staging

The International Federation of Gynaecology and Obstetrics (FIGO) staging is shown in Box 13.2.

Management (Figure 13.2)

Primary surgery

Surgery involves total abdominal hysterectomy (TAH), bilateral salpingo-oophorectomy (BSO), infra-colic omentectomy, peritoneal washings, biopsy of any lesions or adhesions, blind peritoneal biopsies of the bladder, cul de sac, paracolic gutter, hemidiaphragm and pelvic sidewall and pelvic and para-aortic node sampling. Surgical staging is important to guide treatment with chemotherapy and estimate prognosis.

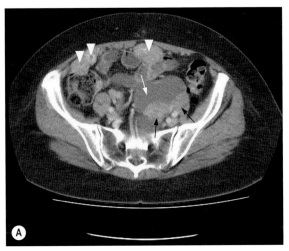 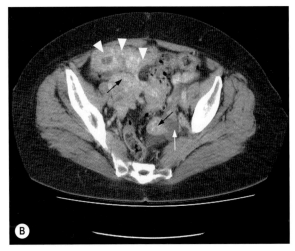

Figure 13.1
A&B, CT scan in ovarian cancer. Contrast enhanced CT in a patient with advanced ovarian cancer demonstrates bilateral solid (black arrows) and cystic (white arrows) adnexal masses and omental cake (white arrow heads). Courtesy of Dr. E Sala, University of Cambridge.

Box 13.2: FIGO staging of ovarian cancer

Stage I – limited to one or both ovaries
IA – involves one ovary; capsule intact; no tumour on ovarian surface; no malignant cells in ascites or peritoneal washings
IB – involves both ovaries; capsule intact; no tumour on ovarian surface; negative washings
IC – tumour limited to ovaries with any of the following: capsule ruptured, tumour on ovarian surface, positive washings

Stage II – pelvic extension or implants
IIA – extension or implants onto uterus or fallopian tube; negative washings
IIB – extension or implants onto other pelvic structures; negative washings
IIC – pelvic extension or implants with positive peritoneal washings

Stage III – microscopic peritoneal implants outside of the pelvis; or limited to the pelvis with extension to the small bowel or omentum
IIIA – microscopic peritoneal metastases beyond pelvis
IIIB – macroscopic peritoneal metastases beyond pelvis less than 2 cm in size
IIIC – peritoneal metastases beyond pelvis >2 cm or lymph node metastases including para-aortic nodes

Stage IV – distant metastases to the liver or outside the peritoneal cavity

---

Early stage disease (stage I and II)

Surgery
Initial management in early stage disease is maximal cytoreductive surgery and surgical staging. Around one-third of patients with apparent stage I–IIA disease will have a higher stage of disease after full staging, mostly stage III (77%). The frequency of lymph node involvement for apparent stage I disease is 20%. There is no evidence that total lymphadenectomy

improves survival. Patients with mucinous tumours should have an appendicectomy, as this may be the site of the primary.

Fertility preserving surgery
In younger patients with stage IA tumours and favourable histology, unilateral salpingo-oophorectomy and staging may be carried out, although data on fertility preserving surgery is limited. Endometrial biopsy should be carried

199

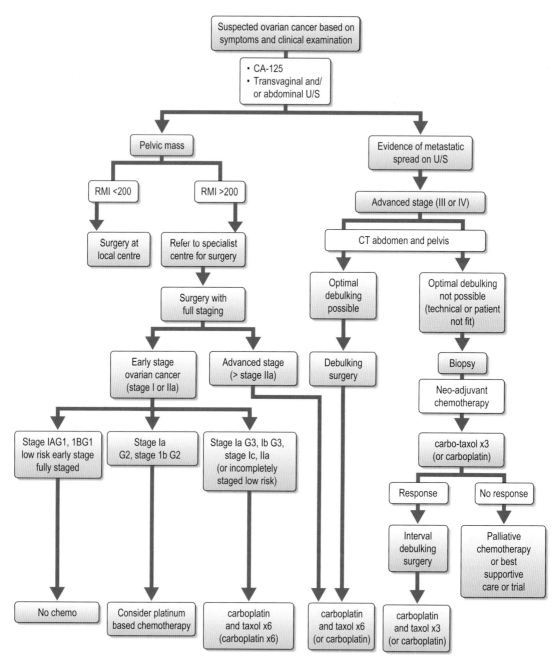

Figure 13.2
Management of ovarian cancer.

out as a synchronous primary is present in 10% of patients. Wedge biopsy of the contralateral ovary should only be taken if it appears abnormal, as the probability of involvement of a macroscopically normal ovary is low (2.5%).

Chemotherapy
For patients with stage IA/B G1 non-clear cell cancer (low risk) 5-year disease free survival is >90% without chemotherapy if optimal surgery has been performed. For patients with high risk

Box 13.3: Chemotherapy regimes in ovarian cancer

First line and platinum sensitive relapse
- Carboplatin
  AUC 5–7 IV; Cycle duration 3 weeks
- Carboplatin + paclitaxel
  Carboplatin AUC 5/6 IV and paclitaxel 175 mg/m^2 IV
  Cycle duration 3 weeks

Second and subsequent lines & platinum resistant relapse
- Caelyx
  40 mg/m^2 every 3–4 weeks
- Topotecan
  1.5 mg/m^2 D1–5 every 4 weeks
- Weekly paclitaxel
  80 mg/m^2 IV

Box 13.4: Thrombosis in ovarian cancer

Patients with ovarian cancer have a relatively high risk of venous thromboembolism. Approximately 5% of ovarian cancer will have either a DVT or PE within in the first 2 years after diagnosis, with 30% of these occurring within the first 3 months. Rates of thrombosis are highest in those with metastatic disease, medical co-morbidities and clear cell histology. Management is with low molecular weight heparin. Vena-caval filters may be considered prior to surgery to prevent pulmonary emboli if the clot extends proximally, is non-resolving, or if the patient develops further emboli despite optimal anticoagulation.

Box 13.5: Stage-wise survival according to surgical cytoreduction at primary surgery

	5-year DFS	5-year OS	Median PFS (months)	Median OS (months)
Microscopic residual	30%	50–60%	29	68
<1 cm residual	10%	30–35%	16	40
>1 cm	5%	20–25%	13	33

features (G3, clear cell, stage IIA disease), 5-year recurrence rates are 25–40% and adjuvant chemotherapy is recommended. In these patients, chemotherapy improves 5-year disease free survival (DFS) by 11% (from 65% to 76%), and 5-year overall survival (OS) by 8% (75% to 82%). Chemotherapy with 6 cycles of carboplatin and paclitaxel is recommended, although 6 cycles of carboplatin is also acceptable (Box 13.3). For stage I G2 tumours the role of chemotherapy is not clear but 6 cycles of carboplatin may be offered.

Advanced stage disease (stage III and IV)

Patients with advanced disease may develop medical complications as a result of their cancer, notably thrombosis which has consequences for further management (Box 13.4).

Surgery

The extent of cytoreductive surgery is the most important prognostic factor after stage. The aim of surgery is to achieve a complete macroscopic debulking, or failing this, an 'optimal debulking'. The definition of 'optimal debulking' is visible residual tumour of <1 cm. Studies have shown that patients with residual >2 cm show no improvement in survival over patients without debulking, and are considered incurable. Outcomes according to cytoreductive surgery are shown in Box 13.5. However, even after a complete response 25–50% will recur later.

Meta-analyses suggest that patients with stage IV disease obtain a survival benefit after optimal debulking surgery. Even in patients with liver metastases, studies indicate an improved survival for those in whom optimal extra-hepatic cytoreduction is achieved (27 vs. 8 months). However, more extensive surgery such as hepatic metastatectomies does not appear to improve the survival of patients. Patients with chemotherapy resistant disease have a poor prognosis, even if optimal extra-hepatic cytoreduction is achieved.

Assessment of operability

Surgery is the primary treatment of choice where a complete debulking is considered possible. Patients with bulky disease or a poor performance status (25%) are treated with neo-adjuvant chemotherapy then reassessed for interval debulking surgery (IDS). Surgery should only be attempted where optimal debulking is possible. In general, debulking is less likely to be successful in patients with bulky upper abdominal disease or fixed tumour. Even if debulking surgery is not possible, palliative bowel surgery may be appropriate to relieve impending or actual bowel obstruction.

Neoadjuvant chemotherapy

A randomized trial (EORTC 55971) has shown that neo-adjuvant chemotherapy has equivalent efficacy with lower morbidity than primary debulking surgery in patients with stage bulky III/IV disease. Neo-adjuvant chemotherapy usually comprises 3 cycles of carboplatin and paclitaxel (or carboplatin alone) followed by interval debulking surgery for patients responding to chemotherapy, then a further three cycles of adjuvant carboplatin and paclitaxel. Approximately 10% of patients will progress on chemotherapy (platinum refractory) and the prognosis for these patients is poor and not improved by surgery. For this group further treatment is with a change of chemotherapy or best supportive care.

Adjuvant chemotherapy

Adjuvant chemotherapy is aimed at improving overall survival. There are no studies comparing best supportive care with chemotherapy. Meta-analyses suggest that adjuvant treatment with platinum compared with non-platinum mono-therapy achieves a 30% relative risk reduction in mortality implying some benefit from platinum based chemotherapy. Four phase III trials have investigated the benefit of adding taxanes to platinum. Two trials (GOG111 and OV10) showed a mean survival benefit of 10–14 months whist other two (ICON3 and GOG132) did not. A meta-analysis of the four trials demonstrates a small survival advantage with the addition of paclitaxel to platinum. Many expert consider the combination of carboplatin and paclitaxel as the standard adjuvant chemotherapy.

The choice between single agent carboplatin and carboplatin with paclitaxel as first line treatment should be made after discussion of the risks and benefits with the patient. Since platinum exerts the major effect, and paclitaxel increases toxicity, single agent carboplatin will be the treatment of choice for patients with poor performance status or co-morbidities.

Intraperitoneal (IP) chemotherapy

A number of studies have investigated intra-peritoneal chemotherapy. Although some have shown a small improvement in PFS and OS (GOG-172), the toxicities were high (p. 38). In the UK, IP chemotherapy is not currently offered outside a clinical trial.

Table 13.1: Prognosis of ovarian cancer

FIGO stage	5-year survival (%)	5-year disease-free survival
I	80–90	70–85
II	65–80	55–65
IIIa	50	45
IIIb	40	25
IIIc	30	20
IV	15	10

Prognosis

Prognosis according to stage is shown in Table 13.1. The most important prognostic variables after stage are in order; degree of differentiation, cyst rupture, substage of disease and age.

Relapse

Despite 70% of patients with advanced disease having a complete clinical response at the end of surgery and chemotherapy (no detectable disease on CT scan and/or normal CA-125), 70% of these will relapse, with a median progression free survival from diagnosis of 16 months. The time from first relapse to death is now around 2 years. There are no studies comparing best supportive care with chemotherapy in relapsed patients, but the recent studies suggest that chemotherapy improves survival.

Presentation of relapse

55–70% of patients present with an asymptomatic rise in CA-125. The median time from this to onset of symptoms is 3 months. 30–45% of patients present with symptoms, of whom 30% relapse in the abdomen, 36% in the pelvis, 14% in abdomen and pelvis, and the remainder have distant metastases (frequently liver metastases).

Relapse may be defined by conventional RECIST criteria (p. 44) or by the gynaecological cancer inter-group (GCIG) CA-125 criteria. CA-125 relapse for those who had elevated pre-treatment value which normalized after first line treatment (60% of all new patients) is defined as ≥2× upper limit of normal on two occasions not less than 1 week apart. Patients in whom CA-125

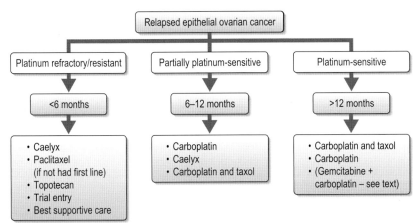

Figure 13.3
Treatment of relapsed ovarian cancer.

was elevated but never normalized (30% of all new patients): relapse is defined as a CA-125 value ≥2× nadir value on two occasions. The definition of relapse in patients with normal CA-125 prior to initial treatment (10% of all new patients) is similar to that of patients with elevated CA-125 which normalized after first line treatment.

Treatment (Figure 13.3)

Chemotherapy for relapsed disease is palliative and aims to prevent or treat symptoms in order to improve quality of life and possibly extend survival. In selected cases with a long disease free interval (exceeding 12 or 18 months) and localized relapse, surgery may be an option and long term disease free survival may be possible.

The probability of response to re-treatment with platinum chemotherapy depends upon the interval between the completion of platinum-based first line therapy to the time of relapse, known as the platinum free interval (PFI). A longer PFI is associated with a higher response rate, longer PFS and improved survival.

Disease relapsing >6 months after platinum treatment is considered 'platinum sensitive', however this group is subdivided into 'relatively' platinum sensitive (PFI 6–12 months) and fully platinum sensitive (PFI >12 months).

Although most of the data about the PFI and its relation to response is taken from first relapse studies, this finding has been extended to second and subsequent relapses. Standard practice is continue re-treating with platinum (or platinum combination) until the patient becomes platinum resistant, regardless of the line of treatment. It

has been suggested that the response rate to platinum can be improved by 'artificially' extending the platinum free interval by using non-platinum agents, but this has not been proven.

Platinum sensitive disease

Patients with a PFI of >18 months show response rates of 60–95% to second line therapy, with a median time to progression of 10–12 months. Those with a PFI of 12–18 months show response rates of 50–60%, and a time to progression of approximately 9 months. Patients with a PFI of 6–12 months show response rates of 25–35% to platinum chemotherapy and a median time to progression of <6 months.

ICON4 showed an improvement in response rate for carboplatin and paclitaxel compared with carboplatin alone (57% vs. 50%), progression free survival (12 months vs. 9 months), and 2-year survival (57% vs. 50%) and median survival (29 vs. 24 months). In relapsed platinum sensitive disease, combination treatment is therefore recommended unless there is significant residual neuropathy. Gemcitabine and carboplatin is sometimes used as combination therapy, as phase III trial results show similar improvements in response rates and progression free survival to carboplatin and paclitaxel.

In patients with a PFI of 6–12 months, the benefits of combination chemotherapy are reduced. Single agent carboplatin is more commonly offered in this group. An alternative that may be considered in this group is peglyated doxorubicin (caelyx), since response rates from non-comparative phase III trials are similar.

Platinum resistant disease

Approximately 25% of patients will progress during, or within 6 months of completion of first line treatment. These patients have a low probability of response to any chemotherapy and should be considered for clinical trials if possible. The response to platinum agents is <10%. The overall median time-to-progression (TTP) is 2–3 months from starting second line treatment. The median OS from time of relapse is 8–10 months, and 2-year survival is 17–21%.

Caelyx, paclitaxel and topotecan are useful; all with response rates are around 6–13%. Rates of stable disease 28–43%, PFS is 2–3 months and OS is 8–10 months. Caelyx is most commonly chosen as the initial treatment because of its favourable toxicity profile. Paclitaxel tends to be used only when patients have not received paclitaxel with 1st line therapy. Recently some centres in the UK have used a weekly carboplatin and paclitaxel regime which has shown favourable response rates. However this regime awaits validation in a prospective RCT. Other agents with activity are oral etoposide, gemcitabine, vinorelbine, ifosfamide and tamoxifen. In this group of patients there is no evidence that combination treatment is superior to single agent.

Hormonal treatment

A proportion of ovarian cancers express the oestrogen receptor (ER) in a percentage of the tumour population. After the use of tamoxifen and aromatase inhibitors in breast cancers, several groups have used these agents in relapsed ER positive ovarian cancers. Compared with breast cancer a lower proportion of tumour cells express ER but the response to aromatase inhibitors has been shown to reflect the percentage of ER positivity. In a phase II study 17% had a response and 26% had stable disease by CA-125 criteria when letrozole was used in patients with significant ER positivity in their tumour at the time of relapse. By RECIST criteria 9% had a PR and 42% achieved stable disease. The responses were greatest amongst those with the highest ER scores.

Future directions

Examples of agents under investigation include anti-angiogenics such as VEGF inhibition with bevacizumab, and PARP inhibitors. Poly (ADP-ribose) polymerase (PARP) is an enzyme involved in the repair of single strand DNA breaks. The involvement of the PARP pathway in ovarian cancer was suggested by the relationship of BRCA positive patients who have an increased incidence of ovarian cancer and a deficiency in homologous repair. In addition 50% of sporadic serous papillary ovarian cancers also have impaired PARP expression. PARP inhibitors have shown some benefit in the prevention of further relapse when used in a maintenance setting after response to chemotherapy.

Palliative care

The most common palliative symptoms in advanced ovarian cancer are ascites, pleural effusion and small bowel obstruction. Permanent ascitic drains can be placed for those with frequent recurrent ascites. The most debilitating symptom is of small bowel obstruction which is frequently recurrent. Treatment of small bowel obstruction consists of minimal oral intake and symptomatic control with anti-emetics (haloperidol or cyclizine), antispasmodics (e.g. buscopan) and steroids (dexamethasone) if not responding to the initial treatment. Pain relief should be added to the syringe driver (e.g. diamorphine). If there is colicky abdominal pain metoclopramide should be avoided as this will exacerbate the symptoms. If secretions remain high, octreotide given via a separate syringe driver can be useful. Intravenous fluids should be given but the use of parenteral nutrition should be reserved for patients with a meaningful chance of treatment to remission, e.g. with bowel obstruction at presentation or at first relapse after a long disease free interval.

Follow-up

Most (approximately 95%) recurrences will occur in the first 3 years and relapse after 5 years is rare. Follow-up is directed at detecting localized relapse which is potentially curable with surgery or radiotherapy, e.g. local vaginal vault relapse. Follow-up should include clinical examination, CA-125 (if elevated at presentation) and intermittent imaging if CA-125 was not informative or with symptoms. A typical follow-up would be 3-monthly for 2–3 years then 6-monthly up to 5 years. Patients with an informative CA-125 can become very focused on their blood result at each appointment so a clear plan of action with a raised CA-125 is recommended as there is no evidence that treatment with an asymptomatic elevated CA-125 improves outcome.

Endometrial cancer

Introduction

Endometrial cancer is the fifth most common female cancer in developed countries. In the UK 6800 new patients are diagnosed every year. The incidence rises steeply to a peak at 64–74, with 75% of cases diagnosed in post-menopausal women. In the UK, women have a lifetime risk of 0.9% of developing endometrial cancer. Endometrial cancer is responsible for 2% of all cancer deaths in women in the UK. Most cases are diagnosed at an early stage and overall 5-year survival is 75%.

Aetiology

Table 13.2 shows the risk factors for endometrial cancer. Less than 5% of endometrial cancers are hereditary, and most of these arise in women with hereditary non-polyposis coli (HNPCC) or Lynch syndrome II (p. 51).

Pathogenesis and pathology

Generally there are two types (type I and II) of endometrial cancer and the characteristics these differ.

Table 13.2: Risk factors for endometrial cancer

Risk factor	Relative risk
Increased age	–
Unopposed oestrogen	2–10
Late menopause (after age 55)	2
Nulliparity	2
Polycystic ovary syndrome	3
Obesity	2–4
Diabetes mellitus	2
Hereditary non-polyposis colorectal cancer	22 to 50% lifetime risk
Tamoxifen	2/1000

- Type I (80%) – related to oestrogen stimulation and associated with obesity, nulliparity, and insulin resistance. Median age at presentation is 59 years. The precursor lesion of endometrioid carcinoma is atypical hyperplasia. These tumours are typically low grade (grade 1/2) endometrioid tumours presenting in early stage and express oestrogen (ER) and progesterone receptors (PR) in 92% of cases. It has an overall survival of 80%.
- Type II (20%) – unrelated to oestrogen stimulation and often occur in elderly thin women. Median age at presentation is 68 years. These tend to be high grade tumours of non-endometrioid histology (including serous, clear cell and high grade endometrial), usually present at a later stage and have a poorer prognosis, with recurrence in 50% of patients. Endometrial intraepithelial carcinoma is proposed as a precursor of serous carcinomas which express ER in 31% of cases and PR in 12%. Clear cell carcinomas do not have a proven precursor lesion and rarely express ER or PR.

Histologic types of endometrial malignancies are as follows:

- Endometrioid carcinomas (75%) – usually low-grade and confined to uterus.
- Uterine serous papillary carcinoma (UPSC – 5–10%) – high-grade, high-risk of metastasis and often presents with extra-uterine disease.
- Clear cell carcinoma (1–5%) – high-grade and high-risk of metastasis.
- Mixed adenocarcinomas (5%) – usually composed of endometrioid and serous papillary carcinoma.
- Mesenchymal tumours include stromal sarcomas, leiomyosarcoma and other types of sarcoma (p. 260, uterine sarcomas). Mixed non-epithelial tumours include carcinosarcomas (previously termed malignant mixed Müllerian tumours).

Presentation

Abnormal vaginal bleeding is the usual presentation. Other presentations include vaginal discharge, pain in advanced disease and symptoms of metastatic disease. Less than 5% are diagnosed incidentally (abnormal smear test).

Diagnosis and staging

Initial investigations

- Trans-vaginal ultrasound scan (TVUSS) is the initial investigation of choice. In the UK, a threshold of 5 mm has been adopted to determine if it is required. Women with an endometrial thickness >5 mm (7–8% probability of endometrial cancer) need further investigation by hysteroscopy.
- Endometrial sampling/hysteroscopy is useful in obtaining histologic confirmation. Pre-menopausal women with significant menstrual abnormality should be investigated by endometrial biopsy with or without hysteroscopy.

Further investigations

Once a diagnosis of endometrial cancer is made, further investigations are indicated to stage and assess fitness for definitive treatment.

- Blood – full blood count, biochemistry and serum CA-125 (raised in extrauterine spread especially in USPC).
- Chest X-ray.
- Magnetic resonance imaging (MRI) (Figure 13.4) – is the imaging of choice to assess the depth of myometrial invasion, and lymph node metastasis.

- CT scan of abdomen and chest is indicated for patients with high risk of distant metastasis such as stages II–IV and histologic types of clear cell, UPSC, and carcinosarcomas.
- PET scan – is not sufficiently sensitive to assess lymph node involvement (60–69%) and therefore at present has no role in the staging of endometrial cancer.
- Examination under anaesthesia (EUA) – when locally advanced tumour is suspected following clinical or radiological examination, EUA is indicated to determine operability.

Staging

The FIGO postoperative surgico-pathological staging system is given in Box 13.6.

Prognostic factors

The most important prognostic factors are stage, age, depth of myometrial invasion >50%, grade 3, serous or clear cell histology and lymphovascular invasion (LVI). Table 13.3 shows the 5-year survival rate according to stage and grade.

Endometrioid cancer presents more commonly with stage I and II (86%) than serous papillary (57%) or clear cell (70%). However, serous papillary and clear cell carcinomas have a poorer prognosis even after their stage at presentation is taken into account (see Table 13.4).

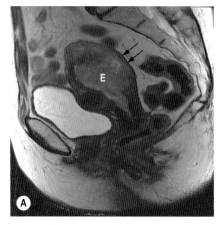
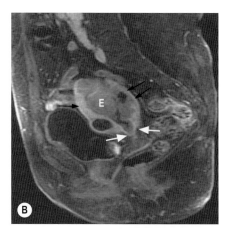

Figure 13.4
MRI in endometrial cancer. Sagittal T2-weighted (A) and sagittal dynamic contrast enhanced T1-weighted (B) images in a patient with stage 1B endometrial carcinoma demonstrate a large endometrial tumour (E) which is invading the outer myometrium (black arrows). The tumour is extending to the endocervix, but the cervical stroma (white arrows) is intact. Courtesy of Dr. E Sala, University of Cambridge.

Box 13.6: FIGO staging of endometrial cancer

Stage I* Tumour confined to the corpus uteri (includes endocervical gland involvement)
IA No or less than half myometrial invasion
IB Invasion equal to or more than half of the myometrium

Stage II Tumour invades cervical stroma, but does not extend beyond the uterus

Stage III Local and/or regional spread of the tumour
IIIA Tumour invades the serosa of the corpus uteri and/or adnexae**
IIIB Vaginal and/or parametrial involvement**
IIIC Metastases to pelvic and/or para-aortic lymph nodes**
IIIC1 Positive pelvic nodes
IIIC2 Positive para-aortic lymph nodes with or without positive pelvic lymph nodes

Stage IV Tumour invades bladder and/or bowel mucosa, and/or distant metastases
IVA Tumour invasion of bladder and/or bowel mucosa
IVB Distant metastases, including intra-abdominal metastases and/or inguinal lymph nodes

*Grade 1–3.
**Positive cytology does not change stage, but reported separately.

Table 13.4: 5-year relative survival rates for endometrial carcinoma according to histology

Stage	5-year relative survival rate (%)		
	Endometrioid	Serous papillary	Clear cell
I	98	74	88
II	86	56	67
III	67	33	48
IV	37	18	18

Table 13.3: 5-year survival rate by stage and grade

	Stage 1A	Stage 1B	Stage 1C	II	III	IV
Grade 1	99	99	99	93	83	60
Grade 2	99	99	95	85	68	45
Grade 3	91	93	77	67	48	17

Treatment (Figure 13.5)

Stage I disease

Surgery

Total abdominal hysterectomy with bilateral salpingo-oophorectomy (TAH-BSO) and peritoneal washings for cytology is the treatment of choice. Vaginal hysterectomy (LAVH) can be considered in some patients.

Controversy exists over the role of staging lymphadenectomy for stage I endometrial cancer. Grade and myometrial invasion are important determinants of lymph node involvement in stage

I cancer. For grade 3 tumours, the risk of lymph node involvement is 15%, and for those with more than ⅔ invasion of the myometrium, the risk is approximately 25%. With both these factors, there is a 34% risk of pelvic node involvement, and a 24% risk of aortic node involvement. North American practice is to perform routine bilateral pelvic lymph node dissection (BPLND) with or without para-aortic lymphadenectomy but there is no clear evidence that lymphadenectomy improves survival. The initial results of the ASTEC trial comparing pelvic lymphadenectomy with no lymphadenectomy in mostly stage I disease showed similar survival and progression free survival with both approach and hence the UK practice is to perform lymph node sampling of clinically suspicious nodes only. The rationale being patients with micrometastases will be identifiable as having a high risk of locoregional relapse and these patients can be stratified to receive radiotherapy. Some UK centres perform lymphadenectomy in stage I patients with a high risk of locoregional relapse, and omitting External beam radiotherapy (EBRT) to those with uninvolved nodes.

Staging lymphadenectomy is useful for better risk stratification of stage I patients with high-risk disease and significant co-morbidity, e.g. inflammatory bowel disease which would increase the risk of radiation related morbidity.

Adjuvant radiotherapy (Box 13.7)
Meta-analyses show that EBRT reduces locoregional recurrence in stage I endometrial cancer by 72% but does not have any benefit on survival. Three quarters of locoregional recurrences are restricted to the vagina, and most of these are

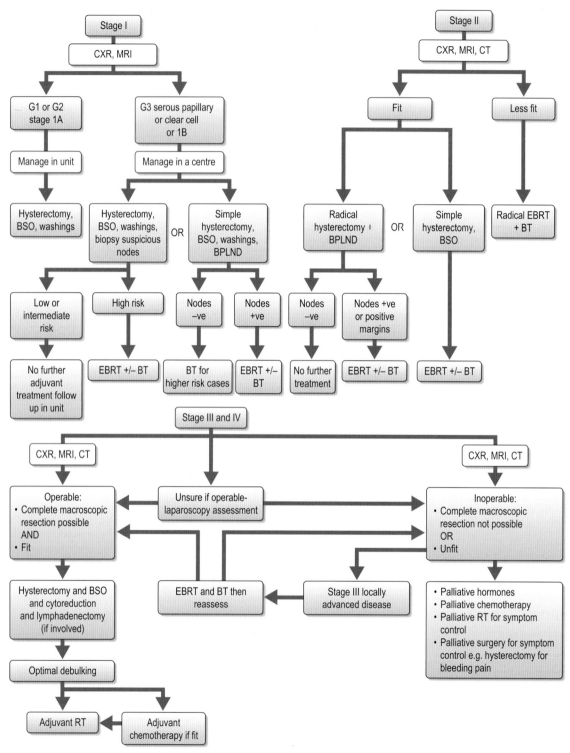

Figure 13.5
Management of endometrial cancer.

Box 13.7: Radiotherapy for endometrial cancer

Indications
- Primary radical radiotherapy (unfit for surgery)
- Postoperative
  - Vaginal brachytherapy (BT) alone
    - Stage IB G2
  - External beam radiotherapy (EBRT) and vaginal brachytherapy
    - Stage I disease – IC/G3/clear cell/UPSC
    - Stage II and above

Technique
Conventional planning
- Superior border: L5/S1
- Inferior border: lower edge of obturator foramen
- Lateral borders: 1 cm beyond pelvic brim
- Anterior: mid-symphysis pubis
- Posterior: 2.5–3 cm anterior to sacral hollow

CT planning
- CTV – vaginal vault and 7 mm margin around the contrast enhancing blood vessels for nodal regions
- PTV – 10–15 mm around vaginal vault, 7 mm around lymph node CTV (10–15 mm for macroscopic disease) and 7 mm around parametrium

Dose
External beam radiotherapy: 45 Gy in 25 fractions

Vaginal brachytherapy
Single modality
HDR   21 Gy in 3 fractions to 0.5 cm from the applicator surface

With EBRT
HDR   7 Gy single fraction to 0.5 cm from the applicator surface

LDR   15 Gy to 0.5 cm

Side effects
EBRT
- Bowel symptoms (22%) – abdominal cramps, urgency and frequency of stool, and diarrhoea
- Bladder toxicity: reduced capacity, urgency, recurrent infections and minor incontinence
- Vaginal narrowing (4%)
- Bone toxicity (1%)

Brachytherapy
Temporary diarrhoea and urinary irritation (9% each), transient vaginal mucositis (17%), vaginal cuff telangiectasia (14%), vaginal atrophy, stricture or adhesions (16%), and dyspareunia (5%).

curable with vaginal radiotherapy. However, it is important to define the risk of loco-regional recurrence to choose patients for adjuvant pelvic radiotherapy is to prevent uncontrolled pelvic disease and to prevent stress and morbidity

associated with a diagnosis and treatment of a relapse. A general consensus is that radiotherapy is considered only if the risk of relapse is >15% (see Box 13.8). Role of adjuvant radiotherapy in patients with intermediate risk remains controversial. In this group, PORTEC-1 identified a subgroup of patients (those aged more than 60 years with 1C or G3 disease) who have an 18% risk of locoregional relapse. The GOG 33 study identified lymphovascular invasion (LVI) as a significant poor prognostic factor for locoregional relapse (HR = 2.4, p = 0.005) Most centres in the UK include LVI as a high risk factor, and would offer patients adjuvant EBRT +/– brachytherapy to patients with 1C or G3 disease if they were either >60 or had LVI, sometimes described as high-intermediate risk. Early results of PORTEC-2 trial suggest that vaginal brachytherapy (BT) alone may be sufficient for this group of patients.

A recent meta-analysis found a 10% statistically significant difference in disease free survival for high risk patients treated with EBRT vs. no treatment (80% vs. 69%). Hence all patients with 1CG3 disease should be offered adjuvant EBRT +/– vaginal brachytherapy.

In the UK, most patients will not have had a staging lymphadenectomy. For those with negative nodes but high risk disease the role of radiotherapy is uncertain. Many would treat patients with 1CG3 disease and >50% myometrial invasion with BT, while some would treat with EBRT +/– BT.

Adjuvant chemotherapy
The high risk of distant relapse for patients with 1CG3 disease suggests a possible role of adjuvant chemotherapy but the evidence is not clear. The incidence of distant metastases is reduced in women receiving chemotherapy compared with pelvic radiotherapy but chemotherapy does not prevent pelvic recurrence. The ongoing PORTEC-3 study randomizes between pelvic radiotherapy or pelvic radiotherapy with concurrent cisplatin followed by carboplatin/paclitaxel chemotherapy.

Stage II

For patients with cervical involvement (clinically or on MRI prior to surgery), a modified radical

Box 13.8: Risk of locoregional relapse

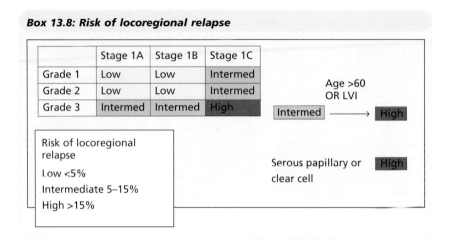

	Stage 1A	Stage 1B	Stage 1C
Grade 1	Low	Low	Intermed
Grade 2	Low	Low	Intermed
Grade 3	Intermed	Intermed	High

Age >60
OR LVI

Intermed → High

Risk of locoregional relapse

Low <5%

Intermediate 5–15%

High >15%

Serous papillary or clear cell   High

hysterectomy with bilateral lymph node dissection is indicated. This involves resection of a parametrial and paracervical tissue, and a cuff of 2 cm of upper vagina. Evidence show that radical hysterectomy results in an improved survival in stage II patients compared to standard hysterectomy (93% vs. 89% at 5 years). For patients with adequate tumour free margins and negative nodes there is no evidence that the addition of radiotherapy improved survival. Those with positive margins or involved nodes should receive adjuvant EBRT and BT.

For some patients, endocervical stromal involvement (stage II) will have been an incidental finding following simple hysterectomy for presumed stage I. These patients would normally receive adjuvant EBRT and BT. In practice, many patients are not fit enough for modified radical hysterectomy and these patients are treated with standard hysterectomy with adjuvant EBRT and BT. There is no proven role for adjuvant chemotherapy for stage II disease yet.

Stage III–IV

The optimal management of patients with advanced stage endometrial cancer is not well defined. Advanced stage endometrial cancers are a heterogeneous group and treatment needs to be individualized.

Surgery

Primary surgery should be considered for all fit patients with stage III disease in whom an optimal cytoreduction appears to be feasible. Several retrospective studies suggest that optimal tumour cytoreduction may improve survival. The definition of optimal cytoreduction varies in different studies from no macroscopic disease to <2 cm. One study found a 5-year survival of 41% in patients with stage III disease had a complete resection of macroscopic tumour compared with 16% for those without. In cases of suspicious operability, a diagnostic laparoscopy should be carried out. In patients with borderline operability, primary radiotherapy may be used to improve chances of subsequent surgery.

Most stage IV tumours will not be considered operable. However, in a subgroup of stage IV patients where complete resection is feasible, a 25% long-term survival can be achieved.

Palliative hysterectomy is useful in controlling local symptoms such as bleeding or pain. Occasionally bowel or urinary diversion may be appropriate, although radiotherapy and/or platinum based chemotherapy may also offer useful palliation.

Radiotherapy (Box 13.7)

Postoperative EBRT and BT should be carried out for patients with a complete macroscopic resection of stage III disease. Patients with stage IIIC disease involving the para-aortic or pelvic nodes may have extended field radiotherapy covering the para-aortic region. The likelihood of local control is related to disease volume. Although radiotherapy reduces the local recurrence rates, there are no data showing improved survival.

> **Box 13.9: Chemotherapy regimes in endometrial cancer**
>
> - Carboplatin (AUC 5–7) IV d1 repeated 3-weekly
> - Paclitaxel (Taxol) 175 mg/m² IV repeated 3-weekly
> - Doxorubicin (Adriamycin) 60 mg/m² IV for 7 cycles + cisplatin (CDDP) 50 mg/m² IV repeated 3-weekly
> - Carboplatin (AUC 5–7) IV d1 + paclitaxel 175 mg/m² IV d1 repeated 3-weekly

Patients with optimal debulking should also be considered for adjuvant chemotherapy based on the results of GOG 122 (see below) followed by radiotherapy for those with a complete clinical response.

For patients with inoperable stage III and IV disease, palliative radiotherapy is an option for local and distant symptom control.

Chemotherapy for Stage III–IV (Box 13.9)

Adjuvant chemotherapy

Adjuvant chemotherapy should be offered to patients with stage III/IV who have had a complete debulking, and may be considered for those with residual tumour <2 cm based on the GOG 122 trial. This phase III trial randomized patients with stage III/IV endometrial cancer, with less than 2 cm of residual disease (87% with no macroscopic disease) to whole abdominal radiation or doxorubicin and cisplatin chemotherapy. Chemotherapy significantly improved progression-free and overall survival compared with WAI. Progression free survival at 5 – years was 50% for those in the chemotherapy arm compared with 38% in the radiotherapy arm, and OS survival was 55% compared with 42% respectively (p < 0.01). Other studies have reported higher pelvic failure rate (40%) in patients with high-risk endometrial cancer treated with adjuvant chemotherapy alone. Hence current practice is to offer adjuvant pelvic radiotherapy in addition to chemotherapy.

Palliative chemotherapy

Patients with unresectable disease may be treated with palliative chemotherapy or hormonal treatment. Generally patients with rapidly progressive or symptomatic disease are treated with chemotherapy, while those with slowly progressing or asymptomatic disease are treated with hormones.

There is limited information available on quality of life or survival data.

The median overall survival for patients with metastatic endometrial cancer following chemotherapy is 6–12 months. The time to progression is generally 4–6 months. The most active single agents in advanced or recurrent endometrial cancer are anthracyclines, platinum and paclitaxel which have similar response rates of 20–35%. The most commonly used combination regimes are carboplatin and paclitaxel and (60–70% response from phase II studies), and cisplatin and Adriamycin (34% response).

Hormonal therapy

It is particularly useful for patients with slowly progressing or asymptomatic disease, and for those unfit for chemotherapy.

Progestogen

Oral progestogen treatment has a response rate of 15–20%. The median duration of response is four months, and survival is approximately 8 to 11 months. Patients with low-grade histology (37% response for G1 compared with 9% for G3), expression of oestrogen (ER) (29% response) and/or progesterone receptors (PR) (39% response) and a long treatment-free interval between initial diagnosis and recurrence have the highest probability of responding. Megestrol acetate is usually given initially at 160 mg daily. Medroxyprogesterone acetate 200–400 mg daily is an alternative. Side effects include weight gain and increased risk of thrombosis. There is no known benefit from using progestogens for adjuvant treatment.

Tamoxifen

Tamoxifen has an overall response rate of 10% and is not generally used as a single agent.

Gonadotrophin-releasing hormone (GnRH) analogues

GnRH analogues may provide benefit in progestogen-refractory advanced or metastatic disease. The response rate is up to 28%. Complete and partial responses to treatment are seen with monthly injections of goserelin acetate 3.6 mg giving a progression free-survival of several months.

Aromatase inhibitors

Reported response rates are approximately 10%. One phase II study reported a disease stabilization rate of 39% for a median of 6.7 months with 2.5 mg letrozole in patients with metastatic or recurrent endometrial cancer.

Recurrent disease

Approximately two-thirds of relapses will either be distant, or locoregional and distant. However the other third will be a pelvic recurrence, of which 75% will be the upper vagina, or 'vaginal vault'.

For patients with a vault recurrence who have not previously received radiotherapy, radical radiotherapy is the treatment of choice (Box 13.8). Those patients who had previously received only BT can have EBRT with a boost if tumour is <0.5 cm. In the PORTEC-1 study 75% of patients with pelvic recurrence could be treated with curative intent and 85% achieved complete remission. The survival rate after relapse was 69% at 3 years in the control group compared with 13% in patients who had received EBRT up-front.

In single recurrence at the vaginal vault, or localized pelvic disease not extending to the sidewall after previous pelvic radiotherapy, surgery may offer a chance of cure. If the bladder and bowels are involved, then a large exenterative procedure may be required for complete resection. The surgical morbidity of exenteration is significant and is suitable only for selected patients, after metastatic disease has been carefully ruled out. Reported 5-year survival is up to of 50% with a complete cytoreduction.

Patients not suitable for salvage surgery or radiotherapy may be treated with systemic therapy.

Special situations

Serous papillary and clear cell carcinoma

Patterns of spread for uterine serous papillary carcinoma (USPC) are similar to epithelial ovarian carcinoma and 50% of recurrences occur in the abdomen alone. Clear cell carcinoma relapses occur more commonly in the pelvis and para-aortic nodes and less commonly in the abdomen than UPSC.

The principles of surgery for both these tumours parallel those for ovarian cancer (p. 198). Optimal therapy of early-stage papillary serous and clear cell carcinomas remains undefined. However the high relapse rates indicate that surgery alone is inadequate. Hence, all women with resected stage IB, IC, and II USPC or clear cell cancers may be offered platinum based chemotherapy (usually with carboplatin and taxol) with postoperative radiotherapy (EBRT+VBT, VBT or EBRT alone) in those with a complete clinical response. Most centres would also offer adjuvant chemotherapy and radiotherapy for stage IA serous papillary carcinoma in which there was any residual disease at hysterectomy following biopsy. Some centres consider whole abdominal radiation for UPSC because of the high rate of abdominal relapse, though the benefit has not been established.

Surgery and chemotherapy for stage III and IV UPSC and clear cell carcinoma is as for ovarian cancer. Radiotherapy is offered to those who have had a complete clinical response.

Synchronous cancers

Synchronous primary cancers of the ovary are found in 5% of patients with endometrial cancer. Management is the combined treatment for each separate cancer. Metastatic disease should be considered where the disease on the ovary is small volume, surface deposits, bilateral with multinodular implants and with lymphovascular invasion of the ovarian cortex.

Follow-up

There is no evidence for best follow-up. The majority of recurrences (80%) occur in the first 18 months to two years. A typical follow up schedule would be outpatient appointments three-monthly for two years, followed by six-monthly to 5-years with full history and physical examination (including pelvic) examination.

Cervical cancer

Introduction and aetiology

Cervical cancer affects 520,000 women each year worldwide. In the UK around 2900 women are diagnosed with cervical cancer per year which represents 2% of female cancer. It is the second most common cancer in women under 35 (after breast cancer). In the UK, the life time risk of developing risk of cervical cancer is 1 in 116.

There are a number of risk factors implicated in the development of cervical cancer such as sexual activity under the age of 20, smoking, immunosuppression, and infection with sexually transmitted diseases. Human papilloma virus (HPV) has emerged as the principal causative agent in the majority of cases of cervical cancer. The most frequent subtypes are 16 or 18.

Pathogenesis and pathology

Most cervical carcinomas arise at the squamo-columnar junction of the ectocervix and endocervix. There is a progression from dysplastic lesions to invasive carcinoma. Dysplastic lesions undergo spontaneous regression in 25–38%, persist in 50–60% and progress to invasive cancers in 2–14%.

Squamous cell and adenocarcinomas account for 90–95% of the cervical cancers. Other histo-logic types are shown in Box 13.10.

Patterns of spread

From the cervix, the tumour may extend locally to the lower uterine segment, vagina, or into the paracervical spaces. It may become fixed to the pelvic wall by direct extension or due to regional adenopathy.

Cervical cancer follows a pattern of metastatic progression, initially to nodes in the pelvis and then para aortic nodes and distant sites. The most frequent sites of distant recurrence are lung, extra pelvic nodes, liver, and bone.

Presentation

Early invasive disease may be asymptomatic. The earliest symptom of invasive cervical cancer is usually abnormal vaginal bleeding, often post-coital. Pelvic pain may result from loco-regionally invasive disease. The triad of sciatic pain, leg

---

Box 13.10: Histopathologic subtypes of cervical cancer

- Squamous carcinoma: keratinizing, non-keratinizing and verrucous
- Endometrioid adenocarcinoma
- Clear cell adenocarcinoma
- Adenosquamous carcinoma
- Adenoid cystic carcinoma
- Small cell carcinoma
- Undifferentiated carcinoma

---

oedema, and hydronephrosis is associated with extensive pelvic wall involvement. Patients with advanced disease may present with haematuria or symptoms of a vesicovaginal fistula. Cachexia, cough, jaundice, and a left supraclavicular nodal mass may occur with distant metastases.

Evaluation and staging

Pretreatment evaluation

- Examination under anaesthesia (EUA).
- FBC, and biochemistry to exclude anaemia and renal impairment.
- Biopsy for histological diagnosis.
- Chest X-ray.
- MRI pelvis (Figure 13.6) is useful in assessing tumour extent and nodal status.
- Cystoscopy/sigmoidoscopy/barium enema/IVU – if there is clinical suspicion of bladder, rectal or ureteric involvement.
- PET/CT has a role in accurate selection of patients for surgery as well as for treatment planning.
- CT scan chest, abdomen and pelvis are indicated in patient with clinically apparent stage IV disease.

Staging

The FIGO staging is given in Table 13.5 which does not take into consideration the findings on imaging.

Management (Figure 13.7)

Choice of treatment is based on tumour size, stage, histology, evidence of lymph node involvement, risk factors for complications of surgery or radiotherapy, and patient preference.

In situ disease (CIN III) can be treated by a number of methods (such as cone biopsy, laser therapy etc.) depending on the extent of disease, age of the patient, and requirement for fertility preservation.

Stage IA disease

Stage IA1
IA1 without lymphovascular invasion (LVI) the treatment options are:

- Cone biopsy or large loop excision of the transformation zone (LLETZ) if patient wishes to preserve fertility.
- Simple hysterectomy.

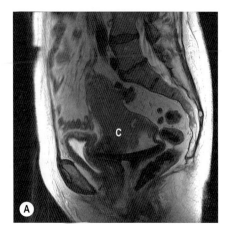
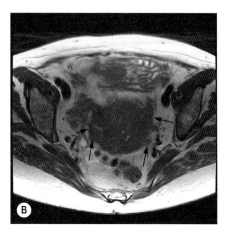
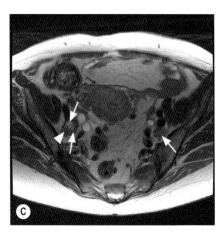

Figure 13.6
MRI scan in cervical cancer. Sagittal (A) and axial (B&C) T2-weighed MRI in a patient with stage 2B squamous cervical cancer demonstrate a large cervical tumour (C) with bilateral parametrial invasion (black arrows) and bilateral enlarged external iliac lymph nodes (white arrows). Note the presence of cystic/necrotic changes within the right external iliac node (white arrow head) which is a common feature of squamous cell cervical cancer. Courtesy of Dr. E Sala, University of Cambridge.

IA1 with LVI is managed with:

- Modified radical hysterectomy with pelvic node dissection or
- Radical trachelectomy with laparoscopic pelvic node dissection if fertility is desired.

Stage IA2
The treatment options are:
- Radical hysterectomy (type II) with pelvic node dissection (3–10% risk of node involvement).
- Radical trachelectomy with laparoscopic pelvic node dissection (if tumour <2 cm and no LVI) if fertility preservation is intended. The 5-year cumulative pregnancy rate was 52.8% with low cancer recurrence rate with this approach.

- Radiotherapy – brachytherapy alone (75–80 Gy equivalent to point A – Box 13.11) or with external beam pelvic in women who are not fit for surgery.

Stage IB and IIA
Similar cure rates are obtained with surgery or radiotherapy for stage IB squamous carcinoma (SCC) of the cervix. The choice between treatments depends upon the age of the patient, desire to preserve ovarian function, co-morbid conditions, and patient choice.

Stage IB1 and IIA1 (<4 cm tumour)
The treatment options are between radical hysterectomy with bilateral pelvic node dissection or radical radiotherapy.

Table 13.5: FIGO cervical cancer staging

Stage I confined to the cervix (extension to the corpus disregarded)

IA Invasive carcinoma diagnosed only by microscopy
IA1 Stromal invasion of ≤3.0 mm in depth and extension of ≤7.0 mm
IA2 stromal invasion of >3.0 mm and not >5.0 mm with an extension of not >7.0 mm
IB Clinically visible lesions limited to the cervix uteri or pre-clinical cancers greater than stage IA
IB1 Clinically visible lesion ≤4.0 cm in greatest dimension
IB2 Clinically visible lesion >4.0 cm in greatest dimension

Stage II Cervical carcinoma invades beyond the uterus, but not to the pelvic wall or to the lower third of the vagina

IIA Without parametrial invasion
IIA1 Clinically visible lesion ≤4.0 cm in greatest dimension
IIA2 Clinically visible lesion >4 cm in greatest dimension
IIB Parametrial invasion

Stage III

IIIA Tumor involves lower third of the vagina, with no extension to the pelvic wall
IIIB Extension to the pelvic wall and/or hydronephrosis or non-functioning kidney

Stage IV extended beyond the true pelvis or has involved (biopsy proven) the mucosa of the bladder or rectum

IVA Spread of the growth to adjacent organs
IVB Spread to distant organs

Surgery involves removal of the uterus, upper third of vagina, bilateral parametria, uterosacral, utero-vesical ligaments and bilateral pelvic lymph nodes. Para-aortic lymph node sampling is indicated if there is clinical suspicion of nodal involvement to plan radiotherapy fields. Radiotherapy is with external beam pelvic irradiation combined with intracavitary applications, which deliver a dose of equivalent to 80–85 Gy to point A (Box 13.11).

Patients with more than two involved pelvic nodes are usually offered postoperative radiotherapy.

Stage IB2 and IIA2 (>4 cm tumour)
The treatment options include:

- Radical hysterectomy and bilateral pelvic lymphadenectomy +/– adjuvant therapy as indicated.
- Concurrent chemoradiation (weekly cisplatin) – deliver 85–90 Gy to point A.
- Radical radiation therapy (when cisplatin is not suitable PS >2 and GFR <50 ml/min) (Box 13.11).

Adjuvant treatment
Adjuvant chemoradiation (EBRT with concurrent weekly cisplatin) is recommended after radical surgery if there are any risk factors such as positive nodes, positive parametria, or close (≤5 mm) or positive surgical margins. Adjuvant concurrent chemoradiation (using 5FU + cisplatin or cisplatin alone) improves survival compared with pelvic irradiation alone in these patients.

Patients with any two of the three factors of deep invasion of cervical stroma, lympho-vascular space invasion, or tumour size >4 cm are classified as intermediate risk. In these patients, adjuvant whole pelvic irradiation reduces the local failure rate and improves progression-free survival.

Concurrent chemoradiation
A recent meta-analysis of 2491 patients in 24 trials suggests that addition of concurrent chemotherapy to radical radiotherapy improves disease-free survival by an absolute 10% and overall survival by 13%. Hence concurrent chemoradiotherapy is the standard of care in patients who have no contraindications for cisplatin.

Stage IIB–IIIB
Concurrent chemoradiotherapy (weekly cisplatin during EBRT) is the treatment of choice. Using a combination of EBRT and brachytherapy a dose of 85–90 Gy to point A and 55–60 Gy to point B is given. Patients with common iliac nodes and para-aortic nodes are treated with extended field radiotherapy.

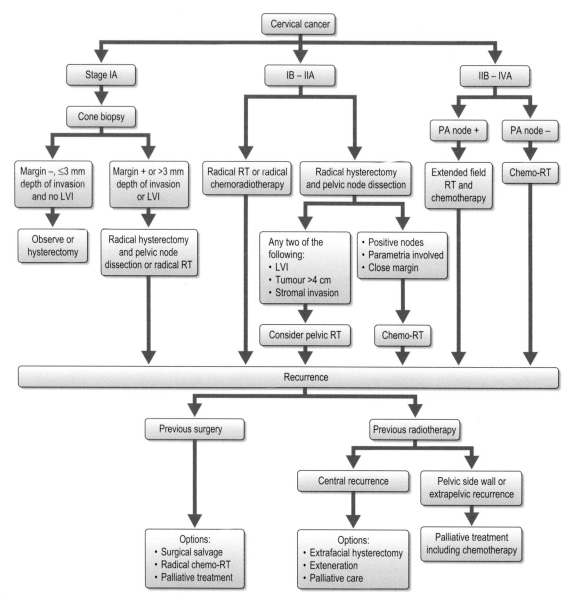

Figure 13.7
Management of cervical cancer.

Stage IV

Stage IVA

The management of patients with stage IVA disease (invasion of bladder and/or rectum) has to be individualized. The treatment options include:

1. Neo-adjuvant chemotherapy or concurrent chemoradiotherapy.
2. Pelvic exenteration.
3. Palliative radiotherapy or chemotherapy.
4. Best supportive care.

   A radical approach with neo-adjuvant chemotherapy or concurrent chemoradiotherapy is suitable for selected patients with good general and renal status and not suitable for surgical exenteration. Surgical exenteration is suitable for selected stage IV patients.

Box 13.11: Radiotherapy in cervical cancer

Principles of cervical cancer radiotherapy

Radical radiotherapy is aimed to delivery 80–90 Gy to point A and 50–60 Gy to point B using a combination of external beam radiotherapy (EBRT) and brachytherapy. Point A in anatomical terms is the point of crossing of uterine artery and ureters and for dosimetry, it is a point 2 cm from central line and 2 cm above ovoids. Point B is 3 cm lateral to point A and receives 20% dose of point A dose from intracavitary radiotherapy.

The maximum tolerated dose of pelvic EBRT is 50 Gy in 1.8–2 Gy per fraction. The rest of radiotherapy is delivered using brachytherapy. The total dose is based on conventional radium treatment over using a dose rate of 0.5 Gy/hour. When medium dose rate (MDR) of >1.5 Gy/hour is used, a 10% reduction of conventional dose is made to account for the reduced treatment time. With high dose rate (1.5 Gy/minute), this reduction is 40–45% from conventional dose.

Indications
Postoperative
- Parametrial involvement
- Positive nodes
- Close or positive margin

Radical radiotherapy
- Stage IB2–IIA
- Stage IIB–IVA
- Isolated pelvic recurrence after previous surgery

Target volume definition
Conventional
- Superior – top of L5 (to cover common iliac nodes)
- Inferior – lower border of obturator foramen/3 cm below inferior aspect of disease (IIIA disease)
- Lateral – 1 cm beyond pelvic brim
- Anterior – mid-symphysis pubis
- Posterior – 2 cm anterior to sacral hollow (1.5–2 cm behind primary disease on MRI)

CT planning (Figure 13.8 A&B)
- GTV – primary tumour and enlarged lymph nodes
- CTV – primary tumour, uterus, cervix, upper vagina, ovaries, parametria, proximal uterosacral ligament + lymph nodes (marked as 7–10 mm margin around blood vessels)
- PTV – 10–15 mm margin around all CTV except for nodal regions and parametria where a 7 mm margin around CTV is used

Dose

Stage	EBRT	Brachytherapy (Figure 13.8 C&D)	
		LDR	HDR
Tumour <4 cm (1B1)	45 Gy in 25	30 Gy to point A	21 Gy in 3 # to point A
IB2, II, IIIB, IVA and pelvic nodal disease	50.4 Gy in 28#**	27 Gy to point A	14 Gy in 2 # to point A
IIIA	50.4 Gy in 28#**	Brachytherapy using line source and dose same as other stages	
Postoperative	45 Gy in 25#		7 Gy in 1# to 0.5 cm depth
Para-aortic node	45 Gy in 25#		

**Given with cisplatin 40 mg/m² (maximum 70 mg) weekly for 5 weeks; # - fractions

When brachytherapy is not possible, additional EBRT (16–20 Gy in 8–10#) may be considered.

Parametrial boost – may be considered in patients with distal parametrial disease at the time of brachytherapy and some centres routines consider this for bulky parametrial disease. A parallel opposed field is used to deliver 6–10 Gy in 3–5 fractions. The medial edge of the half-beam blocked parametrial boost field is placed at the 70–80% brachytherapy isodose.

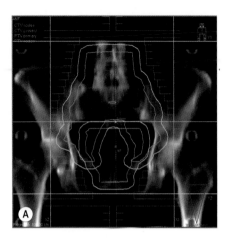

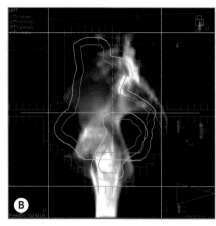

Figure 13.8
A,B – Treatment volumes for external beam radiotherapy in cervical cancer C,D – Brachytherapy dose distribution and dosimetric points (AR – right side point A, AL – left side point A, BR – right side point B, BL – left side point B, ICRU bladder – bladder point and ICRU rectum – rectal point).

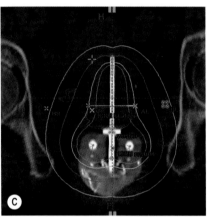

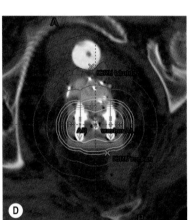

The majority of stage IVA patients are of poor performance status or with many co-morbidities and extensive local disease, and are best treated with palliative treatment (radiotherapy or chemotherapy). Patients with poor general health, or extensive local disease can be offered best supportive care.

Stage IVB
No standard chemotherapy regimen is proven in patients with stage IVB cervical cancer. Radiation therapy can be used for palliation of central disease or symptomatic distant metastasis. The role of systemic therapy is discussed later.

Recurrence

Treatment decisions should be based on the performance status of the patient, the site and extent of recurrence and/or metastases, and prior treatment.

Recurrence after primary surgery

Relapse in the pelvis following primary surgery may be treated by radiotherapy or pelvic exenteration. Radical radiotherapy (+/− concurrent chemotherapy) may cure a substantial proportion of those with isolated pelvic failure after primary surgery. Radiation dose and volume should be tailored to the extent of disease. Where disease is metastatic or recurrent in the pelvis after failure of primary therapy and not curable, a trial of cisplatin chemotherapy with palliative intent or symptomatic care may be considered. The expected median time to progression or death is three to seven months.

Recurrence after primary radiotherapy

Selected patients may be considered for pelvic exenteration, which is the only potentially curative treatment after primary irradiation. Those with resectable central recurrences that involve the bladder and/or rectum without evidence of intraperitoneal or extra pelvic spread and who have a dissectable tumour-free plane along the pelvic sidewall are potentially suitable. Surgery should be undertaken only in centres with appropriate facilities and expertise. The prognosis is better for patients with a disease-free interval greater than six months, a recurrence 3 cm or less in diameter, and no sidewall fixation. The 5-year survival for patients selected for treatment with pelvic exenteration is between 30–60% and the operative mortality should be <10%.

Role of chemotherapy in distant metastasis and recurrent metastatic disease

Chemotherapy has a palliative role after failure of surgery or radiotherapy. There are a number of agents with activity in metastatic or recurrent cervical cancer. Cisplatin is the most active agent, with a response rate of 20–30% and a median survival of 7 months. Recent studies suggest that cisplatin in combination with paclitaxel or topotecan is superior than cisplatin alone.

Prognosis

Stage is the single most important prognostic factor for local control and overall survival. Survival rate after radical hysterectomy for stage IB disease, is around 85–95% for node negative and 45–55% for node positive disease. Survival rates for patients with para-aortic nodal disease treated with extended-field radiotherapy vary between 10% and 50% depending on the extent of pelvic disease and para-aortic lymph node involvement. Other factors associated with a poor prognosis are LVSI, deep stromal invasion (10 mm or more, or more than 70% invasion) and parametrial extension. Stage-wise 5-year survival is as follows:

- Stage I A – 95–97%.
- Stage I B1 – 89%.
- Stage IB2 – 76%.
- Stage IIA – 73%.
- Stage IIB – 66%.
- Stage III – 40%.
- Stage IVA – 22%.
- Stage IVB – 9%.

Treatment toxicities

Significant surgical complications are uretero-vaginal fistula (<2%) and vesicovaginal fistula (<1%). The risk of complications increases with addition of radiotherapy. Extensive pelvic fibrosis can lead to ureteric obstruction and small bowel obstruction.

The late sequelae following radiation therapy commonly affect the rectum, bladder and small bowel. These depend on the duration of follow-up, type of treatment modalities and estimated radiation doses to these organs. The reported grade III/IV late sequelae range from 5–15%.

Palliative care

Palliative care issues include pelvic pain, bleeding, bone pain from metastases and systemic symptoms for advanced cancer.

Follow-up

Optimal follow-up strategy has not been established. A general guideline is for clinical evaluation three monthly for one year, four-monthly for one year, 6-monthly for three years and then annually. Patients are advised to have annual chest X-ray. Other investigations are dictated by clinical indications.

Screening

The main goal of screening is to reduce the incidence and mortality. Screening has been shown to be an effective method of identifying pre-neoplastic disease and reducing mortality. Cervical Cytology (Pap Smear) Screening programs have been found to be successful in reducing cervical cancer incidence. In the UK, women aged 25 years receive the first invitation for screening, those aged 25–49 years have 3 yearly screening, those aged 50–64 years have 5-yearly and those above 65 years have screening test only if they have not had screening since 50 years or have had a recent abnormal test.

Prevention

HPV vaccines have been shown to reduce the number of further pre-invasive lesions and invasive disease in young women with pre-invasive lesions. In the UK, there is a national programme to vaccinate girls aged 12–13 against HPV.

Ovarian germ cell tumours

Introduction and aetiology

Ovarian germ cell tumours (GCTs) have a peak incidence at 15–19 years, due equally to dysgerminoma and teratoma, and a second at age 65–69 mainly due to teratoma. They account for less than 5% of all ovarian malignancies in Western countries, and up to 15% of ovarian cancers in Asian and black patients.

The cause is unknown. Less than 5% are associated with dysgenetic ovaries (unlike their testicular counterparts). The oral contraceptive pill does not confer a protective effect in germ cell tumours as it does in the epithelial ovarian cancers.

Pathology

GCTs are classified as dysgerminomas or non-dysgerminomas based on their origin in primordial germ cells and their ability to differentiate in vivo. Dysgerminomas are the ovarian counterpart of seminomas, whereas the non-dysgerminomatous tumours include all other germ cell tumours and encompass a wide range of differentiated cell types.

- Dysgerminoma – is the most common (30–40%) malignant germ cell tumour. It has the highest rate of bilaterality (10–15%) and is the commonest (20–30%) malignant GCT associated with pregnancy.
- Non-dysgerminoma – composed of immature teratoma, endodermal sinus tumours (yolk sac carcinoma), embryonal carcinoma, non-gestational choriocarcinoma, polyembryoma and mixed germ cell tumour.
  - Immature teratoma (20%) – is sometimes associated with miliary peritoneal implants composed exclusively of mature glial tissue (called gliomatosis peritonei).
  - Endodermal sinus tumour or EST (also called yolk sac tumour – YST) (20%). It usually presents as stage I disease, but rapidly growing with more than 50% of the patients reporting symptoms of less than one-week duration. These tumours invariably express alpha-fetoprotein (AFP). Intraperitoneal spread predominates in this tumour.
- Embryonal carcinoma (3%) – is often associated (60%) with abnormal hormonal manifestations of precocious puberty, irregular bleeding, amenorrhea, or hirsutism due to β-hCG stimulation. It can produce both AFP and β-hCG.
- Mixed germ cell tumours (7%) are composed of at least two different germ cell elements of which at least one is primitive. The most frequent combination is dysgerminoma and EST followed by dysgerminoma and immature teratoma.

Clinical features

Abdominal pain (87%) is the most frequent symptom followed by abdominal mass (85%), but 10% may present with acute abdomen due to torsion, haemorrhage or rupture of the ovarian tumour. Abdominal distension, fever and vaginal bleeding each occur in 10%. Ascites is present in 20% of cases.

Patterns of spread

Spread of tumour occurs by peritoneal, lymphatic and haematogenous routes. Lymphatic spread is predominant in dysgerminoma whereas other modes of spread are equally important in non-dysgerminomas.

Investigations and staging

Initial investigations include estimation of serum tumour markers and imaging.

Tumour markers

Estimation of the tumour markers preoperatively, postoperatively and during follow-up is helpful in predicting the diagnosis, response to the treatment and recurrence respectively.

The two specific markers for GCTs are beta-human chorionic gonadotrophin (β-hCG) and alpha-feto protein (AFP). Up to five percent patients with dysgerminoma can have an elevated β-hCG, which gives rise to a positive pregnancy test in 3% of patients. An elevated AFP or a β-hCG level of >100 IU/L indicates the presence of nondysgerminomatous elements.

Most endodermal sinus tumours secrete AFP. Embryonal carcinomas can secrete both AFP and β-hCG whereas tumour markers are negative in pure immature teratomas.

Other markers include lactate dehydrogenase (LDH) levels in dysgerminomas (88% have raised serum LDH isoenzyme-10) and placental alkaline phosphatase (PLAP) – raised in >95% of dysgerminomas. More than 50% of GCTs express CA-125 but its role in clinical management not known.

Imaging

Dysgerminomas and non-dysgerminomas exhibit different radiological features. On CT (Figure 13.9) and MRI dysgerminoma shows multiloculated solid mass divided by fibrovascular septa. There can be associated abdominal lymphadenopathy. Calcification is rare in dysgerminoma but when present it appears as a speckled pattern.

Non-dysgerminomas are usually unilateral mixed solid and cystic mass. On CT and MRI, there may be a heterogeneous enhancement due to haemorrhage or necrosis. Calcification occurs in up to 40% of the cases.

There are so far no studies examining the role of PET scans in ovarian GCTs, however, in future, it may have the similar clinical application as that of testicular germ cell tumours.

Staging

The GCTs are staged according to the FIGO staging (Box 13.2). 60–70% of GCTs are stage I, 25–30% in stage III and stage II and IV are rare. Distant metastases occur in long standing, recurrent disease or poorly differentiated tumours.

Management *(Figure 13.10)*

Germ cell tumours are potentially curable malignancies with platinum-based chemotherapy.

Surgery

Primary surgery
Principles of surgery follow that of the epithelial ovarian cancer. However, since this disease predominantly affects the young females, conservative surgery to preserve fertility is preferred and the minimal surgery is unilateral oophorectomy. Even in advanced stage (20–30%), the contralateral ovary, fallopian tube and uterus may be left in situ to preserve fertility, and postoperative chemotherapy is given. Although the role of maximal cytoreduction is less defined than for epithelial ovarian cancer, all obvious metastases should be debulked or removed if possible. Even if BSO is necessary, the uterus can be left behind for future assisted reproduction. Routine biopsy of a normal looking contralateral ovary is not advised due to the risk of infertility from peritoneal adhesion or ovarian failure. The role of routine lymphadenectomy is yet to be established.

Secondary cytoreduction and second look laparotomy
A small study suggests that there may be a possible role for secondary debulking in chemo-refractory patients with immature teratoma. Routine second-look surgery is not recommended because of the low incidence of positivity after combination chemotherapy. However, a second-look procedure may be recommended for the subset of patients with a teratoma component in the primary tumour and persistent radiologic abnormalities along with normal serum tumour markers at the end of chemotherapy.

Postoperative management

Dysgerminoma
Adequately staged FIGO IA dysgerminoma has long-term survival of more than 90%, and these patients are observed without any postoperative treatment. The recurrences (rate of 15–25%) in these patients can be effectively salvaged with chemotherapy. All other patients need adjuvant

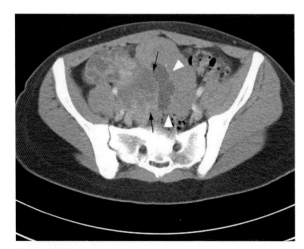

Figure 13.9
Dysgerminoma of the ovary. Contrast-enhanced CT scan shows a large, multilobulated solid mass with highly enhancing fibrovascular septa (arrows) and cystic change (arrowheads).

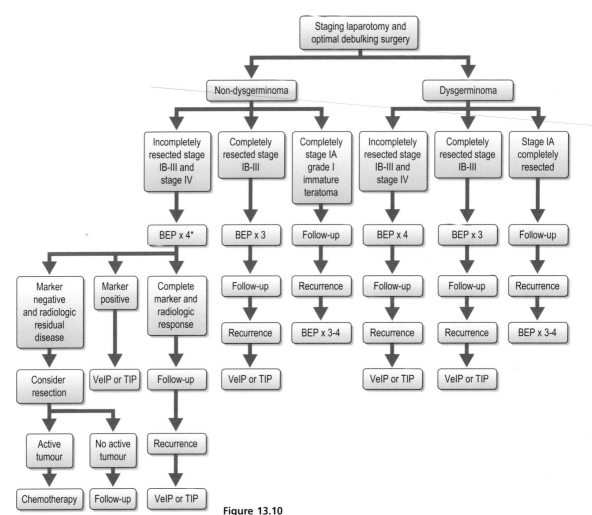

Figure 13.10
Management of malignant ovarian germ cell tumours.

* If adequate marker response may continue up to 5–6 courses

treatment after maximal debulking with or without fertility preservation.

Completely resected stage IB–III and those without staging laparotomy are treated with three courses of standard chemotherapy with BEP regime (Box 13.12). Disease-free survival of completely resected dysgerminoma is very high, approaching 100% and that of advanced disease is in the range of 60–80%. Incompletely resected stage II–IV are treated with 3–4 courses of BEP.

Rarely, radiotherapy may be an option for women with other co-morbid conditions preventing chemotherapy administration or those who decline chemotherapy. Whole abdominal radiotherapy is used which leads to loss of fertility.

Non-dysgerminoma

Surgery alone is adequate for properly staged FIGO Stage IA grade I immature teratoma, which has 80–85% long-term disease-free-survival. All other groups of patients with non-dysgerminoma should receive postoperative chemotherapy.

The optimal number of courses of chemotherapy for GCT is unclear, unlike testicular tumours. One GOG study had shown that three courses of BEP will nearly always prevent recurrence in well-staged patients with completely resected ovarian germ cell tumours. However, those with a raised tumour marker but with no measurable disease should receive two more courses of chemotherapy after normalization of serum markers and those with bulky residual tumour may need 5–6 courses.

The role of carboplatin in place of cisplatin is undergoing clinical trials.

Recurrence

The role of surgery in the management of recurrence has yet to be established. One study reported better survival for patients with immature teratoma who underwent salvage surgery than of those with other tumour cell types.

There is no clear standard for treatment of relapsed ovarian germ cell tumour. Based on experience of testicular tumours, ovarian GCTs can also be divided into those which are platinum resistant and those which are platinum sensitive. Platinum resistant tumours are defined as progressive disease during treatment or during 6–8 weeks of stopping treatment. Prognosis in these cases is dismal and high dose chemotherapy or experimental drugs are advocated. Platinum sensitive tumours are defined as relapses occurring after 6–8 weeks of discontinuation of treatment. Prognosis in these cases is good. They are treated with platinum containing salvage chemotherapy regimens such as VeIP or TIP (Box 13.12).

Prognosis and survival

In spite of high cure rates, 12–20% of patients still die of this disease. Poor prognostic factors include advanced stage, bulky residual disease after surgery, age >22 years, endodermal sinus tumour and AFP of >1000 ng/ml at diagnosis.

In stage I dysgerminoma the long term survival approaches 100%. The stage-wise overall survival long-term survival is stage I 100%, stage II 85%, stage III 79% and stage IV 71%.

Follow-up and survivorship

The majority of case relapses occur within the first two years after completion of treatment, although dysgerminoma can relapse late. Initial follow up should be every 2–3 months for 1–2 years then 3–4 months up to 3 years after which 6-monthly to 5 years. Dysgerminomas should be followed up to 10 years. For those who had raised markers at the time of presentation, these should be followed every 2 months for the first year and 3-monthly for the second year, preferably alongside clinical follow-up. Regular imaging depends upon the nature of the previous tumour. With the risk of radiation from regular CT scanning, USS or MRI is advocated in most cases. Patients without raised markers should be scanned alongside their clinical follow-up.

Limited experience suggests that future fertility is not significantly affected by previous treatment for GCTs and there are no reports of adverse outcome or increased malformations in the fetus.

Future directions

Due to the success of treating most cases, current developments are in optimizing treatment for relapsed disease. This includes high dose chemotherapy.

Sex cord stromal tumours

Ovarian sex cord stromal tumours comprise 5–8% of all primary ovarian tumours. These tumours are generally low grade with no associated BRCA mutations. Many tumours produce steroid hormones and present with features of oestrogen or androgen hypersecretion. These are classified as granulosa cell tumours, thecoma-fibroma, Sertoli–Leydig cell tumours and gynandroblastoma. Inhibin, a protein secreted by these tumours, can be used as a diagnostic marker, particularly for granulosa cell tumour. These tumours are staged similar to epithelial ovarian cancers.

Granulosa cell tumour

There are two subtypes:

- Adult type – 95% of tumours occur in 5th decade of life.
- Juvenile type – 5% of tumours occur in children and young women.

These tumours usually present with large masses with features of increased oestrogen production. These can be associated with endometrial hyperplasia and adenocarcinoma. TAH-BSO is the treatment of choice in those who have completed their family. Unilateral salpingo-oophorectomy is an option for young women with stage I disease. Role of adjuvant chemotherapy after surgery is unknown. The approaches vary from routine chemotherapy for stage II–IV to no treatment until recurrence. Retrospective data suggests that adults with stage III–IV disease have a better progression free survival with adjuvant chemotherapy. The most commonly used chemotherapy is BEP (p. 223). Alternative options include combinations of carboplatin with paclitaxel and cisplatin with etoposide.

Patients with recurrent localized disease may undergo salvage surgery if feasible; otherwise treated with chemotherapy. Radiotherapy may have a role in patients with isolated inoperable pelvic recurrence.

5-year survival of completely resected stage I disease is >90% and advanced stage is 30%. Late relapses are not unusual.

Fibroma/thecoma

Fibromas are treated with oophorectomy, while thecomas are treated with either conservative surgery or TAH-BSO.

Sertoli–Leydig cell tumours

The majority of these tumours (75%) occur in women aged less than 40 years. These can be either benign or malignant (<20%) and only 2–3% have extra-ovarian disease at presentation. The presentation is with abdominal pain or distension or with features of virilization. TAH-BSO is the treatment of choice and conservative surgery is attempted when fertility preservation is intended. The benefit of adjuvant chemotherapy is not known. 5-year survival is 70–90%. Patients with recurrent and metastatic disease are treated with platinum based chemotherapy (usual regime is BEP).

Gynandroblastomas

These are very rare benign mixed tumours with elements of Sertoli–Leydig or granulosa cell elements. Presentation can be either with features of virilization or increased oestrogen production. Unilateral oophorectomy is the treatment of choice.

Gestational trophoblastic disease

Introduction

Gestational trophoblastic disease (GTD) is a rare complication of pregnancy. The gestational trophoblastic tumours include invasive mole, choriocarcinoma and placental site trophoblastic tumour (PSTT). 15% of complete moles develop into an invasive mole and around 3% of complete moles may develop into choriocarcinomas. Risk factors include age (<16 and >40 years), previous molar pregnancy and Asian origin.

Pathology

Persistent GTD can occur after any pregnancy. Invasive mole is composed of diffuse trophoblastic hyperplasia invading underlying tissues. Choriocarcinoma is characterized by absence of chorionic villi with sheets of anaplastic cyto- and syncytiotrophoblasts. PSTT is composed mainly of intermediate trophoblasts.

Clinical features

Up to 20% of patients present with persistent trophoblastic disease after surgical evacuation. The usual presentation is irregular vaginal bleeding and/or persistently elevated serum beta-hCG. Metastatic disease can occur in 4% of patients. The commonest site of metastasis is lung followed by vagina, CNS, liver and pelvis and presentation depends on the site of disease.

All women are followed up with serum beta-hCG estimation after evacuation of a molar pregnancy to identify persistent disease. 5–10% women may need chemotherapy for persistent GTD. The indications for chemotherapy are shown in Box 13.13.

Table 13.6: FIGO-WHO prognostic scoring

Score	0	1	2	4
Age (years)	<40	>40	–	–
Antecedent pregnancy	Mole	Abortion	Term	–
Interval months from index pregnancy	<4	4 –<7	7 –<13	≥13
Pre-treatment serum hCG (IU/L)	$<10^3$	10^3–$<10^4$	10^4–$<10^5$	$≥10^5$
Largest tumour size (including uterus) (cm)	<3	3–<5	≥5	–
Site of metastasis	Lung	Spleen, kidney	Gastrointestinal	Liver, brain
Number of metastasis	NA	1–4	5–8	>8
Previous failed chemotherapy	NA	NA	Single drug	≥2 drugs

Box 13.13: Indications for chemotherapy in persistent trophoblastic disease

- Serum hCG >20,000 iu/l after one or two uterine evacuations
- Static or rising hCG levels after one or two uterine evacuations
- Persistent hCG elevation six months post-uterine evacuation
- Persistent vaginal bleeding with raised hCG levels
- Pulmonary metastasis with static or rising hCG levels
- Metastasis in liver, brain, or GI tract
- Histological diagnosis of choriocarcinoma

Box 13.14: FIGO staging of GTD

- Stage I – Disease confined to uterus
- Stage II – disease beyond uterus but confined to genital structures
- Stage III – lung metastasis with or without genital tract involvement
- Stage IV – distant metastasis other than lung

Box 13.15: Chemotherapy in GTD

Low risk
- Methotrexate with folinic acid
- D-actinomycin

Salvage chemotherapy for low risk and first line chemotherapy in high risk
- MEA (methotrexate, etoposide and dactinomycin)
- EMA/CO (methotrexate, etoposide, dactinomycin/ cyclophosphamide and vincristine)

Salvage chemotherapy for high risk
- EMA/EP (methotrexate, etoposide, dactinomycin/ etoposide, cisplatin)

Assessment prior to chemotherapy

Investigations

Patients need further investigations with FBC, biochemistry, serum beta hCG, chest X-ray and CT scan of thorax and CNS staging in high risk patients (WHO score of ≥7, high risk score, multiple lung metastases and hCG >50,000 iu/l). CNS staging consists of imaging the craniospinal axis and CSF examination (ratio of CSF: serum hCG > greater than 1 in 60 suggests involvement).

Staging and prognostic scoring

FIGO staging (Box 13.14) is mainly used to compare outcome data and the scoring system (Table 13.6) guides treatment. Low risk disease is defined by a total score of ≤6 and high risk score ≥7.

Treatment

Low-risk disease (score ≤6)

Single agent chemotherapy is the treatment of choice and the commonly used agents are methotrexate and dactinomycin (Box 13.15). Methotrexate does not cause alopecia. Around 10–20% patients do not respond to methotrexate, and salvage treatment options are single agent D-actinomycin (if hCG level is low) or combination chemotherapy (if hCG level is high) (Box 13.15). Selected patients are salvaged with hysterectomy.

High risk disease (score ≥7)
Patients with high risk disease are treated with combination chemotherapy with or without surgery. The commonly used combination chemotherapy regimes are shown in Box 13.15. Most of the chemotherapy regimes give an 80–85% complete remission.

Relapse or resistant disease
20–30% of patients will be resistant to treatment or relapse after initial treatment. The commonly used regime is EMA/EP (Box 13.15). There is a role for surgical salvage in selected patients.

Central nervous system disease
Patients with CNS disease are treated with chemotherapy with or without surgery or radiotherapy. Modifying EMA/CO chemotherapy with an increased dose of systemic methotrexate and with the addition of intrathecal methotrexate may improve the dose of methotrexate in CNS.

Placental site trophoblastic tumour (PSTT)

PSTT is less chemosensitive than other GTDs and hence hysterectomy is the treatment of choice for disease limited to uterus. Metastatic PSTT is treated like high risk GTD.

Assessing response to treatment and number of courses of chemotherapy

In patients receiving chemotherapy for low-risk disease, patients are closely monitored after one course of chemotherapy with weekly hCG. Further treatment is withheld as long as serum hCG is falling. A second course of treatment is indicated if the hCG levels are stationary for three consecutive weeks, re-elevates or does not decline by one logarithmic fall within 18 days of completion of the first treatment. If a second course of chemotherapy is necessary, the same treatment is given if there was an adequate response to previous treatment. An adequate response is defined as at least a logarithmic fall in hCG after a course of chemotherapy. If the response is not adequate, another single agent chemotherapy or combination chemotherapy is

given. There is no consensus on when to stop chemotherapy after biochemical remission. Many patients receive 1–3 cycles of chemotherapy after biochemical remission, depending on the risk category and the rate of reduction of hCG.

Follow-up and survivorship

Patients need regular follow-up after completion of treatment. Women are advised not to conceive for at least 12 months after completion of their treatment. Women are advised not to take the oral contraceptive pill until hCG is normal.

There is no evidence that treatment for a previous GTD affects future pregnancy and its outcome. Chemotherapy generally results in an early menopause such that patients are advised to complete their families before the age of 35. There is also a risk of second tumours such as AML.

Vulval cancer

Introduction

Vulval cancer is rare, with 1022 new cases being diagnosed in the UK each year. It predominantly affects older women, with 80% of cases occurring in those over 60. HPV (mainly 16, 18 and 31) has been found to be responsible for approximately 30–50% of vulval cancers and up to 80% of vulval intraepithelial neoplasias (VIN). There is also an increased risk in those with HIV as well as those on immunosuppressions. Other risk factors include smoking and chronic skin conditions such as lichen sclerosus (a 4–7% risk of malignancy), lichen planus and Paget's disease.

Pathology

There are two varieties of intraepithelial neoplasia: squamous cell carcinoma-in-situ (Bowen's disease) or vulvar intraepithelial neoplasia III and Paget's disease.

The majority (90%) of vulval cancers are squamous cell (SCC) in origin, however, melanomas (4%), basal cell carcinomas, adenocarcinomas (1–2%), undifferentiated carcinomas, sarcomas (<2%) and metastatic tumours from a variety of primary sites also occur. Verrucous SCC carcinomas are a slow growing type of squamous cell carcinoma.

Patterns of spread

Vulval cancer spreads by direct extension to involve adjacent structures such as the vagina, urethra and anus, by lymphatic channels to the inguinal and femoral groin nodes, and haematogenously to distant sites including the lungs, liver and bone. The overall incidence of lymph node metastases is approximately 30%. Haematogenous spread tends to occur late, and is rare in the absence of nodal metastases.

Clinical features

The most common symptoms include itch or irritation, pain and soreness, a thickened, raised area of discolouration, ulcer, vaginal discharge or bleeding, or lump.

Diagnosis and staging

The size and location of the lesion should be documented, and any involvement of adjacent structures such as vagina, urethra, base of bladder or anus, should be noted. The diagnosis of vulval cancer is made after biopsy. Vulval cancer is staged using the FIGO classification (Box 13.16).

Management *(Figure 13.11)*

Early-stage disease (Stages I and II)

Surgery is the treatment of choice which involves a wide and deep resection (radical local excision) to obtain surgical margins of at least 1 cm. All patients except stage Ia (depth of penetration <1 mm when the risk of node metastasis is <1%) need an ipsilateral inguinofemoral lymphadenectomy to reduce the risk of recurrence. Bilateral lymphadenectomy is indicated if the tumour is within 1 cm of midline or involving labia minor. Postoperative bilateral pelvic and groin irradiation is indicated in the following setting:

- One macrometastases (>5 mm in diameter).
- Two or more micrometastases (≤5 mm).
- Extracapsular spread.

Radiotherapy field should include inguino-femoral nodes and at least pelvic nodes below the SI joints. Microscopic disease needs 50 Gy in 1.8–2 Gy per fraction, 60 Gy for extracapsular spread or multiple nodes and 60–70 Gy for macroscopic disease.

> **Box 13.16: FIGO staging of vulval cancer**
>
> Stage I – Tumour confined to the vulva
>
> - IA – Lesions ≤2 cm in size, confined to the vulva or perineum and with stromal invasion ≤1.0 mm, no nodal metastasis
> - IB Lesions >2 cm in size or with stromal invasion >1.0 mm
>
> Stage II – Tumour of any size with extension to adjacent perineal structures (⅓ lower urethra, ⅓ lower vagina, anus) with negative nodes.
>
> Stage III – Tumour of any size with or without extension to adjacent perineal structures (⅓ lower urethra, ⅓ lower vagina, anus) with positive inguino-femoral lymph nodes.
>
> - IIIA
>   - (i) With 1 lymph node metastasis (≥5 mm), or
>   - (ii) 1–2 lymph node metastasis(es) (<5 mm)
> - IIIB
>   - (i) With 2 or more lymph node metastases (≥5 mm), or
>   - (ii) 3 or more lymph node metastases (>5 mm)
> - IIIC With positive nodes with extracapsular spread
>
> Stage IV – Tumour invades other regional (⅔ upper urethra, ⅔ upper vagina), or distant structures.
>
> - IVA Tumour invades any of the following:
>   - (i) upper urethral and/or vaginal mucosa, bladder mucosa, rectal mucosa, or fixed to pelvic bone, or
>   - (ii) fixed or ulcerated inguino-femoral lymph nodes
> - IVB – Any distant metastasis including pelvic lymph nodes

Advanced disease

If it is possible to resect the primary lesion with clear margins and without the need for a bowel or urinary stoma, primary surgery is desirable. Surgery involves radical vulvectomy, bilateral groin node dissection and pelvic exenteration, or ano-vulvectomy with formation of end colostomy. The overall 5-year survival rate in women with locally advanced disease treated by radical ano-vulvectomy has been reported to be 62%. Postoperative radiotherapy is indicated if the margin is <5 mm and re-excision is not feasible.

Primary radiotherapy is the treatment of choice in those women with larger, more advanced lesions involving bladder or rectum, or who are considered unsuitable for surgery. Nodal disease may be dissected prior to management of

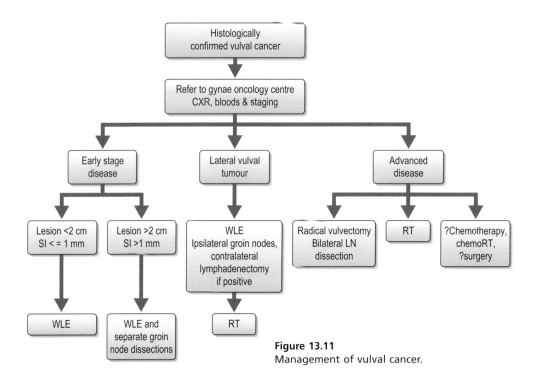

Figure 13.11
Management of vulval cancer.

primary tumour. Initial treatment involves 50 Gy at 1.7–1.8 Gy per fraction to include pelvis, inguinal nodes and primary tumour. The second phase of treatment is to the gross disease to deliver a total dose of 60–70 Gy. The exact role of the combination of chemotherapy (cisplatin alone or in combination with 5-FU) with radiotherapy is not fully explored.

Prognosis

Prognosis depends on nodal status and the size of the primary lesion. In the absence of lymph node involvement, the 5-year survival is >80%. This decreases to approximately 50% with inguinal node involvement, and to 10–15% with pelvic node metastases.

Post-treatment issues

Lymphoedema is a late complication, with an incidence of 62–69% following groin node dissection. When it occurs, the onset of lymphoedema is apparent within three months in 50% of women, and within 12 months in 85% of women.

Complications following radiotherapy include vulval soreness, skin blistering, diarrhoea, urinary frequency, and the formation of fistulae (recto-vaginal, vesico-vaginal and entero-vaginal). The incidence of developing lower limb lymphoedema is also greater in those women who have been treated by surgery including lymphadenectomy, and adjuvant radiotherapy (groin and pelvis).

Recurrence and management

15 and 33% of vulval cancers recur and the most common sites of recurrence are the vulva (69.5%), groin nodes (24.3%), the pelvis in 15.6% and distant metastases in 18.5%.

Local vulval recurrences are treated by surgery when possible. Groin recurrences are more difficult to manage. Radiotherapy is the preferred treatment, but surgery should be considered in patients who have already received groin irradiation.

Cancer of the vagina

Introduction

Primary vaginal cancer constitutes 2% of female genital tract cancers, and 240 new cases are diagnosed annually in the UK. It causes approximately 100 deaths in the UK each year.

Aetiology

The incidence of vaginal cancer is greatest in women between the ages of 60–70 years, with more than 70% of cases occurring in this group. Risk factors include fetal exposure of diethylstilboestrol (vaginal clear cell carcinoma), persistent HPV infection especially 16, a history (in up to 30%) of in-situ or invasive cervical cancer treated in the preceding 5-years, and a previous history of chronic vaginal irritation, use of ring pessaries, and previous treatment with radiotherapy. Vaginal cancer is also common in less well educated women, those with lower income, with five or more lifetime sexual partners, an early age at first intercourse, and smokers.

Pathology

The common histologic types are:

- Squamous cell carcinoma – 80% of vaginal cancers are due to direct extension of adjacent tumours (e.g. cervical) or metastases (e.g. endometrial) and 20% originate in the vagina, the most common histological type is squamous cell (over 90% of cases).
- Adenocarcinoma – tends to occur in women over the age of 50, with the exception of clear cell carcinoma. Clear cell adenocarcinoma is rare, almost always associated with an exposure to diethylstilboestrol in utero, and most commonly presents between 17 and 22 years of age.
- Papillary adenocarcinoma tends to arise from the connective tissue surrounding the vagina, and is less likely to spread via the lymphatics.
- Adenosquamous carcinomas (2%) tend to be more aggressive.
- Malignant melanomas of the vagina (2%) – develop in women in the 5th decade of life, and in the lower third of the vagina.

Presentation

Patients generally remain asymptomatic (20%) in both the pre-invasive and early stages of vaginal cancer, and early lesions are most commonly detected during routine cervical screening. 80–90% of women will present with bleeding, discharge, dyspareunia, vaginal irritation, or a vaginal mass. In more advanced disease, women

Box 13.17: FIGO staging of vaginal cancer

Stage	
Stage I	Tumour limited to vaginal wall
Stage II	Tumour involving the subvaginal tissue but not extending to pelvic side wall
Stage III	Tumour extending up to pelvic side wall
Stage IVa	Spread to adjacent organs and/or direct extension beyond true pelvis
Stage IVb	Distant

may also complain of pelvic pain, constipation, difficulty in micturition and lower limb oedema.

Diagnosis and staging

The diagnosis of primary vaginal cancer is made by histology and clinical examination. Tumours extending to the external cervical os are classified as cervical cancers, while tumours involving the vulva as vulval cancers. MRI scan is useful in assessing local extension of tumour. FIGO staging for vagina is given in Box 13.17.

Principles of management

Factors to be considered when planning treatment for vaginal cancer are the stage, size and location of the lesion, previous pelvic irradiation and performance status.

Surgery

Surgery can be curative in selected women with early stage (I, small stage II) disease, and in women with stage IV disease in whom exenteration is planned. Surgery is the treatment of choice if clear excision margins (at least 1 cm) are achievable.

Superficial lesions may be treated by wide local excision. Stage I lesions at the apex, particularly on the posterior vaginal wall may be treated with a partial vaginectomy or extension of a radical hysterectomy. Lesions that lie in the upper part of the vagina can be treated by radical hysterovaginectomy with removal of the parametria and paracolpos. In women who have had a previous hysterectomy, an upper vaginectomy and parametrectomy can be performed. Both procedures should also include bilateral pelvic node dissection.

In stage II disease with lesions in sites that would allow a less aggressive procedure than a radical vaginectomy and with minimal extension outside the vaginal wall, surgery may be considered.

Pelvic exenteration is useful in stage IVa disease without extension of the lesion to the pelvic side walls, and distant sites of metastases.

In young patients requiring radiotherapy, laparotomy is done to transpose ovaries.

Radiotherapy

Radiotherapy is the treatment of choice unless clear resection margins (at least 1 cm) can be obtained. The proximity of the vagina to the bladder and rectum can potentially limit treatment options and increase the risk of complications to these organs.

In early stage disease (stage I and II), intracavitary radiation may be used, while both intracavitary and external irradiation are required for larger and more advanced lesions. The use of both external irradiation and brachytherapy in treating vaginal cancer has been shown to achieve excellent results, and allows vaginal preservation. If the lower one-third of the vagina is involved groin nodes should be irradiated or dissected.

Women with advanced disease tend to be treated with chemoradiation rather than radiotherapy alone.

Chemoradiotherapy

Most of the evidence for chemoradiotherapy in vaginal cancer originates from studies in cervical cancer using cisplatin or cisplatin with 5-FU. Chemotherapy alone appears to offer little benefit in the management of advanced (stage III and IV) disease.

Prognosis

The overall 5-year survival rate for vaginal cancer is 44%, which is poorer than that for both cervical and vulval cancer. Women over 60 years of age, lesions in the middle and lower third of the vagina, and poorly differentiated tumours, are poor prognostic factors.

Recurrence and management

The main site of relapse is the pelvis. In central recurrence, there may be a role for pelvic exenteration or further radiotherapy. The 5-year survival rate following recurrence is approximately 12%. There is no proven benefit for chemotherapy.

Follow-up

Follow-up is important in addressing the issues of treatment-induced morbidities. Vaginal scarring and stenosis are the main problems leading to depression and sexual dysfunction. Late bladder and bowel toxicities and early menopause due to radiation also need attention.

Further reading

Colombo N, Peiretti M, Castiglione M. Non-epithelial ovarian cancer: ESMO clinical recommendations for diagnosis, treatment and follow-up. Ann Oncol. 2009;20 Suppl 4:24–26.

Han LY, Kipps E, Kaye SB. Current treatment and clinical trials in ovarian cancer. Expert Opin Investig Drugs. 2010;19:521–534.

Amant F, Moerman P, Neven P et al. Endometrial cancer. Lancet. 2005;366:491–505.

Gehrig PA, Bae-Jump VL. Promising novel therapies for the treatment of endometrial cancer. Gynecol Oncol. 2010;116:187–194.

Goonatillake S, Khong R, Hoskin P. Chemoradiation in gynaecological cancer. Clin Oncol. 2009;21:566–572.

Taylor A, Powell ME. Conformal and intensity-modulated radiotherapy for cervical cancer. Clin Oncol. 2008;20: 417–425.

del Campo JM, Prat A, Gil-Moreno A et al. Update on novel therapeutic agents for cervical cancer. Gynecol Oncol. 2008;110:S72–S76.

Koulouris CR, Penson RT. Ovarian stromal and germ cell tumors. Semin Oncol. 2009;36:126–136.

Crosbie EJ, Slade RJ, Ahmed AS. The management of vulval cancer. Cancer Treat Rev. 2009;35:533–539.

Gray HJ. Advances in vulvar and vaginal cancer treatment. Gynecol Oncol. 2010 May 13. [Epub ahead of print] PMID: 20471671

Cancers of the skin

14

HM Hatcher and TV Ajithkumar

Cutaneous melanoma

Epidemiology

Melanoma is the most aggressive form of skin cancer which is increasing in incidence. In Europe, its incidence has risen by 3–8% per year since the 1960s. The lifetime risk of melanoma in the UK is 1 in 147 for men and 1 in 117 for women. In Australia the risks are significantly higher with lifetime risks of 1 in 25 for men and 1 in 35 for women. Overall survival rates have improved due to early detection but survival of higher stage disease has improved very little in the past 10 years.

The peak incidence of melanoma occurs in middle age (40s) with less than 10% occurring in childhood, although the rates in those under 20 have increased by over 3% in the past 10 years.

Aetiology

Ultraviolent sun radiation (especially UVB) is the main risk factor for the development of cutaneous melanoma. People with a history of blistering sunburns have a 2.5 times higher risk of melanoma. Other surrogate makers of sun sensitivity such as freckling (RR 2.5), burn without tanning (RR 1.7), red hair (RR 2.4) and blue eyes (RR 1.6) also have an increased risk.

Other risk factors are:

- Genetic – people with a strong family history and multiple atypical moles are at the greatest risk of melanoma. Those with an inherited mutation in the *CDKN2A* and *CDK4* genes have 60–90% lifetime risk of melanoma.

- Naevi – Multiple benign naevi (>100) as well as multiple aypical naevi increases the risk of melanoma (RR 11)
- Immunosuppression – Transplant recipients (RR 3) and patients with AIDS (RR 1.5) have increased risk of melanoma
- Previous melanoma – those with a previous melanoma have a 2–10% risk of a further melanoma which increases further with two previous melanomas.

Pathology

There are four histological variants of cutaneous melanoma:

- Superficial spreading is the most common type. This often arises within a pre-existing naevus and is surrounded by a zone of atypical melanocytes that may extend beyond the visible border of the lesion.
- Nodular melanoma (10–15%) presents as symmetrical, uniform dark blue-black lesions. Amelanotic nodular melanomas are often misdiagnosed.
- Lentigo maligna melanoma (10–15%) usually occurs on the sun-exposed areas of head and neck and hands. Clinically these are large (often >3 cm) flat lesions with areas of dark brown or black discolouration. These lesions arise from the premalignant lesion called Hutchinson's freckle.
- Acral-lentigenous melanomas, as the name suggests (acral – distal), occur on the palms, soles and subungual regions. These lesions occur with the same frequency in whites and non-whites (2–8% of melanoma in whites and 40–60% melanoma of non-whites). These

© 2011, Elsevier Ltd
DOI: 10.1016/B978-0-7234-3458-0.00019-1

Box 14.1: Prognostic factors in cutaneous melanoma

- Breslow thickness
- Ulceration
- Presence of satellite lesions
- LDH
- Vascular invasion
- Surgical margin
- Clark's level
- Nodal disease
- Extranodal metastases
- Mitotic count

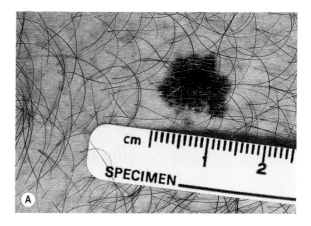

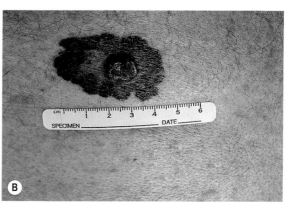

Figure 14.1
Early melanoma showing ABCD signs (A) and advanced plaque like melanoma (B) with nodule which also exhibits ABCD signs. From Darrell Rigel: Cancer of the Skin (Saunders) with permission.

lesions can be easily misdiagnosed as sub-ungual haematoma.

Other forms of melanoma include ocular, mucosal and vulval (p. 236).

The histology of melanomas is very variable depending on the specific subtype and primary site. Many of the features assessed by histology have prognostic value (Box 14.1). In addition to these the pathologist should report the type of melanoma, greatest thickness, radial or vertical growth phase, excision margins and immuno-histochemical stains. Immunohistochemical stains used in melanoma include S100 (the most frequently used but also stains benign melanocytes), HMB-45, Mitf, MART-1 and tyrosinase.

Presentation

Patients usually present with new skin lesions or change in existing skin lesion. It is important to get a detailed history of:

- How long lesion has been present?
- When did it start changing?
- Whether it arose from a pre-existing lesion?
- Previous history of sun exposure, sun burns, skin cancers and immunosuppressive treatment.
- Family history of melanoma.

Initial assessment

Initial assessment of patients with suspected melanoma includes detailed examination and a clinical photograph of the lesion, full skin examination and examination for lymphadenopathy and hepatomegaly. Clinical signs of melanoma

include itching, bleeding, ulceration or changes in a pre-existing mole. ABCDE features (Figure 14.1) help to distinguish early melanoma from a benign mole:

- A – Asymmetry.
- B – Border irregularity.
- C – Colour variation.
- D – Diameter of >6 mm.
- E – Evolution (change in lesion).

Investigations

In the absence of clinical evidence of metastatic disease in regional lymph nodes at presentation, there is no indication for any staging investigations. In patients with thick primary tumours (>4 mm), CT scan may be useful prior to rule out metastatic disease. Studies show that a routine chest X-ray revealed metastasis in only 0.1% whereas 15% showed false positivity. Similarly CT scan showed metastasis in 1.3% while false positivity was 16%.

Patients with >4 mm thick lesion and evidence of nodal metastasis (including micrometastasis) need staging investigations with full blood count, liver function tests, serum lactate dehydrogenase (LDH), chest X-ray and CT scan of chest, abdomen and pelvis.

Tissue diagnosis

Excision biopsy to include 2–5 mm of clinical margin of normal skin with a cuff of subdermal fat is the standard procedure. This helps to confirm diagnosis and provide guidance for subsequent management based on Breslow thickness. Full thickness incisional biopsy from the thickest part of the lesion is acceptable as a mode of diagnosis in certain anatomical areas (e.g. face, ear, palm/sole) and for large lesions. Shave and punch biopsies are not recommended.

Staging

Breslow thickness, ulceration and mitotic count are most important prognostic factors of localized disease whereas Clark level is an independent prognostic factor for melanoma of <1 mm thickness (Box 14.1). Staging is by TNM AJCC system and is related to prognosis (Table 14.1). M1a includes distant skin, subcutaneous or nodal metastases with a normal LDH. M1b is lung metastases with a normal LDH and M1c is with any other metastases or with a raised LDH level.

Management

Non-metastatic disease

Primary surgery
Surgical excision with an adequate margin is primary treatment of choice for patients with no distant metastasis. The margin is the clinically measured margin during surgery rather than histopathological margin. The extent of the margin depends on the depth of the melanoma and may need to be adjusted for cosmetic or functional reasons. The recommended margins are: 1 cm for lesions less than 1 mm in depth, 1–2 cm for lesions 1–2 mm in depth, and 2 cm for lesions >2 mm in depth.

Management of regional lymph node
The role of elective lymph node excision for node negative patients has being debated for several years. Although initial retrospective studies showed a survival benefit with this approach, four randomized studies failed to show any survival advantage. Debate on the role of elective node dissection has been subsumed by emergence of the sentinel node concept.

The sentinel node (SN) is the node to which the lymph initially drains from a tumour before passing to the other regional nodes. In theory the sentinel node is most likely to contain the tumour cells and if none are present in this node, it is unlikely that other lymph nodes are involved.

The risk of sentinel node metastasis depends on the thickness of lesion. A tumour less than 0.8 mm thick has 1% SN positivity, 0.8 to 1.5 mm has 8%, 1.5–4 mm thickness has 23% and more than 4 mm thickness has 36% risk. Although, sentinel node positivity is proven to have strong correlation with survival (90% 5-year survival for SN negative vs. 56% for SN positive), the role of lymph node dissection for SN positive disease is still evolving. Many agree that there is no proven overall survival benefit from the routine application of SN to patients with cutaneous melanoma. However, there is some suggestion that it may increase the disease free survival.

Patients with >4 mm thick lesions have a predicted incidence of SN positivity of 30–40%. Hence it is reasonable to offer SN in this group of patients to provide prognostic information and selection into clinical trials.

The ongoing MSLT-II trial aims to examine the benefit of complete dissection on survival by randomizing patients with SN positive melanoma to undergo either complete nodal dissection or observation.

Adjuvant treatment
No trial has shown a survival benefit for adjuvant chemotherapy in localized malignant melanoma. Due to the activity of immune treatment in advanced melanoma several trials have examined the role of interferon and vaccines in the adjuvant treatment of melanoma. A pooled analysis of three ECOG studies showed that adjuvant high dose interferon improves relapse-free – survival (about 10% at 5- years) but not overall survival

Table 14.1: *TNM staging & 5-year survival of cutaneous melanoma*

Staging		5-year survival (%)
Stage IA		95
T1aN0M0	≤1 mm thickness without ulceration and mitosis <1/mm^2	
Stage IB		91
T1bN0M0	≤1 mm thickness with ulceration or mitosis ≥1/mm^2	
T2aN0M0	1.01–2 mm thickness without ulceration	
Stage IIA		77–79
T2bN0M0	1.01–2 mm thickness with ulceration	
T3aN0M0	2.01–4 mm thickness without ulceration	
Stage IIB		63–67
T3bN0M0	2.01–4 mm thickness with ulceration	
T4aN0M0	>4 mm thickness without ulceration	
Stage IIC		45
T4bN0M0	>4 mm thickness with ulceration	
Stage IIIA		
T1-4aN1aM0	Micrometastasis* in 1 node	70
T1-4aN2aM0	Micrometastasis in 2–3 nodes	63
Stage IIIB		
T1-4bN1a/2aM0		50–53
T1-4aN1bM0	Macrometastasis** in 1 node	46–59
T1-4aN2bM0	Macrometastasis in 2–3 nodes	46–59
T1-4aN2cM0	in-transit metastases/satellites without nodes	
Stage IIIC		24–29
T1-4bN1b/2b/2cM0		
Any T N3M0	metastasis in >3 nodes or matted nodes or in-transit or satellites with metastatic nodes	
Stage IV		
Any T, any N, M1	distant metastasis	7–19%

*micrometastases after sentinel node biopsy; **macrometastases are clinically detectable pathologically confirmed nodes.

in patients with a high-risk resected melanoma. This group included patients with ≥4 mm thick with no nodal involvement and melanoma involving regional nodes or in-transit metastasis. However, high dose interferon is associated with a number of side effects such as acute constitutional symptoms, chronic fatigue, headache, weight loss, nausea, myelosuppression and depression and most patients will require dose modifications during treatment.

A trial examining the role of a ganglioside vaccine in the adjuvant treatment of high risk melanoma showed no benefit and there were concerns that patients may have done worse than with no treatment.

Management of positive nodes
Patients with metastatic lymph node disease are treated with regional node dissection if feasible and up to 13–59% of these patients do not

develop metastatic disease. There is a significant risk of lymphoedema (especially with groin dissections) and patients should wear compression stockings for many months. Some trials are examining the role of adjuvant treatment, such as bevacizumab, after groin dissection. A randomized study has evaluated the role of postoperative radiotherapy (48 Gy in 20 fractions) in patients with a high risk (>25%) of regional recurrence after lymphadenectomy. The two-year lymph node field relapse-free rate was significantly improved with adjuvant radiotherapy compared with observation (82 vs. 65% HR 0.47, 95% CI 0.28–0.67); but without no improvement in 2-year overall survival. The long term toxicity of radiotherapy yet to be reported.

Management of metastatic disease

Metastatic melanoma has a poor prognosis. Most patients with non-visceral metastases survive up to 18 months whereas the median survival of those with visceral involvement or an elevated serum LDH is 4–6 months. Lymph node and skin metastases in the absence of other metastases have the best prognosis (up to 18 months). Those with lung metastases in the absence of other visceral disease have an intermediate prognosis (up to 12 months median survival). Those with other visceral disease have a median survival of less than 6 months which is limited further in the presence of a high and rapidly increasing LDH. Patients with liver metastases from a primary uveal melanoma have a particularly poor prognosis usually limited to less than 3 months.

Treatment of melanoma metastases depends on the site of disease, whether or not it is localized and the overall fitness of the patient. Treatment can be with surgery, radiotherapy, systemic therapies or best supportive care.

Role of surgery

In the presence of an isolated metastasis, especially if the patient has a long disease free interval, e.g. 1 year, surgery may be the best option. The most common sites for surgical resection are skin, brain and lung. Resection of liver metastases is not usually performed as liver metastases are associated with such a poor prognosis. Appropriate staging is important in these patients who undergo surgical resection. PET scans have been used to exclude further distant disease, especially if complex surgery is planned, e.g. resection of cerebral metastases.

Patients with up to three visceral metastases are candidates for surgical resection and the 5-year survival can be more than 20% after complete resection of lung metastases and 28–41% after complete resection of gastrointestinal metastases. Similarly patients with solitary brain metastases can also be candidates for resection. Adjuvant radiotherapy is often used in some of these patients, especially after resection of cerebral metastasis.

Role of radiotherapy

Radiotherapy can also be given after surgical resection of a solitary metastasis and this is particularly the case after resection of a solitary brain metastasis. The treatment options include whole brain radiotherapy (20 Gy in five fractions or 30 Gy in 10 fractions), stereotactic radiosurgery or a combination of both. The optimal radiotherapy in this situation is yet to be defined.

Palliative radiotherapy is useful in bone metastasis and spinal cord compression not amenable to surgical decompression (p. 328). Skin metastases which are rapidly enlarging and about to ulcerate can also be treated with palliative radiotherapy.

Chemotherapy and other systemic treatments in metastatic disease

Dacarbazine is the standard intravenous chemotherapy drug for metastatic melanoma with a response rate of 10–20% and a median duration of response of 3–6 months. It is given 3–4 weekly at doses of 850–1000 mg/m^2 with nausea as the main side effect. Temozolamide is an oral analogue of dacarbazine and crosses the blood–brain barrier but is more expensive and has no improvement in response rates compared with dacarbazine (Table 14.2). There is no evidence that combination chemotherapy regime is superior to single agent drugs in terms of response rates or survival.

Immunotherapy with high dose interleukin-2 (IL-2) or interferon alpha has shown response rates of 10–21%. Toxicities include hypotension, capillary leak syndrome, sepsis and renal failure.

A recent study of ipilimumab, a monoclonal antibody against cytotoxic T-lymphocyte antigen 4 (CTLA-4), showed improved overall survival in previously treated patients with unresectable

Table 14.2: Response rates (%) for single agents in metastatic melanoma

Agent	% Response rate (CR + PR)
Dacarbazine	20
Temozolamide	21
Carmustine (BCNU)	18
Lomustine (CCNU)	13
Cisplatin	23
Carboplatin	16
Vinblastine	13
Paclitaxel	18
Docetaxel	15

stage III/IV melanoma who were positive for HLA-A*0201. Side effects of this treatment included rash, colitis, diarrhoea and hepatitis.

Combining chemotherapy with an immune modulator has been assessed in several clinical trials. A meta-analysis showed that this improved response rates, but did not translate into a survival benefit.

In summary no drug or combination of drugs has shown a significant response rate and survival benefit over single agent dacarbazine. It remains the standard drug in metastatic melanoma but patients should be entered into clinical trials where possible.

Isolated limb perfusion

In some cases widespread metastases do not occur but there may be disseminated skin metastases in a limb which cover an area too large for radiotherapy. In these patients, if systemic treatment is not feasible, isolated limb perfusion with TNF-alpha and melphalan can establish good local control. This is only performed in a limited number of centres but can provide good clinical benefit.

Radiofrequency ablation

For some patients with limited systemic disease but in whom surgery is not possible, radiofrequency ablation (RFA) has been used for liver and lung metastases. In general they should be less than 5 cm in size and accessible to the RFA catheter used. Complications include bleeding and pneumothorax.

Newer agents

Given the risk of recurrence and poor outcomes with systemic treatment in metastatic disease, new agents are being developed to target specific pathways involved in melanoma. Examples include VEGF, BRAF and bcl-2. Studies are ongoing to assess the potential benefit of bevacizumab in resected stage III and stage IV disease and the role of other anti angiogenics. Sorafenib which is a TKI which has activity against BRAF has been shown to improve response rates when combined with chemotherapy, although no survival benefit was observed. Agents with a more specific BRAF activity are being developed.

Prognostic factors and survival

Prognostic factors are highlighted in Box 14.1. Survival according to stage is included in Table 14.1.

Follow-up

After surgery all patients should be followed up due to the risk of further melanomas as well as nodal or systemic recurrence. Full skin and nodal examination should be carried out and abdominal examination to exclude hepatomegaly. For high-risk patients (>IA) blood tests to examine LDH, liver function tests and FBC may be carried out. At the point of nodal recurrence reassessment with CT is suggested prior to surgery and 6–12 months later. For those who have had metastatic disease resected a CT several months later is recommended along with close follow-up. All patients, especially who have had nodal disease or metastases, should be warned about the symptoms of spinal cord compression.

Non-cutaneous melanoma

Ocular melanoma

Ocular melanoma is a rare subtype of melanoma which can occur in many areas of the eye. Most commonly it occurs in the choroid but less than 5% occur in the iris. The aetiology is uncertain; some studies suggest a link with UV radiation. The risks are higher in those who have had cutaneous melanoma, pale iris colour or who have a family history of ocular melanoma. The staging system differs to that of cutaneous melanoma.

Poor prognostic factors include age over 60, size and involvement of the ciliary body. Although often localized at presentation they have a high risk (10–80% depending on number of prognostic factors) to spread to the liver, often several years after successful treatment of the primary. Long-term survival is less than 35% even with successful treatment of the primary. Surgery used to be the standard treatment but radiotherapy has replaced this in most cases. Radiotherapy can be administered as external beam, as a radio-active plaque (e.g. iridium-192) or with protons or other charged particles. Local control rates are similar with each technique. The vision is often lost in the irradiated eye with the list of complications including cataracts, glaucoma, retinopathy and vitreous haemorrhage.

Treatment of metastases in ocular melanoma has shown that they tend to have a reduced response rate to chemotherapy and immunotherapy than cutaneous melanoma and are more rapidly progressive.

Due to their propensity for metastases (especially liver and lung) which can be delayed, follow-up includes imaging of the liver and lungs in addition to LDH and liver function tests. Combined follow-up with ophthalmology is required.

Mucosal melanoma

Mucosal melanomas constitute less than 2% of all melanomas. The most common sites of presentation are head and neck (up to 50%), female genital tract (25%) and anorectal (20%). The remainder occur in very rare sites such as other areas of the gastrointestinal tract, Eustachian tube and salivary glands. They occur later in life (50–70s) than cutaneous melanoma, are more common in non-Caucasians and slightly more common in men than women. They tend to present late as they are essentially hidden from sight and have a very poor prognosis. For head and neck tumours 5-year survival is less than 30% which reduces to <20% with involved lymph nodes. The most common presentation is with bleeding, anaemia or local symptoms such as pain. There is no specific staging system. The treatment of choice is surgical resection with clear margins but this is often difficult due to location of the tumour. Radiotherapy has been used to try to improve local control but has not shown an improvement in survival and is not a standard

practice. A study using carbon ions to minimise local morbidity showed good local control but 5-year survival was still less than 30%. Chemotherapy with standard drugs for cutaneous melanoma has been tried with similar success. Nodal disease occurs to a greater extent than in ocular melanoma so regional lymph nodes should always be examined at follow-up.

Basal cell carcinoma

Introduction

Basal cell carcinoma (BCC) is a slow growing, locally invasive (hence called rodent ulcer) malignant epidermal skin tumour. The exact incidence is difficult to obtain; though there is a worldwide trend in increasing incidence.

The most significant aetiological factors appear to UV exposure and genetic predisposition. BCC is common in the sun-exposed area of head and neck. Multiple BCC is a feature of Gorlin's syndrome. Other risk factors include increasing age, male, fair skin, immunosuppression, vaccination scars and arsenic exposure. Sunscreen use and low fat diet are thought to be protective.

Pathology

The common histologic subtypes are superficial, nodular and morphoeic (sclerosing). Other variants include micronodular, infiltrative and basosquamous BCC which are aggressive with high local recurrence. Perivascular and perineural invasion is associated with aggressive tumours. BCC infiltrate tissues in a three dimensional fashion. Lymph node metastasis is extremely rare except in those with multiple recurrences or uncontrolled primary tumour.

Clinical features

The common growth patterns are superficial, multifocal, nodular and morphoeic (Figure 14.2). The sites affected are head and neck (52%), trunk (27%), upper limb (13%) and lower limb (8%).

- Superficial BCC occurs on the trunk or limbs of young people. It presents as a well-defined, erythematous, scaling or slightly shiny macular lesion. Stretching the lesion causes an increase in the degree of erythema, highlights the shiny surface and reveals a peripheral thread-like pearly rim or island of pearliness

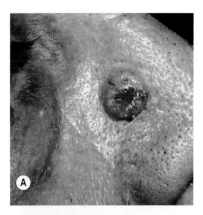

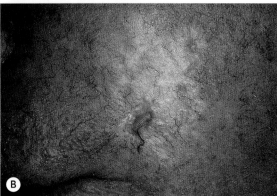

Figure 14.2
Nodular BCC with rolled borders with telangiectasia (A) and a morphoeic BCC characterized by a white plaque with telangiectasia and ill-defined borders (B). From Darrell Rigel: Cancer of the Skin (Saunders) with permission.

distributed throughout the lesion. These lesions will progressively enlarge and may reach 5–10 cm in diameter. Biopsy is needed prior to definitive treatment.

• Nodular BCC occurs on the head and neck region of elderly patients. It presents as a shiny, pearly, telangiectatic papule or nodule. The pearly appearance becomes more obvious during skin stretching. Radially arranged dilated capillaries are often seen across the surface of lesion. With ongoing growth, tumour ulceration can occur which leads to central umbilication of lesion with a raised rolled border. Islands of pigments can also be seen.

• Morphoeic SCC typically presents as a pale scar and palpation reveals firm induration which extends more widely and deeply than is evident on inspection. It slowly enlarges to reach a large size. Biopsy is necessary.

Other histolological subtypes are uncommon and do not have any characteristic clinical presentation.

Examination

Clinical examination should be done in a well-lit area with the aid of a magnifier. Whole skin examination and regional nodal examination is necessary.

Diagnosis

Diagnosis is often clinical. Biopsy is indicated when there is clinical suspicion of an alternative diagnosis or histologic subtype may influence treatment decision. Punch or shave biopsy may be appropriate. Imaging of the local area, e.g. by CT, may be indicated when there is suspicion of bone involvement and deep infiltration (particularly for a lesion close to the embryonic fusion lines such as the nasal vestibular region, or pre- and post-auricular regions).

Treatment

Treatment is aimed at eradication of tumour with acceptable cosmetic and functional outcome. A number of treatment options are available (Box 14.2) and the choice of treatment in small BCC depends on various factors (Box 14.3). Radiotherapy is indicated when cosmetic and/or functional outcome is better with radiotherapy compared with surgery and when there is a need to avoid complex plastic surgery.

Surgery and radiotherapy (RT) are effective treatment for small and less invasive tumours. Large and deeply invasive lesions are treated with surgery with or without postoperative radiotherapy.

RT favoured in:

- Mid-face, nasal , inner canthus, lower eye lid, lip commissures (better function)
- Multiple superficial lesions difficult to excise (better cosmesis)
- Patients >70 years (long-term toxicity is less of an issue)
- Patients who wish to avoid surgery
- Patients prone to keloid formation

Surgery is the choice in:

- Readily excisable lesions in those <70 years
- Lesions in hair-bearing areas or overlying lacrimal gland
- Recurrence after radiotherapy
- Multifocal disease especially with dysplastic skin
- Upper eyelid tumours (better function)
- Dorsum of the hand (better function)
- Below knee and other sites of poor vascularity (problem with healing and function)
- Invasion to bones and joints*

*Cartilage invasion is not an absolute contraindication to radiotherapy. Radiotherapy is, however, avoided in large pinna lesions with extensive, inflamed or painful cartilage invasion.

Surgery

Wide excision (WE)

WE of simple lesions need a 2–3 mm margin whereas complex lesions or clinically poorly defined lesions need a margin of 3–5 mm. An adequate microscopic margin is 0.5 mm. The most appropriate management after incomplete excision is debatable. The treatment options include re-excision, radiotherapy or observation. Adjuvant radiotherapy improves 5-year survival from 61 to 91%. Observation is an option for elderly patients where further surgery and radiotherapy may not be appropriate.

Mohs' micrographic surgery

During this procedure, the tumour is excised and the entire peripheral and deep margins are examined by frozen section for residual tumour. Mapping and staining of excised tissue and a specialized tissue sectioning procedure enables precise localization of residual tumour and the process of excision continues until the margin is tumour free. This is more appropriate for tumours with poorly defined borders, recurrent tumour and extensive disease.

Radiotherapy

Radiotherapy results in 93–95% 10-year control rate for BCC of ≤2 cm. Radiotherapy details are given in Box 14.4.

Recurrence

Recurrence is common with mid face and pre-auricular lesions, tumours >2 cm and aggressive subtypes. Two-thirds of recurrences occur within 2 years of primary treatment and 20% occur in 2–5 years. Recurrences after non-surgical treatment are generally treated with surgical resection followed by plastic surgical repair. Recurrence after surgical treatment can be treated with surgery or radiotherapy.

Prognosis

Overall 10-year control rate is >90%. A number of factors influence prognosis. The important prognostic factors are size, depth of invasion, histological subtype (morphoeic, infiltrative and basosquamous have higher recurrence), completion of excision (incomplete excisions have a 30% recurrence rate), site of disease (disease around nose, eyes and ears have higher recurrence rates) and presence of perineural spread.

Squamous cell carcinoma

Introduction

Squamous cell carcinoma (SCC) is the second most common skin cancer constituting 20% of skin malignancies. The incidence appears to be increasing and males are more commonly affected.

Risk factors include exposure to ionizing or ultraviolet radiation, immunosuppression, scars, chronic wounds, smoking and arsenic exposure. Congenital conditions such as oculocutaneous albinism and xeroderma pigmentosum are also associated with increased risk of SCC. It is common in sun-exposed areas and hence sun screen is protective.

Pathology

In situ (Bowen's disease) SCC is limited to epidermis which presents as a flat scaling pink lesion with irregular borders. There is no risk of

Box 14.4: Radiotherapy for skin cancer

Consent
- Acute reactions involve dermatitis and mucositis which resolve by 6 weeks following treatment.
- Late effects involve thinning of skin, alopecia, loss of sweating, change in colour, telangiectasis and fibrosis.

Position and immobilization
Depends on the site.

Type of radiation
Depends on depth of penetration needed and type of underlying tissue.

Depth of penetration
- ≤5 mm deep lesion – superficial X-ray.
- >5 mm–2 cm deep lesion – deep X-ray or low energy electrons (6 MeV).
- >2 cm tumour – high energy electrons or photons.

Underlying tissue
- Bone – electrons are preferable to avoid increased absorbed dose from deep X-rays.
- Air cavities (e.g. near sinuses) – X-rays or photons preferred as dosimetry is difficult with electrons.

Treatment volume
- Well-defined BCC – 5 mm margin around macroscopic tumour.
- Ill-defined BCC and SCC – 10 mm margin.

Beam shaping – custom made lead cut out for X-rays and end frame cut-out for electron. Crenallation of the margin of a round cut out gives a better cosmesis by blurring the edge of radiation reaction.

Radiotherapy dose
BCC is thought to be more radiosensitive than SCC. Equivalent doses for BCC and SCC and rough guide for selection of fractionation regime are as follows:

BCC	SCC
60 Gy/30 fractions/6 weeks*	60–66 Gy/30–32 fractions
50 Gy/20 fractions/4 weeks*	55 Gy/20 fractions
40 Gy/15 fractions/3 weeks	40 Gy/10 fractions
40.5 Gy/9 fractions/3 weeks	45 Gy/9 fractions
32.5 Gy/5 fractions/1 week	32.5 Gy/5 fractions
32 Gy/4 fractions/4 weeks**	32 Gy/4 fractions/4weeks
12–15 Gy/1 fraction**	12–15 Gy/1 fraction

*fractionation used in patient aged <70 years and/or tumour of >3–4 cm; **used in frail patients.

Special considerations

Electron planning
- Electron beam field is defined by 50% isodose and the 90% isodose is 3–5 mm inside the field. Hence, in order to enclose the PTV within 90% isodose, a 5 mm larger electron applicator than defined by PTV is needed.
- At higher energies, isodoses close to the surface bows inwards which necessitates 1 cm larger applicator diameter than the defined PTV to ensure homogenous dose to the tumour (p. 18, Figure 3.2B).
- Surface dose increases with electron energy; a bolus is needed for lower energies to bring up 90% isodose to the skin surface (p. 18, Figure 3.2A).
- Bolus is also used to bring up high dose to surface to avoid radiation to underlying critical structures.
- Stand off effect – fill the area with bolus/calculate correction

Normal tissue shielding
- Lower eyelid and canthi tumours need corneal shielding.
- Lip tumours need buccal shields. Shields should be coated with wax to absorb scattered radiation.
- Tumours in the pinna and nasal regions when treated with electrons need wax coated lead plugs in the external auditory canal and nose respectively to avoid normal tissue damage.

metastasis, although progression to invasive SCC occurs in 3–11% of cases.

In situ SCC of the glans penis (erythroplasia of Queyrat) has 20% risk of metastasis and 30% can progress to invasive disease.

Invasive SCC is composed of a collection of atypical keratocytes which invade the dermis and deeper structures. Other histologic variants are:

- Adenoid SCC – can metastasize in 3–19% and associated with rapid local growth.
- Adenosquamous SCC – shows squamous appearance superficially and glandular appearance deeply. These are aggressive tumours.
- Spindle cell SCC – appears as ulcerated nodules or exophytic tumours and may be difficult to distinguish from sarcoma histologically. These tumours are aggressive with a tendency to perineural invasion and metastasis (25%).
- Verrucous SCC – appears like a large wart. These are slow growing, locally invasive and do not metastasize.
- Keratoacanthoma – appears as a rapidly growing nodule with a central keratin plug. True lesions can undergo spontaneous regression but most are now viewed as SCC.

Clinical presentation

Typical presentation is a raised pink papule or plaque with erosion or ulceration (Figure 14.3). In advanced cases it presents as large ulcerated

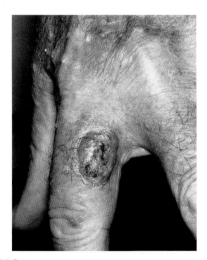

Figure 14.3
Digital squamous cell carcinoma. From Darrell Rigel: Cancer of the Skin (Saunders) with permission.

masses and bleeding. Metastasis is primarily to the regional nodes (2–6%). The head and neck region is the commonest site in men whereas the upper limb followed by head and neck are the commonest sites in females. Only 8% of SCC arise on the trunk.

Examination

Examination should be of the whole skin and regional lymph nodes.

Diagnosis

Tissue biopsy is essential for diagnosis. CT scan helps to detect regional lymph nodes. FNA of the enlarged lymph node under radiological guidance is advised. Open surgical biopsy should be avoided. The role of sentinel node biopsy is evolving.

Staging

T1 – ≤2 cm in greatest dimension.
T2 – >2 to 5 cm in greatest dimension.
T3 – >5 cm in greatest dimension.
T4 – tumour invades deep extradermal structures.
N1 – regional nodal metastasis.
M1 – distant metastasis.

Treatment

Three factors that influence treatment of SCC are: the need for removal of tumour locally, the possibility of 'in-transit' metastasis and regional nodal metastasis. Treatment options include:

- Cryotherapy (for small tumours with well defined borders).
- Curettage and electrodessication (for well differentiated tumours of <1 cm size).
- Radiotherapy (see Box 14.3) – used as a primary treatment and adjuvant after surgery.
- Surgical excision (see Box 14.3) and Mohs' micrographic surgery.

Surgery

Surgery is aimed at complete removal of the tumour and of any metastasis. Low-risk tumours of <2 cm are excised with a minimal margin of 4 mm whereas tumours of >2 cm size, high risk tumours (grade 2–4, in high risk locations such as ear, lip, scalp, eyelids and nose) and those extending into subcutaneous tissue need a minimum margin of 6 mm or more. Depth of excision should be through normal underlying fat. The accepted minimal microscopic margin is >1 mm.

Mohs' micrographic surgery is indicated in high risk tumours and recurrences.

Management of lymph nodes

The treatment of metastatic lymph nodes is primary surgery. Elective lymph node dissection is not routinely advised. There is some evidence that it may have a role in tumours of >8 mm in depth. Patients with recurrent thick (>4 mm) lesions in the vicinity of the parotid (temple, forehead and preauricular area) may also be considered for elective nodal treatment.

Radiotherapy

Principles of primary radiotherapy and treatment guidelines are same as that of BCC (Boxes 14.3 and 14.4). 5-year control rate with radiotherapy is comparable with surgery with >93% for T1 lesions, 65–85% with T2 and 50–60% with T3–4 lesions. Radiotherapy is indicated after incomplete excision when further surgery is not contemplated, as incomplete excision leads to 50% local recurrence.

Postoperative radiotherapy to the primary tumour site is considered for patients with high risk disease after complete excision. High risk disease includes: tumour invasion beyond subcutaneous tissue (T4), recurrent disease, margin <5 mm, perineural invasion (major or minor nerve), lymphovascular invasion, in-transit metastases and nodal metastasis. Indications for postoperative radiotherapy after primary surgical management of metastatic lymph nodes are:

- ≥3 cm node.
- ≥2 positive nodes in neck and ≥3 nodes in axilla and groin.
- Extranodal extension.
- Close or positive margin.
- Skin involvement.
- Major nerve involvement.
- Parotid node metastases.
- After salvage surgery for recurrent nodal metastases.

The role of postoperative chemo-radiotherapy for high risk SCC is being evaluated. Palliative radiotherapy is used in metastatic disease to obtain symptom relief.

Chemotherapy

In patients with distant metastasis from SCC, cisplatin based chemotherapy is the most effective regime. A commonly used combination is cisplatin with adriamycin, which has an overall response rate of >80% with complete response rate of 30%. However, survival is generally less than 2 years.

Recurrence

Most recurrences occur within 2–3 years. Treatment is individualized based on the extent of recurrence and previous treatment.

Prognostic factors

- Grade of differentiation – grade 3–4 lesions are twice as likely to recur and three times as likely to metastasize than grade 1–2 lesions.
- Histologic type – spindle cell carcinoma and adenosquamous carcinoma have high risk of recurrence and metastasis.
- Location of tumour – scalp, lips, pinna, nose and genital lesions have a high risk of metastasis.
- Tumour size – risk of recurrence and metastasis increases with size of the tumour. Risk of recurrence is twice (15% vs. 7%) and risk of metastasis is three-fold (30% vs. 9%) in tumours >2 cm compared with tumours of <2 cm.
- Depth of invasion – tumours with depth <2 mm seldom metastasize whereas those with >4 mm have high risk of recurrence and metastasis.
- Perineural invasion – occurs in 2.5% of tumours and its presence indicates a high risk of local recurrence (up to 50%) and distant metastasis (up to 35%).
- After lymphadenectomy, prognosis depends on number of positive nodes and presence of extranodal spread.
- Recurrence – local recurrence increases rate for further recurrence (25%) and lymph node metastasis (30%).
- Tumours in immunosuppressant patients and those arising from scars have a poor prognosis.

Outcome

Local control rate for SCC is 10–15% lower than a similarly sized BCC.

Bowen's disease (in situ SCC)

Presents as a slow-growing erythematous plaque. Surgery, topical treatment and radiotherapy are the options of treatment. Radiotherapy involves 40–50 Gy in 10–20 fractions using 100–150 kV superficial X-rays resulting in 95–100% local control.

Keratoacanthoma

Presents as a rapidly enlarging lesion with central keratin plug. Histologically, it is difficult to distinguish this from SCC. In up to 20% of patients spontaneous regression can occur over 6–12 weeks. Treatment options include early excision and radiotherapy (similar to SCC).

Squamous cell carcinoma of lip

Lesions involving <30% of lip can be treated with wedge excision and repair. When >30% of the lip is involved, surgery results in functional disability and hence radiotherapy is a treatment option. Treatment is with orthovoltage X-rays or electrons with an intraoral lead shield to protect the mandible or teeth or by implantation. Typical radiation dose is 50–55 Gy in 20–25 fractions.

Merkel cell carcinoma

Introduction

Merkel cell carcinoma (MCC) is a rare aggressive neuroendocrine tumour of the skin. The exact aetiology is not known. The reported risk factors include ultraviolet exposure, previous skin cancers and haematological malignancies, immunosuppression and HIV infection. The average age at presentation is 69 years. Males are more commonly affected.

Pathology

Histologically these are small blue cell neoplasms which express neuroendocrine and cytokeratin markers.

Clinical features

MCC present as red or violaceous nodules with a shiny surface, often with overlying telangiectasia (Figure 14.4). Spread through dermal lymphatics can result in the development of satellite lesions. The most common site of disease is the head and neck region, followed by extremities and trunk. One-third of patients have regional nodal metastases at presentation and 50%

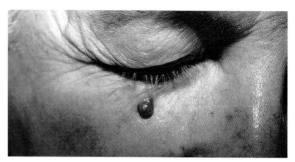

Figure 14.4
Merkel cell carcinoma. From Darrell Rigel: Cancer of the Skin (Saunders) with permission.

develop distant metastasis. Liver, lung, bone and brain are the sites of distant metastases.

Diagnosis and staging

Initial evaluation includes clinical examination of the whole skin surface and regional nodes. Imaging includes CT scan of the relevant nodal region as well as chest and liver. Blood tests include full blood count and biochemistry.

70–80% patients present with local disease (stage IA ≤2 cm and IB >2 cm), 10–30% with regional nodal disease (stage II) and 1–4% with distant metastasis (stage III).

Treatment

Stage I disease is usually treated with wide excision of the primary tumour (2.5–3 cm margin) and sentinel node biopsy. All patients receive postoperative radiotherapy to the primary site with a generous margin of 3–5 cm (to ensure dermal lymphatics are treated). Regional lymph nodes are generally treated electively due to the high risk of recurrence (46–76%) when nodes are not treated. Radiotherapy dose ranges from 45–60 Gy using 1.8–2 Gy per fraction. The role of adjuvant chemotherapy is unknown. Recent studies indicate that primary radiotherapy (60 Gy) is an appropriate alternative which yields a better cosmesis.

Stage II disease is treated with surgery of the primary lesion and nodal dissection. All patients receive postoperative radiotherapy (50–60 Gy). Adjuvant chemotherapy may be considered. Chemotherapy regime mirrors those used for small cell lung cancer.

Stage III disease has a median survival of 9 months. Platinum based chemotherapy yields a short lived complete response of 44% and partial response of 11%.

Prognosis

Stage is an important prognostic factor. The median survival of node negative patients is 40 months whereas that of node positive patients is 11 months. Other poor prognostic factors include tumour >2 cm, age >60 years and lack of adjuvant radiotherapy.

Skin adnexal carcinoma

Skin adnexal carcinomas are eccrine and apocrine sweat gland carcinomas, sebaceous gland carcinoma and microcystic adnexal carcinoma. These represent 0.2% of skin cancers and usually exhibit aggressive behaviour and local recurrence. There are a number of histological subtypes.

Eccrine sweat gland carcinoma is common in the head and neck region, trunk and extremities and apocrine carcinoma is common in the axilla. These tumours exhibit an initial indolent growth followed by rapid progression including distant metastasis. Surgery is the treatment of choice which involves wide excision and elective lymph node dissection. Postoperative radiotherapy is advisable in the presence of tumour of >5 cm, deep infiltration, close (<1 mm) or positive margin, high-grade tumours, perineural infiltration, dermal lymphatic invasion, ≥4 positive nodes and extranodal invasion. Radiotherapy management is same as that of SCC.

Sebaceous carcinoma commonly occurs in the upper lid, scalp or face and is common in women. Surgery is the treatment of choice; either wide excision or Mohs' micrographic surgery. Radiotherapy may be indicated for high risk patients such as those with a positive margin and extensive nodal involvement. However, the risk of potential damage to ocular structures needs to be considered. Elderly patients may be treated with primary radiotherapy delivering >55 Gy. 36% patients develop local recurrence and 20–25% patients die of this cancer.

Microcystic adnexal carcinoma is a locally destructive carcinoma often present as a sclerotic or indurated plaque with an intact dermis. The usual sites of involvement are mid face and lip. Wide local excision or Mohs' surgery is the treatment of choice. Surgery is associated with a local recurrence of 50–60%. These are thought to be radioresistant tumours.

Cutaneous lymphoma

The role of radiotherapy is essentially palliative in cutaneous lymphoma, the exceptions being primary cutaneous B cell lymphoma (CBCL) and selected patients with cutaneous T-cell lymphoma especially mycosis fungoides. In CBCL, radiotherapy of 36–40 Gy results in an 85–100% control rate. Selected patients with mycosis fungoides can be treated with total skin electron radiotherapy to a dose of 36 Gy over 9 weeks. This is a complex treatment and is only possible in specialist centres.

Kaposi's sarcoma

See p. 295.

Further reading

Garbe C, Peris K, Hauschild A et al. Diagnosis and treatment of melanoma: European consensus-based interdisciplinary guideline. Eur J Cancer. 2010;46:270–283.

Mouawad R, Sebert M, Michels J et al. Treatment for metastatic malignant melanoma: old drugs and new strategies. Crit Rev Oncol Hematol. 2010;74:27–39.

Thompson JF, Scolyer RA, Kefford RF. Cutaneous melanoma in the era of molecular profiling. Lancet. 2009;374:362–365.

Miller AJ, Mihm MC Jr. Melanoma. N Engl J Med. 2006;355:51–65.

Telfer NR, Colver GB, Morton CA. Guidelines for the management of basal cell carcinoma. Br J Dermatol. 2008;159:35–48.

Veness MJ. The important role of radiotherapy in patients with non-melanoma skin cancer and other cutaneous entities. J Med Imaging Radiat Oncol. 2008;52:278–286.

Neville JA, Welch E, Leffell DJ. Management of nonmelanoma skin cancer in 2007. Nat Clin Pract Oncol. 2007;4:462–469.

Rockville Merkel Cell Carcinoma Group. Merkel cell carcinoma: recent progress and current priorities on etiology, pathogenesis, and clinical management. J Clin Oncol. 2009;27:4021–4026.

Eng TY, Boersma MG, Fuller CD et al. A comprehensive review of the treatment of Merkel cell carcinoma. Am J Clin Oncol. 2007;30:624–636.

Senff NJ, Noordijk EM, Kim YH et al. European Organization for Research and Treatment of Cancer and International Society for Cutaneous Lymphoma consensus recommendations for the management of cutaneous B-cell lymphomas. Blood. 2008;112:1600–1609.

Willemze R, Dreyling M. Primary cutaneous lymphoma: ESMO clinical recommendations for diagnosis, treatment and follow-up. Ann Oncol. 2009;20 Suppl 4:115–118.

Cancers of the musculoskeletal system

HM Hatcher and TV Ajithkumar

Overview

Cancers of the musculoskeletal system or sarcomas can be divided into primary tumours of bone and soft tissue sarcomas. Each of these can be subdivided into specific subgroups. This results in a large number of tumours which are often grouped together, but which have different responses to treatment. Due to their rarity, sarcomas should be treated in a centre with appropriate expertise.

Primary bone tumours

Epidemiology and incidence

Primary malignant tumours of bone are rare. The most common subtypes are osteosarcoma, the Ewing's family of tumours and chondrosarcoma.

In the UK, osteosarcoma accounts for up to 35% of all primary bone tumours. There are two peaks of incidence: in those aged 15–19 and a smaller second peak occurs over the age of 65 associated with Paget's disease.

Ewing's sarcomas and their soft tissue counterpart, primitive neuroectodermal tumour (PNET), are the second most common bone malignancy. The median age at diagnosis is 14 although they can occur at any age. There is a male predominance with a 1.5:1 male:female ratio.

Chondrosarcomas comprise less than 12% bone tumours and are the third most common malignant bone tumour. It is common over the age of 40 with the peak incidence in those over the age of 70.

Aetiology

Most primary bone tumours arise spontaneously without a predisposing risk factor. However for each subgroup there are recognized risk factors.

For osteosarcoma the most important risk factor is prior radiotherapy which accounts for only 3% of cases, with a time interval of 14 years (range 4–40 years). It is the most common secondary malignancy following treatment for childhood cancer. Other factors include chemotherapy with alkylating agents, Paget's disease, chronic osteomyelitis, and hereditary conditions such as hereditary retinoblastoma and Li–Fraumeni syndrome (p. 53, 55). In hereditary retinoblastoma, the relative risk (RR) of osteosarcoma is 500 for limb osteosarcomas and 2000 for skull osteosarcomas following irradiation for retinoblastoma. Li–Fraumeni syndrome patients have a RR of 15 for osteosarcoma at all sites.

There are few risk factors for Ewing's sarcoma but treatment for a primary cancer in childhood is a known association.

For chondrosarcoma, there is an increased risk is those with hereditary multiple exostosis or enchondromatosis syndromes, in whom it tends to present at an earlier age.

Pathogenesis

Ewing's tumours consistently have reciprocal chromosomal translocations, usually between the EWS gene on chromosome 22 and FLI-1 on chromosome 11. In 85% of cases this is t(11;22)

Box 15.1: Clinical features seen in many types of bone tumour

- Localized bone pain, usually present for several months
- Pain at night or at rest
- In some cases localized swelling and overlying erythema
- Often a previous injury to the region has been noted and can result in delay in diagnosis

In advanced disease systemic symptoms may be present. These include

- fever
- weight loss and
- lethargy

(q24;q12). Other variants place EWS with other genes such as t(21;22)(q22;q12) EWS-ERG translocation which occurs in up to 10%.

Unlike Ewing's sarcomas there are no characteristic chromosomal translocations in osteosarcomas, although loss of heterozygosity in the regions of both the retinoblastoma gene and p53 have been described. A significant number of osteosarcomas express insulin-like growth factor receptor-1 (IGFR-1) which is being explored as a therapeutic target.

Clinical features

There are some features which are common to many types of bone tumour (Box 15.1).

Systemic symptoms occur more often in Ewing's sarcoma than any other bone sarcoma. Ewing's sarcomas which can have a significant soft tissue component may be mistaken for infection and can also occur in areas of long standing infection. These factors can also lead to significant delays which can impact on the prognosis and psychological impact for the patient.

Diagnosis

An X-ray of the affected area may be suggestive of a diagnosis but a diagnostic biopsy is required to make an accurate diagnosis and direct further treatment. A biopsy should only be performed by a specialist sarcoma surgeon who will take into account possible future surgery and will minimize the risks of tumour spread to the skin or adjacent structures. Fine needle biopsies are not suitable for primary diagnosis but can be used to confirm metastatic disease. The biopsy tract is often marked by clips to ensure it is removed at the time of definitive surgery.

Due to the consistency of chromosomal translocations in Ewing's tumours these are used in diagnosis, either with cytogenetics, FISH or PCR.

Staging

Adequate staging includes optimal imaging of the primary site (MRI) and the entire bone to exclude intra-medullary skip metastases, which occur in osteosarcomas and Ewing's tumours. A CT scan of the chest should be done to assess for possible pulmonary metastases. For PNETs arising in the lower half of the body a CT of the pelvis and abdomen can be considered as there may be lymph node involvement. A bone scintigram, or in some centres a CT-PET, will assess for bone metastases. A whole body MRI on STIR sequence has shown to be effective in detection of bone metastases which may not be visible with other forms of imaging, particularly in Ewing's tumours. A bone marrow aspirate should be performed in patients with a Ewing's tumour to exclude bone marrow involvement. Staging is according to the AJCC bone tumour staging (Table 15.1).

Patients should also undergo investigations which will be relevant to the further management of their individual sarcoma. LDH has prognostic value in Ewing's tumours and ALP in osteosarcomas.

Principles of surgical management in bone tumours

Complete surgical resection of the tumour by specialist sarcoma orthopaedic surgeons is required for the best outcome. Surgery is the major component of management in chondrosarcomas but is also essential for local control in Ewing's and osteosarcomas. Limb sparing surgery has evolved significantly in the past 30 years such that amputation is used less often and should be avoided if possible. Extending endoprostheses have also been developed to minimize the number of surgeries a growing child or young adult may require.

Osteosarcoma

Several subtypes of osteosarcoma exist. Over 90% are high-grade intramedullary tumours,

Table 15.1: AJCC 2002 TNM staging for primary bone tumours

Primary tumour (T)	
TX	Primary tumour cannot be assessed
T0	No evidence of primary tumour
T1	Tumour 8 cm or less in greatest dimension
T2	Tumour more than 8 cm in greatest dimension
T3	Discontinuous tumours (skip lesions) in the primary bone site

Regional lymph nodes (N)	
NX	Regional lymph nodes cannot be assessed
N0	No regional lymph node metastasis
N1	Regional lymph node metastasis

Distant metastasis (M)	
MX	Distant metastasis cannot be assessed
M0	No distant metastasis
M1	Distant metastasis
M1a	Lung
M1b	Other distant sites

Histological grade (G)	
GX	Grade cannot be assessed
G1	Well-differentiated – low-grade
G2	Moderately differentiated – low-grade
G3	Poorly differentiated – high-grade
G4	Undifferentiated – high-grade

Note: Ewing's sarcoma is classified as G4

Stage grouping				
Stage IA	T1	N0	M0	G1, 2 Low-grade
Stage IB	T2	N0	M0	G1, 2 Low-grade
Stage IIA	T1	N0	M0	G3, 4 High-grade
Stage IIB	T2	N0	M0	G3, 4 High-grade
Stage III	T3	N0	M0	Any G
Stage IVA	Any T	N0	M1a	Any G
Stage IVB	Any T	N1	Any M	Any G
	Any T	Any N	M1b	Any G

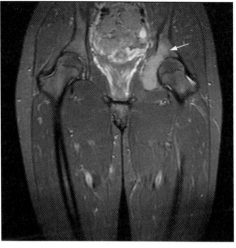

Figure 15.1
Coronal MRI of pelvis and thighs showing osteosarcoma of the left acetabulum (arrow). Note the change in bone texture compared with the normal side.

half of which are osteoblastic and the other half are split equally between fibroblastic and chondroblastic osteosarcomas. The remaining 10% are made up of small subgroups including telangiectatic osteosarcoma, extraosseous osteosarcoma, juxtacortical osteosarcoma and malignant fibrous histiocytoma of bone which is treated in the same way as intramedullary osteosarcoma.

Figures 15.1 and 15.2 show imaging features of osteosarcoma. Box 15.2 shows prognostic factors in osteosarcoma. An overview of management is shown in Figure 15.3.

Localized osteosarcoma

Localized osteosarcoma is treated with neoadjuvant chemotherapy followed by surgery (Figure 15.4) and adjuvant chemotherapy.

Chemotherapy
Prior to the 1980s all patients with apparently localized disease had surgery (usually amputation) but only 20–30% survived over 5 years. Most died of disseminated disease suggesting the presence of micrometastases in apparently early disease. A pivotal study showed that giving adjuvant chemotherapy improved survival from 17% to 66%, and neoadjuvant chemotherapy was subsequently implemented. The most frequently used drugs are cisplatin and doxorubicin. Methotrexate at doses up to 12 g/m² is used in

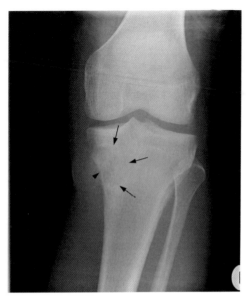

Figure 15.2
X-ray of left knee showing characteristic features of an osteosarcoma of the medial proximal tibia with bone destruction due to an expansile lesion (arrows) and periosteal elevation (arrow head). (Courtesy of Mr Rob Grimer, Royal National Orthopaedic Hospital, Birmingham.)

Box 15.2: Factors predicting a poor prognosis

- Age <14 years or >40 years
- Poor response (<90% necrosis) to neoadjuvant chemotherapy
- Pathological fracture
- Large tumour volume, which is also associated with lung metastases
- Metastases at presentation with bone metastases having a worse prognosis than lung metastases
- Primary tumours which are axial or extraosseous. Secondary osteosarcoma
- Raised ALP or LDH
- Increased cadherin 11 expression

---

addition to cisplatin and doxorubicin in younger patients and has been found to increase tumour necrosis. The degree of tumour necrosis after neoadjuvant chemotherapy is of prognostic value. Less than 90% necrosis is associated with a poorer prognosis. Whether prognosis can be improved by changing chemotherapy after surgery is one of the roles of the international EURAMOS trial.

Box 15.3: Chemotherapy for metastatic osteosarcoma

- In younger patients: cisplatin, doxorubicin and methotrexate (PAM)
- In older patients the methotrexate is often omitted due to increased toxicity
- If the patient has relapsed with metastases within 1–2 years of original treatment, ifosfamide with or without etoposide can be effective
- High-dose methotrexate with folinic acid rescue can be effective if previously treatment was with cisplatin and doxorubicin alone

---

Recently a study with the bacterial cell wall mimic muramyl tripeptide (MTP) when added to combination chemotherapy showed an improvement in 6-year survival to 78% in primary osteosarcomas.

Radiotherapy

Radiotherapy is markedly inferior to surgical resection of the primary tumour for osteosarcomas in terms of overall survival but has been used in patients who decline or who are unable to have surgery.

Metastatic osteosarcoma

In one study 11.4% osteosarcoma patients had metastases at the time of presentation. Metastases can occur in the lungs, bone and bone marrow. Lymph node and brain metastases are exceptionally rare. Isolated pulmonary metastases have the best prognosis and bone metastases the worst prognosis. Overall survival at 5 years ranges from 10–50%. Up to 30% of patients with lung metastases survive over 10 years with a combination of surgery, combination chemotherapy and occasionally radiotherapy. Although the chance of cure is small, patients particularly with limited and potentially resectable lung metastases should be treated aggressively with chemotherapy and surgery.

Chemotherapy

As in the adjuvant setting, the most effective agents are cisplatin, doxorubicin, methotrexate and ifosfamide (Box 15.3). Response rates are between 20–40% although some tumours and metastases may not reduce in size. Apparent calcification of lung metastases can occur (Figure 15.5). If the presentation is with metastases,

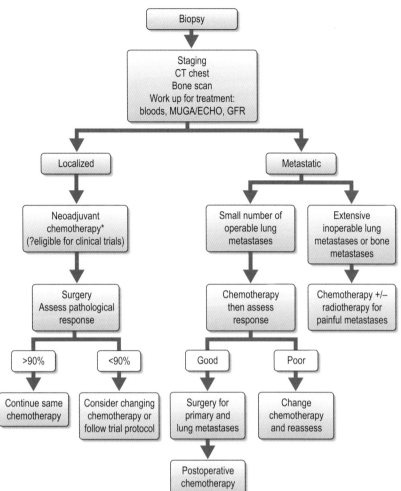

Figure 15.3
Management of osteosarcoma.

* Neoadjuvant chemotherapy PAM (cisplatin, doxorubicin and methotrexate) for young fit patients and cisplatin/doxorubicin for older patients

combination chemotherapy should be the primary treatment.

High-dose treatment with stem cell rescue has shown no improvement in survival. Trials are underway to evaluate biological agents such as insulin like growth factor 1 receptor (IGF1-R) antagonists. Immunotherapy may have a role and the use of liposomal muramyl tripeptide-phosphatidyl-ethanolamine has been shown to produce a survival benefit in the adjuvant setting.

Surgery

Surgery in the metastatic setting should either be aimed at palliation of symptoms, e.g. resection of a large primary extremity tumour with low volume lung metastases, or with the intention of cure, e.g. resection of lung metastases.

Radiotherapy

Although osteosarcomas are relatively radio resistant tumours, radiotherapy has been successfully used in a number of clinical situations such as to control bone pain. It has also been used in addition to chemotherapy and surgery, e.g. following resection of lung metastases some groups advocate whole lung radiotherapy in addition to chemotherapy. It may provide local control for some patients with advanced metastatic disease for whom resection of the primary is inappropriate.

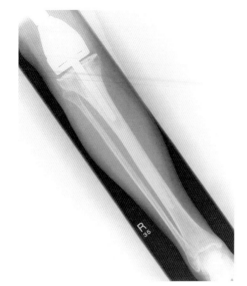

Figure 15.4
X-ray of knee showing endoprosthetic replacement for osteosarcoma of the right tibia.

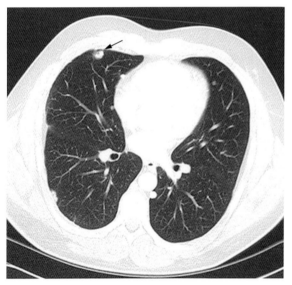

Figure 15.5
Axial CT of chest showing pleurally based and calcified metastases characteristic of osteosarcoma (arrow). These lung metastases can bleed giving rise to bloody pleural effusions.

Recurrent osteosarcoma

Approximately 40% of patients treated with a primary osteosarcoma will recur either locally or with metastatic disease. Management of local recurrence can involve chemotherapy, surgery or

> **Box 15.4: Poor prognostic factors in Ewing's sarcoma**
> - Age over 14 years
> - Metastases at presentation (especially non-pulmonary metastases)
> - Pelvic or axial primary site
> - Size greater than 8 cm
> - Raised LDH

radiotherapy. Chemotherapy drugs are the same as those used for metastatic disease. Surgery may be possible but limb sparing surgery is less likely for local recurrence of extremity tumours. Radiotherapy may be useful for local control but is less effective than surgery.

Ewing's sarcoma

Presentation

Unlike osteosarcomas which present most often in the epiphyses of long bones, Ewing's sarcomas occur within the diaphysis and are often associated with a soft tissue mass. The soft tissue reaction may be confused for infection and contribute to delay in diagnosis. The median delay from symptoms (Box 15.1) to diagnosis is 6–9 months. The most common sites are long bones (53%) or the axial skeleton (47%). 25% have a soft tissue primary. Systemic symptoms (fever, anorexia, weight loss, and lethargy) may be present and are associated with advanced disease. 25% patients have metastases at presentation. Subclinical metastases are present in 80–90% with apparently localized disease, necessitating multimodality treatment even in apparently small volume localized disease. Prognostic factors are listed in Box 15.4.

X-ray may show a characteristic destructive lesion within the bone with surrounding periosteal reaction known as an onion skin appearance (Figure 15.6). A soft tissue reaction may also be seen on X-ray and a pathological fracture is seen in 15%. Ewing's sarcomas, like osteosarcomas, show intense tracer uptake in bone scan (Figure 15.7). Staging is given in Table 15.1 and Figure 15.8 shows an overview of management.

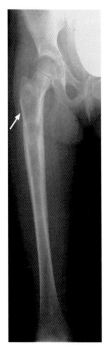

Figure 15.6
X-ray of Ewing's sarcoma of right proximal femur with destructive lesion and onion skin appearance of periosteal reaction. Courtesy of Mr Rob Grimer.

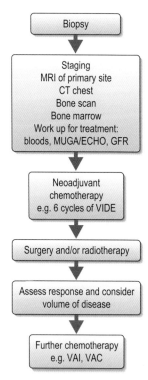

Figure 15.8
Management of Ewing's sarcomas (VIDE – vincristine, ifosfamide, doxorubicin & etoposide; VAI – vincristine, actinomycin-D & ifosfamide; VAC – vincristine, actinomycin-D & cyclophosphamide).

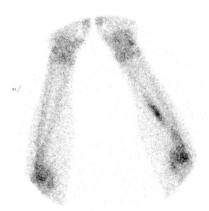

Figure 15.7
Bone scintigram of Ewing's sarcoma of left proximal radius showing localized uptake at the site of the tumour.

Management of localized disease

Chemotherapy

Combination chemotherapy is usually given pre- and postoperatively. Alkylating agents have the highest response rate and have been combined with doxorubicin, vincristine, actinomycin D and etoposide. Trials such as IESS-III showed that alternating ifosfamide and etoposide with vincristine, doxorubicin and cyclophosphamide (VAC) improved survival from 54 to 69% in localized disease. High-dose treatment in localized low-risk disease has not been shown to improve survival. Response to chemotherapy at the time of surgery reflects prognosis.

Stratifying treatment according to risk is under investigation in the EUROEWING99 trial (Figure 15.9). Low-risk patients are randomized between standard treatment and less intense treatment. High-risk/metastatic patients are randomized between standard treatment and high-dose with stem cell rescue.

Surgery

Surgery is performed if possible after neoadjuvant chemotherapy to assess response and reduce risk of relapse. Pelvic tumours are the most difficult to resect, especially if they involve the sacrum, due to the risk of sacral nerve involvement.

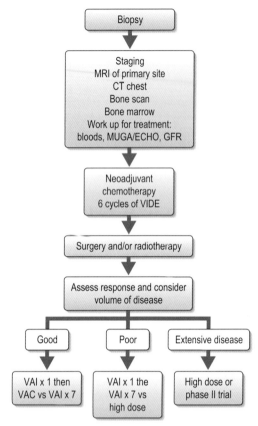

Figure 15.9
Management of Ewing's sarcoma Euro Ewing 99 Protocol.

Radiotherapy

Unlike osteosarcomas, Ewing's tumours are radio-sensitive and, radiotherapy used to be the principle method of achieving disease control. Studies have shown radiotherapy without surgery has a worse outcome than surgery for local control but there may be some selection bias. However, radiotherapy still remains a primary method of local control in unresectable tumours when doses of 45–55 Gy have been used (Box 15.5).

Management of metastatic disease

Some patients with limited pulmonary metastases at presentation may still be cured with combination treatment.

Chemotherapy

The same combination chemotherapy agents are used in advanced disease as in localized disease.

Surgery

Surgery of the primary lesion may still be appropriate with limited pulmonary metastases if these respond to initial chemotherapy. Surgery may also be necessary for local control, especially if highly symptomatic.

Radiotherapy

Radiotherapy can be used to treat either the primary tumour or metastatic lesions in advanced disease. The dose (radical or palliative) used for the primary will depend on the extent of other disease. Bilateral low-dose lung radiotherapy can be used as an adjunct to chemotherapy for patients with lung metastases who have had a good response to treatment. Unilateral lung irradiation is used for symptomatic bulky chest wall lesions. Palliative radiotherapy is used for painful bony metastases.

Prognosis of Ewing's sarcoma

Prognosis in localized disease has improved significantly since the introduction of chemotherapy. Poor prognostic features are listed in Box 15.4. With combination chemotherapy and surgery or radiotherapy 5-year survival is 70%. With limited lung metastases and treatment with chemotherapy plus surgery or radiotherapy 5-year survival of 20–40% can be expected. With more extensive disease 5-year survival falls to less than 25%.

Recurrent Ewing's sarcoma

Recurrence usually occurs within the first 2–5 years and the prognosis for these patients is poor. Relapse after 5–10 years is associated with a survival similar to that of advanced disease at presentation.

After 10 years very few patients relapse but it does occur. Treatment depends on the nature of relapse (local/systemic), nature of initial chemotherapy and time from the end of primary treatment. Isolated lung metastases after a long treatment interval may be suitable for surgical resection and further chemotherapy. To date high-dose regimens remain experimental in this group. The type of chemotherapy depends on the initial regimen but high-dose ifosfamide with etoposide has shown some activity. Trials of new agents such as insulin growth factor 1 receptor antagonists are underway.

Box 15.5: Radiotherapy in sarcomas

Indications
- Radical radiotherapy – inoperable Ewing's sarcoma
- Postoperative adjuvant – deep, >5 cm or high-grade soft tissue sarcoma. Positive margins and further surgery is not contemplated. Local recurrence after a repeated resection
- Preoperative – soft tissue sarcoma and Ewing's sarcoma progress during chemotherapy
- Palliative radiotherapy
- Whole lung radiotherapy – Ewing's sarcoma with lung metastases and good response to chemotherapy

Position & immobilization – depends on site of tumour

Tumour localization – with CT scan or co-registered CT/MRI

Clinical target volume
- Ewing's sarcoma:
  - Long bones – pre-treatment tumour with 5 cm margin superoinferior and 2 cm axial for phase 1 and 2 cm margin for phase II. Whole bone if extensive intramedullary involvement with sparing of epiphyseal plate
  - Flat bones and soft tissue – pre-treatment tumour with 2 cm circumferential
  - Pelvis and chest wall – post-chemotherapy residual volume in areas of non-infiltrative tumour near critical organs with 2 cm margin
- Soft tissue sarcoma
  - CTV – surgical bed and possible areas of spread with 5 cm margin supero-interiorly and 2 cm circumferentially for phase I and 2 cm margin for phase II. Include scars and biopsy sites

Planning target volume – 5–10 mm to CTV depending on immobilization

Dose
- Ewing's tumour – 54.4 Gy in 30 fractions in two phases
- Soft tissue sarcoma – Phase I and preoperative 50 Gy in 25 fractions; phase II: 10–14 Gy in 5–7 fractions
- Whole lung radiotherapy for Ewing's sarcoma – 15–18 Gy as 1.5 Gy per fraction per day

Special notes
- Keep radiation dose to the critical organs near an area being treated within the tolerance.
- Always leave a strip of skin unirradiated over the limbs to avoid fibrosis.
- If joints are in the treatment volume keep dose below <45 Gy.

Chondrosarcoma

The most common sites are pelvis (Figures 15.10 and 15.11), axial skeleton and proximal limbs. As with other bone tumours axial tumours have a worse prognosis than extremity tumours. It presents with a mass which may be painful or painless or with symptoms due to local disease. Systemic symptoms are rare. Diagnosis may be suggested from plain X-rays but MRI should be undertaken for suspected sarcomas.

Chondrosarcomas frequently exhibit calcification. MRI can also assess soft tissue extension. The lesion often has a cauliflower appearance. 5-year survival is over 90% for a localized grade 1 (well-differentiated) tumour but reduces to 25% for a grade 3 (poorly differentiated) tumour.

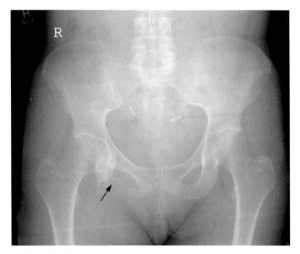

Figure 15.10
X-ray of pelvis showing destructive lesion around right pubic ramus (arrow).

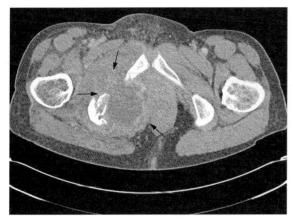

Figure 15.11
T1 weighted MRI of same patient showing extensive chondrosarcoma (arrows) with some calcification and soft tissue extension either side of the pubic ramus.

The primary modality of treatment is surgery. Chemotherapy and radiotherapy have limited role except for palliation.

Giant cell tumours of bone

These represent less than 5% of primary bone tumours and only around 10% are malignant and 5% develop lung metastases. Malignant tumours are usually secondary to radiotherapy. The most frequently affected sites are distal femur, proximal tibia and distal radius. Presentation is usually due to pain which increases with activity. Typical radiological feature is an expansile lytic lesion (soap bubble appearance) near the epiphysis. MRI is used to assess soft tissue and intramedullary extension. Staging should include chest CT due to possibility of lung metastases. A bone scintigram will show increased tracer uptake in the region of the tumour. Giant cell tumours have a different staging system.

Surgery is the most effective treatment but complete resection without leaving a residual deficit in the bone is often difficult. Adding bone cement to the bone graft may reduce the risk of recurrence from 45% to less than 30%. Additional local treatments include cryotherapy. Embolization is often used prior to surgery, especially for sacral tumours, to prevent excessive blood loss at the time of surgery. Radiotherapy can be used for these tumours but there is a risk of secondary malignancy.

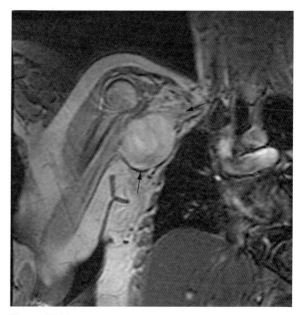

Figure 15.12
Coronal MRI showing MPNST of right brachial plexus (arrows) in a patient with NF1.

Soft tissue sarcomas

Soft tissue sarcomas (STS) represent a collection of heterogeneous tumours characterized by the malignant growth of mesenchymal tissue. The different subgroups can be divided by genetics, pathology, anatomical location and clinical behaviour.

STS comprise less than 1% of malignant tumours and the median age at presentation depends on histological subtype.

Aetiology

The majority of cases arise de novo. Known predisposing factors include familial cancer syndromes, prior radiotherapy and/or chemotherapy, chronic lymphoedema or infection. Familial cancer syndromes include Li–Fraumeni, hereditary retinoblastoma and familial GIST tumours. Malignant peripheral nerve sheath tumours (MPNST) are more common in neurofibromatosis due to inherited mutations in NF1 associated with a 10% lifetime risk of MPNST (Figure 15.12). Desmoid tumours and aggressive fibromatosis occur in those with APC gene mutations associated with familial adenomatous polyposis.

Pathology

There are over 80 subtypes of soft tissue sarcoma. The most common are leiomyosarcoma, liposarcoma, synovial sarcoma, rhabdomyosarcoma, fibrosarcomas (several subtypes), and malignant peripheral nerve sheath tumour. Many soft tissue sarcomas are characterized and classified according to specific translocations and gene rearrangements (Box 15.6).

Presenting features

Presentation depends on the stage and site of disease as well as the histological subtype of sarcoma. The majority of soft tissue masses will be benign but risk factors for malignancy include

Box 15.6: Examples of soft tissue sarcomas which have characteristic chromosomal translocations

Translocations associated with sarcomas

Translocation	Genes	Type of fusion gene
Ewing's family of tumours		
t(11;22)(q24;q12)	EWSR1-FLI1	Transcription factor
t(21;22)(q22;q12)	EWSR1-ERG	Transcription factor
t(7;22)(p22;q12)	EWSR1-ETV1	Transcription factor
t(17;22)(q21;q12)	EWSR1-ETV4	Transcription factor
t(2;22)(q33;q12)	EWSR1-FEV	Transcription factor
Clear-cell sarcoma		
t(12;22)(q13;q12)	EWS-ATF1	Transcription factor
Desmoplastic small round-cell tumour		
t(11;22)(p13;q12)	EWSR1-WT1	Transcription factor
Myxoid chondrosarcoma		
t(9;22) (q22-31;q11-12)	EWSR1-NR4A3	Transcription factor
Myxoid liposarcoma		
t(12;16)(q13;p11)	FUS-CHOP	Transcription factor
t(12;22)(q13;q12)	EWSR1-CHOP	Transcription factor
Alveolar rhabdomyosarcoma		
t(2;13)(q35;q14)	PAX3-FKHR	Transcription factor
t(1;13)(p36;q14)	PAX7-FKHR	Transcription factor
Synovial sarcoma		
t(X;18)(p11;q11)	SYT-SSX	Transcription factor

size >5 cm, deep to the deep fascia, rapid growth and pain. Systemic symptoms (fever, weight loss, anorexia, breathlessness) may be present in advanced disease, particularly if associated with extensive chest disease.

Diagnosis

Correct diagnosis requires an adequate biopsy which, like bone tumours, should not compromise later surgery. Samples should be sent to microbiology if infection is suspected. Pathology should be reviewed by an experienced sarcoma pathologist. Due to the difficulty of diagnosis even with immunohistochemistry, specialist techniques such as cytogenetics and polymerase chain reaction (PCR) may also be necessary to identify translocation specific sarcomas.

Staging

Staging should include evaluation of the primary tumour and a CT of the chest to exclude lung metastases. In certain rare subgroups (rhabdomyosarcoma, synovial sarcoma, clear cell and epithelioid sarcomas) nodal disease may occur so regional CT scanning may be appropriate. The role of bone scintigraphy is less established in soft tissue sarcomas than bone sarcomas. PET has not been fully evaluated (except for GIST) in soft tissue sarcomas. Several staging systems exist, one of the most frequently used is AJCC (Table 15.2) which does not include histology and site, and should not be used for non-extremity sarcomas.

General management principles of soft tissue sarcoma

The overall management is shown in Figure 15.13.

Localized disease

Surgery

Resection has to extend beyond the tumour to a wide margin as an involved resection margin is the most important factor which predicts risk of recurrence. Margins have to be defined in terms of compartments and fascial or skin borders as well as distance. Surgery should be discussed within a sarcoma multidisciplinary team to ensure morbidity is minimized with the use of radiotherapy if required.

Table 15.2: AJCC staging system for soft tissue sarcomas. This uses four criteria of tumour size, nodal status, grade, and metastasis (TNGM)

Grade and TNM definitions		Grade and TNM definitions	
Tumour grade (G)		*AJCC Stage Groupings*	
GX	Grade cannot be assessed	Stage I	
G1	Well differentiated	Stage I tumour is defined as low-grade, superficial, and deep	
G2	Moderately differentiated		
G3	Poorly differentiated	G1, T1a, N0, M0	
G4	Poorly differentiated or undifferentiated	G1, T1b, N0, M0	
Primary tumour (T)		G1, T2a, N0, M0	
		G1, T2b, N0, M0	
TX	Primary tumour cannot be assessed	G2, T1a, N0, M0	
T0	No evidence of primary tumour	G2, T1b, N0, M0	
T1	Tumour 5 cm or less in greatest dimension:	G2, T2a, N0, M0	
	• T1a: Superficial tumour • T1b: Deep tumour	G2, T2b, N0, M0	
		Stage II	
T2	Tumour 5 cm or larger in greatest dimension:	Stage II tumour is defined as high-grade, superficial, and deep	
	• T2a: Superficial tumour • T2b: Deep tumour	G3, T1a, N0, M0	
		G3, T1b, N0, M0	
[Note: Superficial tumour is located exclusively above the superficial fascia without invasion of the fascia; deep tumour is located either exclusively beneath the superficial fascia, or superficial to the fascia with invasion of or through the fascia, or both superficial yet beneath the fascia. Retroperitoneal, mediastinal, and pelvic sarcomas are classified as deep tumours.]		G3, T2a, N0, M0	
		G4, T1a, N0, M0	
		G4, T1b, N0, M0	
		G4, T2a, N0, M0	
		Stage III	
Regional lymph nodes (N)		Stage III tumour is defined as high-grade, large, and deep.	
NX	Regional lymph nodes cannot be assessed	G3, T2b, N0, M0	
N0	No regional lymph node metastasis	G4, T2b, N0, M0	
N1	Regional lymph node metastasis [Note: Presence of positive nodes (N1) is considered stage IV.]	Stage IV	
		Stage IV is defined as any metastasis to lymph nodes or distant sites.	
Distant metastasis (M)		Any G, any T, N1, M0	
MX	Distant metastasis cannot be assessed	Any G, any T, N0, M1	
M0	No distant metastasis		
M1	Distant metastasis		

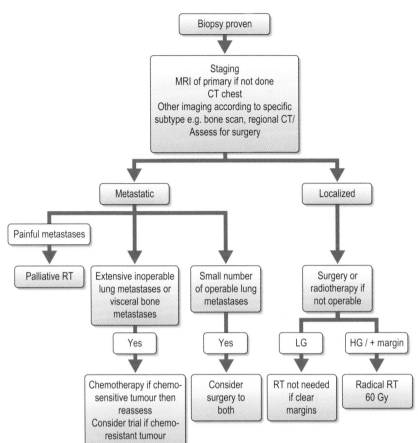

Figure 15.13
Management of limb soft tissue sarcomas (LG-low grade; HG-high grade).

Radiotherapy

Surgery is the primary curative modality for soft tissue sarcomas; radiotherapy has a significant role in the prevention and treatment of local recurrence although there is no evidence that radiotherapy improves overall survival. Many soft tissue sarcomas are radiosensitive. A dose of >60 Gy is needed and the radiotherapy details are shown in Box 15.5.

For some patients who are unfit for surgery or in whom resection is technically not feasible, radiotherapy may be considered as a primary treatment modality. However, unless the tumour is very small and superficial, local control will not be as good as with surgery.

Limb sarcoma radiotherapy presents several challenges including positioning and immobilizing the limb to ensure consistent placement and accurate dose to the tumour bed with a margin. An adequate dose must be delivered to the tumour bed but must not cross the fascial compartment to avoid lymphoedema and delayed fibrosis which significantly affects mobility.

Chest wall sarcomas may be close to the heart or spinal cord making planning complex and potentially limiting doses delivered. They may follow the pleural contour of the chest wall making it difficult to avoid significant lung volumes within the treatment field.

Preoperative and postoperative radiotherapy

Radiotherapy is usually planned postoperatively in two phases to take into account possible tumour spillage at the edge of the surgical procedure then to focus on the central tumour bed. Planning must take into account preoperative scans to estimate tumour location, but should also encompass the surgical edges. Preoperative radiotherapy allows a single phase approach. An ongoing trial, VORTEX, is examining the possibility of reducing the volume of the postoperative treatment comparing a single phase treatment with a standard 2-phase approach.

Radiotherapy has traditionally been given postoperatively but the potential benefits of giving preoperative radiotherapy include a smaller treatment volume, tumour visible on planning scan, reduction of tumour prior to surgery allowing a less morbid and complete operation and reduction in significant late toxicity such as limb oedema, joint restriction and fibrosis. Concerns about using preoperative radiotherapy are effect it may have on interpretation of histology and its associations with wound complications postoperatively.

Adjuvant chemotherapy

The use of adjuvant chemotherapy in soft tissue sarcomas remains controversial and is compounded by different histological subtypes of sarcoma with varied chemo-sensitivities being included as a group in the majority of studies. There are some sarcomas, which tend to predominate in the paediatric setting, in which adjuvant treatment has been shown to be useful, e.g. rhabdomyosarcomas and the extraskeletal Ewing's sarcoma. However, for the majority there is no consensus concerning the use of adjuvant chemotherapy (Box 15.7). A meta-analysis showed a statistically significant improvement in local and distant recurrence if adjuvant chemotherapy was given. There was a trend towards an improved overall survival of 4% at 10 years, but this was not statistically significant. A multi-centre international EORTC study randomized 351 patients to standard treatment versus ifosfamide with doxorubicin. A preliminary analysis has shown no statistically significant difference between the two groups in either local recurrence rates or overall survival.

Treatment recommendations

Surgical resection with wide margins remains the mainstay of treatment for soft tissue sarcoma. This should be performed by specialist sarcoma surgeons. Radiotherapy is recommended for the majority of cases except low-grade tumours which have been excised with a wide margin. Radiotherapy is indicated for low grade tumours with involved resection margin when further surgery is not contemplated. The role of adjuvant chemotherapy for most subgroups remains controversial but could be considered within the context of a clinical trial (Box 15.8).

Advanced and metastatic soft tissue sarcomas

Many sarcomas present with locally advanced or metastatic disease. In the majority of cases this presentation carries a very poor prognosis. Prognostic factors are listed in Box 15.9. The median survival with metastatic disease is 12–14 months.

In other cases, presentation with limited metastatic disease occurs several years after their initial treatment for localized sarcoma and the prognosis may be slightly better in this situation, if the disease is operable. In all these situations treatment options depend on performance status, co-morbidities and histological subtype of sarcoma.

Chemotherapy

Systemic treatment with chemotherapy can be useful but its role is more complex than in other malignancies. There is little evidence that chemotherapy prolongs survival but it can provide significant benefits in symptom control. Response rates as determined by RECIST criteria often do not reflect symptomatic benefit or disease control, especially in response to certain agents such as trabectedin. Different tumour types show different responses to chemotherapy in general and to specific drugs (Box 15.10).

Doxorubicin is a standard first agent with response rates of 20–25%. Doses below 60 mg/m^2

Box 15.7: Adjuvant chemotherapy

The use of adjuvant chemotherapy is not routinely recommended outside a clinical trial, but the studies should be discussed with patients along with their particular situation.

Box 15.8: Sensitivity to chemotherapy of soft tissue sarcomas

The most chemosensitive tumours are synovial sarcoma, myxoid liposarcoma and childhood rhabdomyosarcoma. Extraskeletal Ewing's tumours, discussed under bone tumours, are also chemosensitive. The most chemoresistant tumours are dedifferentiated liposarcoma, alveolar soft part sarcoma, GIST, low-grade liposarcoma and clear cell sarcoma.

Box 15.9: Prognostic factors in soft tissue sarcomas

Different prognostic factors predict for local and systemic recurrence:

- Size and grade best predict distant recurrence and overall survival.
- Other factors which predict survival include age, anatomical site and histological subtype.
- Retroperitoneal and visceral tumours carry a worse prognosis than extremity tumours as, like pelvic Ewing's, they can grow to a very large size before they are detected.
- Specific tumour subtypes such as MPNST and leiomyosarcoma have a poorer overall survival.
- Increased proliferative activity as assessed by immunocytochemical stains has shown a correlation with poorer survival in at least three studies.
- In synovial sarcomas, several studies have shown a poorer prognosis with the *SYT-SSX1* combination rather than *SYT-SSX*, but this has not been confirmed in other studies.
- Involved resection margins and age >50 are worst for local recurrence.
- Specific histological tumour types with a higher rate of local recurrence include MPNST and fibrosarcomas.
- Nomograms have been developed, and validated, which help to predict survival based on these features. The best known is the MSK nomogram which can be found at http://www.mskcc.org/mskcc/html/443.cfm

Box 15.10: Specific chemotherapy and histology

Recent studies have shown that some chemotherapy agents are more effective in some tumours:

- Taxanes and liposomal doxorubicin have been shown to be effective in angiosarcomas.
- Gemcitabine and docetaxel initially showed activity in uterine leiomyosarcomas but also have a response rate up to 30% in other leiomyosarcomas.
- Trabectedin has been shown to be effective in the treatment of liposarcomas, especially myxoid liposarcomas. It also has over a 30% response rate in previously treated leiomyosarcomas and some activity in other sarcomas.

Box 15.11: When to use the combination of ifosfamide and doxorubicin

There are a few special circumstances in which combined chemotherapy may be used first line:

- Life-threatening progressive disease
- Preoperatively to downstage and aim for resection
- Unassessable advanced disease (e.g. diffuse peritoneal metastasis)

Box 15.12: Criteria for resection of lung or intra-abdominal metastases in metastatic soft tissue sarcoma

- No other sites of disease, including primary site
- A long disease-free interval of at least a year
- The disease should be slowly progressing or stable
- Complete resection must appear possible
- Low numbers of metastases although some centres have removed multiple metastases

with no improvement in PFS or overall survival and with increased toxicity. Combination chemotherapy does have a role in the childhood and adolescent tumours such as rhabdomyosarcoma and extraskeletal Ewing's sarcoma (Box 15.11).

Surgery

Despite the poor median overall survival with metastatic disease a small group of patients have a prolonged survival most of whom have disease which is amenable to surgery, e.g. lung metastases or isolated intra-abdominal recurrence. No randomized trial has evaluated the benefit of surgical resection of lung metastases but the 5-year survival of patients selected using strict criteria (Box 15.12) is up to 40%.

Resection of liver metastases, other than for GIST, is performed rarely and there is little evidence that it is of benefit either in terms of survival or symptom control.

Radiotherapy

The majority of soft tissue sarcomas are radio-sensitive and radiotherapy can be an effective tool in symptom control. Doses used are in the range of 35–54 Gy.

Isolated limb perfusion

Some patients present with a massive inoperable limb sarcoma, often accompanied by significant

have been shown to be ineffective and above 75 mg/m^2 to have increased toxicity without clinical benefit. Ifosfamide is often used as a second line agent and has a response rate of 25% overall. In general combination chemotherapy has been shown to improve response rates up to 46% but symptoms, and too large to be encompassed within a radiotherapy field. For some there may be an option of isolated limb perfusion therapy (ILP) with melphalan and recombinant TNF-alpha within specialist centres.

Treatment recommendations

Metastatic soft tissue sarcomas should be managed by a multidisciplinary team of sarcoma specialists who can discuss all available options. Where appropriate, surgery should be performed for isolated recurrence or metastasis. Chemotherapy can provide effective symptom control in many sarcomas but an understanding of the specific differences in histological subtypes is required. There is no evidence that combination chemotherapy improves survival but it is useful in special situations and in adolescent sarcomas.

Specific soft tissue sarcoma subtypes

Leiomyosarcoma

These are smooth muscle tumours and can occur at any site in the body and can be any grade of tumour. The most common sites of metastases are in the lung, except in uterine leiomyosarcomas in which they frequently occur within the liver. Soft tissue and bone metastases also occur. The response to chemotherapy is variable but they have a high response rate to gemcitabine and docetaxel, especially the uterine tumours.

Liposarcoma

Liposarcomas represent a range of tumours with different subtypes having considerable differences in behaviour and management.

Myxoid or round cell liposarcomas arise in the limbs and spread to soft tissues (retroperitoneum, mediastinum) but can occur as a primary retroperitoneal tumour. They have a propensity for bone metastases (especially spine) in up to 17% which may only be visualized on MRI. They are chemo-sensitive, especially to trabectedin. They have a characteristic balanced translocation t(12;16) which gives rise to the TLS-CHOP fusion gene.

Well-differentiated liposarcomas are often abdominal. They tend to recur locally rather than systemically. They are resistant to chemotherapy and radiotherapy.

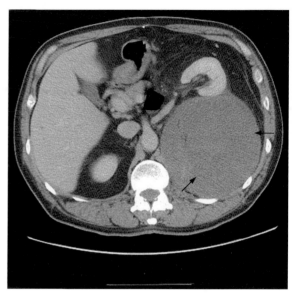

Figure 15.14
Axial CT showing a large retroperitoneal dedifferentiated liposarcoma (arrows) displacing the left kidney.

Dedifferentiated liposarcomas usually occur in the retroperitoneum or abdomen (Figure 15.14). They are high-grade, chemoresistant tumours. They have characteristic genetics with abnormalities in CDK4/MDM2.

Synovial sarcoma

Synovial sarcomas predominate in children and younger adults and prognosis is related to age. Those aged 1–10 years have the best prognosis. The common sites are limbs and trunk. The lungs are the major site of metastasis. They are one of the most chemo-sensitive sarcomas with relatively high response rates, particularly to ifosfamide. They have a balanced translocation t(X;18) between SYT and SSX1 or SSX2.

Uterine sarcomas

The most common histologies are leiomyosarcoma (LMS) and endometrial stromal sarcoma (ESS). Many are found unexpectedly at the time of hysterectomy. A significant proportion of uterine sarcomas express oestrogen (ER) or progesterone (PgR) receptors. Staging is currently according to the FIGO staging system. In ESS pelvic recurrence is more common although distant relapses to the lungs can occur. In LMS pelvic and extra pelvic recurrences can occur. Extra pelvic metastases in LMS can occur in the liver, lung, lymph nodes and bone. Extra pelvic relapse has been shown to be more frequent in those who have had adjuvant radiotherapy.

The prognosis in uterine sarcomas is significantly worse than epithelial endometrial cancer of comparable stage. In one study 5-year survivals of 75.8% for stage I, 60.1% for stage II, 44.9% stage III and 28.7% for stage IV were described. Low-grade ESS have a 5-year survival of 80% but an increased risk of long-term relapse even 20 years after diagnosis. Undifferentiated uterine sarcoma (previously termed high-grade ESS) have a very aggressive course with a 5-year survival around 30%.

In the advanced setting chemotherapy has an established role in the treatment of most uterine sarcomas. Agents used include ifosfamide and doxorubicin. The combination of germcitabine/docetaxel has shown response rate up to 53% in pre-treated LMS with improvement in overall survival up to 18 months. In low-grade ESS chemotherapy is rarely effective with response rates less than 10%. Many of these respond to hormonal manipulation. In undifferentiated (high-grade ESS) sarcomas ifosfamide has the highest response rate (33% in a phase II GOG study) although the duration of response is limited to a few months. There are reports of activity with aromatase inhibitors.

Retroperitoneal sarcoma

Retroperitoneal sarcomas represent 13% soft tissue sarcomas. The most common histologies at this site are liposarcoma (Figure 15.14) and leiomyosarcoma. Many are found incidentally. When they occur symptoms are due to a large mass (abdominal swelling, leg swelling distal to the mass, pain).

If operable a biopsy may not be performed and the tumour resected en masse to prevent tumour seeding the biopsy tract. If not operable a biopsy must be obtained to ensure correct management of an unsuspected alternative diagnosis. Sufficient material must be obtained to perform immunohistochemistry to exclude lymphoma, carcinoma and germ cell tumours.

Adjuvant chemotherapy is not standard treatment in these tumours and in one retrospective study was associated with worse outcome. In advanced disease chemotherapy has been used to aim for operability but there is no evidence it improves overall survival.

In metastatic disease or inoperable recurrence chemotherapy may have a role but is dependent upon histology.

In those cases where postoperative resection margins are involved radiotherapy may be considered although the presence of vital structures (kidney, small bowel) may limit the ability to deliver a sufficient dose. The presence of a large tumour provides some protection to these critical surrounding tissues (kidney, small bowel) if radiotherapy is given preoperatively. This allows higher doses to be administered to the tumour and is technically easier to plan with the tumour in situ. In general, retroperitoneal tumours have a worse prognosis than other soft tissue sarcomas of the same histology.

Gastrointestinal stromal tumour (GIST)

GISTs are a rare subgroup of soft tissue sarcomas which can occur anywhere in the gastrointestinal tract. A small number are associated with a familial GIST syndrome in which there are germline mutations in the KIT gene. Rare paediatric cases are usually wild type with no KIT mutation and tend to have a more indolent course.

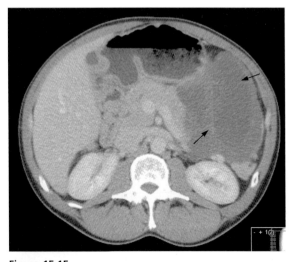

Figure 15.15
Large gastric GIST (shown by arrows) arising from the greater curvature of the stomach.

The most common sites are stomach (50%) (Figure 15.15) and small bowel (25%) but they can occur in the colon (10%), and other sites. Presentation is commonly with anaemia or abdominal mass but abdominal pain can occur with larger tumours. Patterns of spread include liver metastases (most common) and peritoneal metastases. Bone metastases occur rarely and late, often after years of treatment. Lung metastases are exceptionally rare. Nodal metastases are also uncommon.

Pathology and genetics

The morphology can be spindle cell (70%), epithelioid (20%) or mixed type (10%). 95% of GISTs express c-KIT or the CD117 antigen. Mutations in the KIT gene occur in over 90% cases involving exon 11 (in 66%), 9 (in 13%), 13 (in 1.2%), and 17 (0.6%). GIST with mutations within the PDGFRA gene (7% cases) are more frequently associated with an epithelioid morphology, usually occurs in the stomach and tends to be indolent.

The malignant potential of GISTs has been shown to be related to size of the tumour, mitotic rate and location of the primary as described in the NIH consensus criteria (Table 15.3 and Box 15.13).

Management

Definitive curative treatment is only possible with resection of the primary tumour in the absence of metastases. High risk (and intermediate risk) tumours are at risk of relapse after a clear resection. Several trials are examining the use of the drug imatinib in the adjuvant setting. Imatinib is an oral tyrosine kinase inhibitor (TKI) which blocks signalling via KIT by binding to the ATP-binding pocket which is essential for phosphorylation and activation of the c-KIT receptor (p. 370 and Box 15.14). Patients with inoperable primary tumours who do not have metastases may be rendered operable by the use of imatinib. Patients with metastatic disease should be treated initially with imatinib 400 mg per day.

The median time to progression for metastatic disease on imatinib is 2 years. Imatinib should be continued without a break (except for toxicity) until progression. It has been shown that interrupting treatment is associated with progression.

Table 15.3: Risk of aggressive behaviour in GISTs according to NIH consensus criteria

Risk	Size of tumour	Mitotic count
Very low risk	<2 cm	<5 per 50 hpf*
Low risk	2–5 cm	<5 per 50 hpf
	<5 cm	6–10 per 50 hpf
Intermediate risk	5–10 cm	<5 per 50 hpf
	>5 cm	>5 per 50 hpf
High risk	>10 cm	Any mitotic rate
	Any size	>10 per 50 hpf

*hpf – high power field

Box 15.13: Other features which predict aggressive behaviour of GISTs

- Primary site. Duodenal and small bowel GISTs are more aggressive than those arising in the stomach.
- Location of the c-KIT mutation has been evaluated in several studies. Some have shown mutations in Exon 9 to have a more aggressive course than Exon 11. Mutations within codons 562–579 in one study and 557–558 in another were associated with a higher risk of metastases.

Box 15.14: Location of mutations and response to TKIs

There is a correlation between location of c-KIT or PDGFR mutation and response to imatinib or sunitinib.

- Patients with an exon 11 mutation have a greater chance of response to imatinib (67–84%) than those with an exon 9 (40–48%) or no (0–39%) mutation at a dose of 400 mg per day.
- Exon 11 responses were also of a longer duration (576 days) than exon 9 (308 days) or those without a mutation (251 days).
- Higher dose imatinib (800 mg per day) has been shown to be of greater benefit in progression free survival in patients with exon 9 mutations.
- Of the 7% patients with PDGFRA mutations, the commonest is resistant to imatinib (D842V) but others may respond.
- Sunitinib has been shown to be more effective against exon 9 mutant GIST than standard dose imatinib and also appears to be effective against wild-type disease. Secondary mutations that confer resistance to imatinib occur more commonly after prolonged exposure (hence in exon 11 mutant tumours) and may respond to sunitinib.

At progression dose escalation to 800 mg per day may enable temporary control of disease in 30–35% cases with a median time to progression of 4 months. For patients with an isolated liver metastasis who have responded to imatinib, local hepatic resection or radiofrequency ablation may be considered.

Sunitinib malate is a multi targeted TKI which has shown activity in GISTs which have progressed on imatinib. The median progression free survival in this clinical situation is 6 months. 68% patients achieved a partial response or stable disease on sunitinib.

Assessment of response

Assessment of response in GIST may be with CT scan but it has been shown that RECIST criteria may not be the only measure of response in these tumours. FDG-PET can detect reduction in tumour activity within days of commencing imatinib or can visualize small liver metastases which may not be visible on CT. Similarly it can detect increased activity should the tumour develop resistance (new mutations) once on imatinib. Choi described alternative criteria to evaluate GIST response. A 15% reduction in tumour density or 10% unidimensional reduction in tumour size was a better predictor of response than RECIST and these criteria have been shown to correlate better with survival than RECIST.

Further reading

Federman N, Bernthal N, Eilber FC, Tap WD. The multidisciplinary management of osteosarcoma. Curr Treat Options Oncol. 2009;10:82–93.

Ferrari S, Palmerini E. Adjuvant and neoadjuvant combination chemotherapy for osteogenic sarcoma. Curr Opin Oncol. 2007;19:341–346.

Balamuth NJ, Womer RB. Ewing's sarcoma. Lancet Oncol. 2010;11:184–192.

Riedel RF, Larrier N, Dodd L et al. The clinical management of chondrosarcoma. Curr Treat Options Oncol. 2009;10:94–106.

Reynoso D, Subbiah V, Trent JC et al. Neoadjuvant treatment of soft-tissue sarcoma: a multimodality approach. J Surg Oncol. 2010;101:327–333.

Katz SC, Brennan MF. Randomized clinical trials in soft tissue sarcoma. Surg Oncol Clin N Am. 2010;19:1–11.

Verweij J. Soft tissue sarcoma trials: one size no longer fits all. J Clin Oncol. 2009;27:3085–3087.

Judson I. State-of-the-art approach in selective curable tumours: soft tissue sarcoma. Ann Oncol. 2008;19 Suppl 7:vii166–169.

Nam JH, Park JY. Update on treatment of uterine sarcoma. Curr Opin Obstet Gynecol. 2010;22:36–42.

Katz MH, Choi EA, Pollock RE. Current concepts in multimodality therapy for retroperitoneal sarcoma. Expert Rev Anticancer Ther. 2007;7:159–168.

Rubin BP, Heinrich MC, Corless CL. Gastrointestinal stromal tumour. Lancet. 2007;369:1731–1741.

Central nervous system tumours

16

TV Ajithkumar

Introduction

Primary central nervous system (CNS) tumours can arise from any structures in the cranial vault. Around 4000 new patients with malignant brain tumours are diagnosed per year in the UK and 22,000 new patients in USA. There is a bimodal distribution with small peak in children (p. 323) and a steady increase starting at the age of 20 years. Males are more commonly affected, particularly with malignant tumours, whereas women have a higher rate of non-malignant tumours, particularly meningiomas.

Aetiology

The majority of brain tumours are sporadic with an unknown cause. A small proportion of tumours are associated with genetic syndromes and other factors.

1. Genetic syndromes – fewer than 5% patients with glioma have a family history of brain tumours:
   - Neurofibromatosis type I – neurofibromas, optic nerve glioma and pilocytic astrocytoma.
   - Neurofibromatosis type II – meningioma, gliomas and bilateral acoustic neuroma.
   - Tuberous sclerosis – subependymal giant cell astrocytoma, hamartomas.
   - Turcot syndrome – glioblastoma and medulloblastoma.
   - Li–Fraumeni syndrome – astrocytoma and PNET.
   - Basal naevus syndrome – medulloblastoma.

2. Prior radiotherapy increases the risk of a second intracranial tumour, particularly meningiomas and gliomas with a typical latent period of 10 years. Immunosuppression increases the risk of primary CNS lymphoma.
3. Brain tumours are not associated with smoking, alcohol intake or mobile phone use.

Pathology

Box 16.1 shows WHO classification of brain tumours. WHO grading system (Box 16.2) is important in deciding management and prognosis. Molecular features can be incorporated in this grading system to yield important prognostic information. Clinico-pathological features of individual tumours are discussed later.

Presentation

Brain tumour can present with non-specific as well as specific features. Non-specific features are headache (50%) and vomiting due to raised intracranial pressure. Specific features are due to location of the tumour. Lateralizing signs (50%) include hemiparesis, aphasia and visual field defects. Seizure, generalized, partial or focal, can be the presenting symptom in 50% of high-grade and 25% of low-grade gliomas. Stroke-like presentations occur mainly due to bleeding associated with the tumour. It can occur in 5–8% of high-grade and 7–14% of low-grade tumours. Altered mental status can be a presenting feature of primary brain tumour, but is more commonly a presentation of multiple brain metastases.

Box 16.1: WHO classification of brain tumours

Tumours of neuroepithelial tissue

1. Astrocytic tumours
   - Pilocytic astrocytoma (grade 1)
   - Diffuse astrocytoma (grade 2)
   - Anaplastic astrocytoma (grade 3)
   - Glioblastoma (grade 4)
2. Oligodendroglial tumours
   - Oligodendroglioma (grade 2)
   - Anaplastic oligodendroglioma (grade 3)
3. Ependymal tumours
   - Ependymoma (grade 2)
   - Anaplastic ependymoma (grade 2)
4. Mixed glioma
   - Oligoastrocytoma (grade 2)
   - Anaplastic oligoastrocytoma (grade 3)

Choroid plexus tumours
- Papilloma and carcinoma

Embryonal tumours
- Medulloblastoma and its variants (grade 4)
- Supratentorial primitive neuroectodermal tumour (PNET) (grade 4)

Pineal tumours

Neuronal tumours
- Ganglioglioma
- Anaplastic ganglioglioma
- Neurocytoma

Tumours of cranial/spinal nerves

Tumours of the meninges
- Meningioma (grade 1–3)

Tumours of uncertain histogenesis

Haematopoietic neoplasms

Germ cell tumours

Tumours of sellar region
- Pituitary adenoma and carcinoma
- Craniopharyngioma

Metastatic tumours

Box 16.2: WHO grading of primary CNS tumours

Grade 1 – tumours with low proliferative potential and tumour growth by expansion. Generally curable by surgery alone.

Grade 2 – tumours with low proliferative potential but exhibit infiltration. Surgery alone is rarely curative and these tumours can progress to grade 3–4 tumours.

Grade 3 – tumours with cytological evidence of malignancy such as nuclear atypia, endothelial proliferation and mitotic activity. These are rarely curable.

Grade 4 – highly malignant tumours often with necrosis. These are aggressive.

Investigations

Imaging

CT scan

Contrast enhanced CT scan is usually the initial investigation in patients suspected to have a brain lesion. CT scan is not an ideal investigation for low-grade tumours or tumours in the posterior fossa. CT scan may also show features of oedema, hydrocephalus, haemorrhage and calcification depending on the histological variant of brain tumour. Table 16.1 shows radiological appearance of common tumours.

MRI scan

MRI scan with gadolinium and FLAIR (fluid-attenuated inversion recovery) sequence is the standard investigation for brain tumours. T1W imaging demonstrates anatomy and areas of contrast enhancement and T2W and FLAIR images are useful in demonstrating oedema. Appearance of tumour on T1W image is similar to that on CT, but better delineated on MRI. Tumour and oedema demonstrate increased signal on T2 and the area of increased T2 signal on MRI usually includes the hypodense area on CT (Figure 16.1).

Various MR imaging techniques are being evolved to improve the diagnostic ability in the imaging of brain tumours.

Magnetic resonance spectroscopy (MRS)

MRS is clinically useful in distinguishing high-grade glioma and metastases from abscess, assessing tumour recurrence and radiation necrosis, and identification of atypical meningioma as a true meningioma.

Diffusion tensor imaging (DTI)

In radiotherapy planning for high-grade gliomas, conventional methods of imaging cannot distinguish oedema from peritumoural white matter infiltration, resulting in large target volumes. DTI shows white matter abnormalities resulting from tumour infiltrating, and thereby reducing the

Table 16.1: Radiological appearance of common brain tumours

Type of tumour	Imaging characteristic
Pilocystic astrocytoma	Well-circumscribed, contrast enhancing tumour with a cystic or enhancing mural nodule.
Grade II astrocytoma	Isodense or hypodense on CT. Hypointense on T1W image and hyperintense on T2W and FLAIR images. No contrast enhancement and if present suggest malignant transformation. No associated cerebral oedema.
Oligodendroglioma	Same CT/MRI as grade II astrocytoma; but can be associated with areas of contrast enhancement, calcification and haemorrhage.
Anaplastic astrocytoma and GBM	CT – irregular hypodense lesions with varying degree of contrast enhancement and associated oedema and pressure effect. Ring-like enhancement surrounding an irregular shaped necrosis suggests GBM. Some of the high-grade tumours can be non-enhancing particularly in the elderly. MRI – irregular hypointense on T1W and irregular contrast enhancement and hyperintense on T2W and FLAIR, representing tumour and oedema.
Anaplastic oligodendroglioma	Contrast enhancing heterogeneous mass with frequent cystic components, calcifications and necrosis.
Medulloblastoma	CT – hyperdense midline mass with associated hydrocephalus. Marked contrast enhancement. Sometimes show calcification cysts, haemorrhage and nodular seedling. MRI – heterogeneous hypo or isointense on T1W with slightly heterogeneous contrast enhancement. Iso-hyperintense on T2W.
Ependymoma	Heterogeneously enhancing lesion with cystic component. There may be associated calcification and haemorrhage.
Primary CNS lymphoma	Solitary or multiple periventricular homogenously enhancing diffuse lesions ('cotton wool' appearance). Ring enhancement common in immunocompromised patients.
Meningioma	Homogenously contrast enhancing lesion arising from the dura. There is little associated brain oedema. There will be enhancement of dura ('dural tail' sign).
Craniopharyngioma	Solid and cystic lesion on CT scan. MRI appearance depends on the composition of tumour. T1W can be hypo, iso or hyperintense with variable contrast enhancement. T2W can also be hypo, iso or hyperintense.
Pituitary	Contrast enhancing seller/suprasellar lesion on CT. T1W iso-hypointense and T2W hyperintense.
Metastasis	Solitary or multiple irregularly contrast enhancing lesion which may be solid or cystic at the junction of grey and white matter. Location and characteristic depends on type of tumour.

target volume, which would allow significant dose escalation to the tumour with acceptable damage to the normal tissue.

Evaluation of the craniospinal axis

MRI of the craniospinal axis and CSF evaluation is needed for tumours with a high risk of CSF dissemination such as medulloblastoma, germ cell tumours, CNS lymphoma, PNET and ependy-moma (Figure 16.2). CSF evaluation includes CSF biochemistry (typically elevated protein >40 mg/dL and reduced glucose <50 mg/mL), cytology and in cases of suspected germ cell tumours, the estimation of tumour markers (AFP and beta hCG) in CSF and serum. Evaluation of the craniospinal axis is best done prior to surgery or >3 weeks after surgery to avoid false positive results.

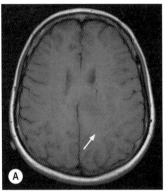 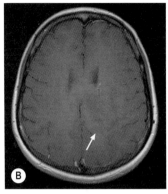 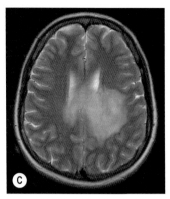

Figure 16.1
MRI scan of diffuse astrocytoma. Scan shows hypointense lesion on left parieto-occipital region (A) without contrast enhancement (B) on T1W image. T2W image (C) shows a hyperintense lesion. Since low-grade tumours are not associated with oedema, this hyperintense lesion represents just the tumour.

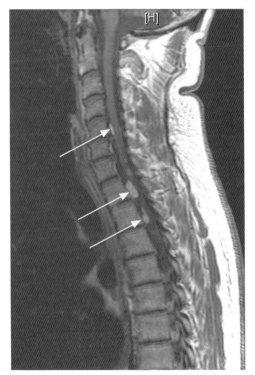

Figure 16.2
Multiple contrast-enhancing tumour nodules in ependymoma suggesting leptomeningeal disease.

Tissue diagnosis

Histologic confirmation is necessary in all patients prior to definite treatment. Biopsy is obtained by either stereotactic guided techniques or open biopsy. In intrinsic brainstem tumours, biopsy may cause neurologic damage and hence may be avoided. Biopsy is avoided in patients with multiple brain metastases from a known primary, optic meningioma and CNS lymphoma in HIV positive patients showing typical radiological findings.

Prognostic factors

The outcome of brain tumours depends on the following factors:

1. Pathology – outcome depends on pathologic type and grade. High-grade tumours have poor prognosis. Recently molecular factors are shown to be important in certain tumour types.
2. Age – increased age is associated with poorer outcome.
3. Performance status – is an important factor in outcome and guiding treatment.
4. Extent of surgical resection – based on observational studies, patients with less residual disease after surgery have a better prognosis.

Principles of management

General medical management

Steroids

Steroids may improve symptoms by reducing intracranial pressure. The most commonly used agent is dexamethasone which is started at a dose

267

of 2–16 mg daily (low doses given once daily and higher doses as 2–4 equally divided doses) and titrated against the patient's symptoms. The optimal dose is just above that at which symptomatic deterioration occurs. If there is no symptomatic improvement, steroids should be stopped.

Anti-epileptics

All patients who have had a seizure should be treated with an anti-epileptic drug (AED); prophylactic use of anti-epileptics is not recommended. Many anti-epileptics are enzyme-inducers, and hence should be carefully monitored when they need to be used concurrently with drugs metabolized by cytochrome p450 enzyme system.

Analgesics

Patients requiring pain control are managed according to the WHO analgesic ladder (p. 66).

Surgical management

Surgery in brain tumours helps in pathological diagnosis, symptom control and definite treatment.

Biopsy can be either stereotactic guided or an open biopsy. Surgery is useful in relieving pressure symptoms as well as decreasing the frequency and intensity of seizures. Surgical resection is constantly evolving in brain tumours. It is common practice to confirm the diagnosis with an intraoperative frozen section or smear prior to attempting a full resection. Complete or maximal resection with minimal injury to neighbouring critical structures is the aim of surgery. The importance of surgical resection in specific tumours is discussed later. The various resection techniques are:

1. Image guided stereotactic resection – is useful in technically challenging locations such as the peri-thalamic region, to minimize critical structure injury.
2. Neuronavigation guided resection – distortion of brain anatomy by tumour and oedema makes surgical resection according to conventional landmarks difficult. Neuronavigation systems allow registration of stored imaging data which can be incorporated with real time intra-operative imaging using intra-operative ultrasound or MRI. This helps surgeons to guide resection based on real time shift of structures during operation.
3. Cortical mapping awake craniotomy – is useful in resection of tumours inside or adjacent to functional brain areas. Intraoperative cortical or subcortical stimulation helps to map functional areas. Initial craniotomy and preliminary stimulation are done with the patient asleep. After arousal, under sedative/hypnotic anaesthesia, the patient responds to motor or language commands but with subsequent amnesia.
4. Fluorescent guided surgery – an evolving technique for malignant gliomas.

Radiotherapy in brain tumours

Radiotherapy has a major role in the management of CNS tumours. Radiotherapy is proven to improve local control and/or survival in grade 3–4 tumours whereas its role in grade 2 tumours is doubtful and has limited role for grade 1 tumours. Radiotherapy is delivered by the following methods:

1. External beam radiotherapy is commonest mode of delivery of radiotherapy to the brain. Immobilization and proper localization is important in the delivery of EBRT. Target volume depends on the type of tumour and intention of treatment.
2. Stereotactic technique – this technique involves improved localization of tumour and precision. Treatment is delivered either as multiple fractions using linear accelerator (called stereotactic radiotherapy) or as single fraction (called radiosurgery) using gamma knife, a special machine for cranial radiosurgery.
3. Charged particle radiotherapy – mainly protons, which deposit the energy only at a depth and hence useful in skull base tumours.

A summary of radiotherapy details for common tumours are given in Table 16.2.

Radiation tolerance and reactions

Radiation to the brain can cause structural damage to critical structures if attention is not paid not to exceed the tolerance dose of individual structures.

Acute radiation reactions may manifest up to 6 weeks following completion of irradiation.

Table 16.2: Radiotherapy for common brain tumours

Tumour	Intent of treatment	GTV*	CTV+ (margin added to GTV)	Dose
Low-grade glioma	Radical	Abnormality on T2W image on fused image	1.5 cm	54 Gy in 30#
Grade III glioma	Radical	Contrast enhancing abnormality on co-registered image	Phase I – 2.5 cm Phase II – 1.5 cm	45 Gy in 25# 9 Gy in 5#
Grade IV glioma	Radical	Contrast enhancing abnormality on co-registered image	Phase I – 2.5 cm Phase II – 1.5 cm	50 Gy in 25# 10 Gy in 5#
	Palliative	Contrast enhancing tumour	2.5 cm	30 Gy/6# or 35 Gy/10#
Brainstem glioma	Radical	Abnormality on T2W/FLAIR on co-registered image	1–1.5 cm	54 Gy/33#
Medulloblastoma	Adjuvant	CT planning for craniospinal RT Abnormality on fused image for phase II	Phase I – whole craniospinal axis Phase II – posterior fossa or visible tumour + 1.5 cm Phase II – spinal metastasis boost	35 Gy/21# 20 Gy/12# 15 Gy/9#
Ependymoma	Adjuvant/radical	Contrast enhancing lesion or surgical cavity in case of complete resection on fused image	1.5–2.5 cm	55 Gy/33# or 54 Gy/30#
Germinoma	Radical	Phase 1 – CT planning Phase 2 – primary and other metastatic sites on fused image	Phase 1 – whole craniospinal axis Phase 2 – plan before start of treatment. Contrast enhancing tumour + 1–2 cm	25 Gy/15# 15 Gy/9#
Non-germinoma	After chemotherapy – meningeal disease	CT planning	Phase 1 – craniospinal RT Phase 2 primary tumour + 2 cm	30 Gy in 20# 24 Gy/12#
Acoustic neuroma	Residual disease	Abnormality on co-registered image	Primary + 2 cm	54 Gy/33#
	Progressive disease	Contrast enhancing mass on co-registered image		
Craniopharyngioma	Postoperative/progressive	Residual tumour on fused image	No margin needed	50 Gy/30#
		Residual tumour on fused image	Preoperative GTV + margin for doubtful margin	50 Gy/30#
Pituitary adenoma	Postoperative or progressive	Visible tumour on co-registered image	No margin	45 Gy/25#
Meningioma	Radical/postoperative	Contrast enhancing tumour on co-registered image. The practice of including dural tail in GTV is variable; many studies fail to show any meningioma in dural tail	0–0.5 cm	50 Gy/30# or 55 Gy/33#

*GTV is outlined on MRI co-registered with planning CT scan. T2W MRI is used for co-registration in low grade glioma, whereas contrast enhanced T1W is used for high-grade glioma, meningioma, craniopharyngioma and pituitary adenoma.

+CTV needs to be edited to confine to skull or skull base. PTV depends on immobilization device: for Perspex shell add 5 mm to CTV and for relocatable stereotactic frames add 2–3 mm to CTV.

Normal tissue tolerance doses (at ≤2 Gy per fraction): brain 60 Gy; brainstem 54 Gy; optic nerve and chiasm 50–54 Gy; pituitary gland <40 Gy; middle and inner ear <40 Gy; lacrimal gland <20 Gy; lens <10–15 Gy as fractions; permanent alopecia 43 Gy.

These reactions are generally those of raised intracranial pressure, fatigue and worsening of neurology. Vomiting is particularly common in patients receiving radiotherapy to the brainstem region.

Early delayed (intermediate) side effects usually appear from 6 weeks to 6 months following radiotherapy and are due to changes in capillary permeability and transient demyelination. Symptoms include headache, somnolence syndrome, lethargy and frequently recurrence of the original presenting features. Recovery is spontaneous but can be accelerated by steroids.

Delayed radiation reaction develops 6 months after radiotherapy. This is thought to be due to white matter injury secondary to vascular injury, demyelination and necrosis. The most serious form of this is radiation necrosis which peaks at 3 years. Conventional imaging fails to distinguish this from recurrent tumour and special imaging is therefore needed (p. 265). Treatment is with steroids and debulking. Other late effects include, depending on the area irradiated, memory problems, pituitary failure, hearing loss, visual changes and second malignancies.

Chemotherapy in brain tumours

Chemotherapy has an established role in paediatric brain tumours mainly as a substitute for radiotherapy. The role of chemotherapy in adult brain tumours is increasing. The active agents are nitrosoureas (carmustine and lomustine), procarbazine, temozolomide, platinum and vincristine. The role of chemotherapy in specific brain tumours is discussed later in this chapter and the commonly used chemotherapy regimens are given in Box 16.3.

New agents in brain tumours

A number of biological agents have been tried recently in the management of brain tumours, particularly in gliomas. Since gliomas exhibit marked neovascularization, anti-angiogenesis inhibitors are an attractive option. Bevacizumab has been studied alone and in combination with chemotherapy in recurrent GBM.

Since EGFR are frequently amplified and overexpressed in GBM, agents such as cetuximab and tarceva seem to be attractive agents. Other target molecules under investigation include PDGF

antagonists (e.g. imatinib) and farnesyltransferase inhibitors (e.g. tipifarnib).

> **Box 16.3: Chemotherapy regimes in brain tumour**
>
> **PCV (glioma)**
> - Procarbazine 100 mg/m^2 (max 200 mg) oral Day 1–10
> - CCNU 100 mg/m^2 (max 200 mg) oral Day 1
> - Vincristine 1.5 mg/m^2 (max 2 mg) IV Day 1
>
> Cycles repeated every 6 weeks for 6 cycles
>
> **Temozolomide (glioma)**
> - Concomitant – 75 mg/m^2 D1–D42 oral, 1 hour prior to radiotherapy & morning dose on weekends
> - Adjuvant and palliative – 150 mg/m^2 D1–5 oral for first cycle, then 200 mg/m^2 D1–D5 total 6 cycles (adjuvant starting 4 weeks after radiotherapy)
>
> **Packer regime (medulloblastoma and PNET)**
> - Concurrent with radiotherapy – vincristine 1.5 mg/m^2 (max 2 mg) weekly with radiotherapy, then 6 weeks of rest followed by:
> - A combination of:
>   - CCNU 75 mg/m^2 every 6 weeks and cisplatin 68 mg/m^2 every 6 weeks and vincristine 1.5 mg/m^2 (max 2 mg) for 3 consecutive weeks. Cycle repeated every 6 weeks for total of 8 cycles

---

Follow-up

Follow-up consists of clinical evaluation with attention to neurological examination and assessment of seizure control. MRI is the image of choice whenever imaging follow-up is indicated. Visual field and hormonal function assessments are important in sellar tumours.

Clinico-pathological features and management of specific tumours

Glioma

Astrocytomas diffusely infiltrate surrounding brain. Pilocytic astrocytoma (grade 1) occurs in children and young adults and are located in the optic tract, hypothalamus, basal ganglia and posterior fossa. These tumours grow slowly and stabilize spontaneously. Diffuse astrocytoma (grade 2) is a low-grade tumour. Anaplastic astrocytoma (grade 3) and glioblastoma multiforme

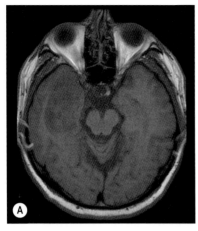 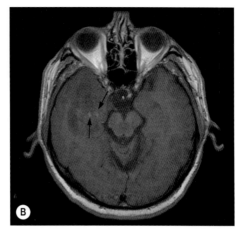

Figure 16.3
MRI scan of oligodendroglioma in right temporal area. MRI scan of oligodendroglioma will exhibit the same features of astrocytoma (A); however oligodendroglioma can have subtle contrast enhancement (arrows on B) and calcification.

(grade 4-GBM) are high grade tumours. Anaplastic astrocytoma is distinguished from low-grade tumours by greater cellular differentiation and hyperchromasia, more frequent mitoses and prominent small vessels lined by epithelioid endothelial cells. Glioblastoma is distinguished by increased cellularity, pleomorphism, giant cells, abnormal mitotic figures and endothelial cell proliferation. Necrosis surrounded by nuclei aligned in pseudopalisading pattern is characteristic. Astrocytomas stain for glial fibrillary acidic protein (GAFP).

Oligodendroglial tumours have typical histological appearance of evenly distributed cells with uniform and rounded nuclei with perinuclear halo. Mixed tumours are composed usually of an oligodendroglial component and an astrocytic component. Their overall prognosis and treatment is dictated by the most aggressive component.

Treatment of pilocytic astrocytoma

Complete surgical resection alone is adequate which results in a 20-year survival of 80%. In patients for whom a complete resection is not possible, maximal safe resection should be attempted followed by observation. In the majority of these patients the tumour does not progress. A second surgery may be attempted during progression, if feasible, followed by non-surgical management. Patients with unresectable tumours with progressive neurological deficit are treated with radiotherapy and carboplatin-based chemotherapy.

Treatment of low grade glioma (WHO grade 2)

Diffuse astrocytoma, oligodendroglioma (Figure 16.3) and mixed oligoastrocytoma are grouped together as low-grade glioma. These tumours mainly affect the young adults (mean age of 35 years for astrocytoma and 45 years for oligodendroglioma). Patients generally present with seizures and in the majority adequate seizure control with serial MRI monitoring will be sufficient. Many of these patients have slow growing tumours. There are two main patterns of progression – secondary gliomatosis cerebri and malignant transformation. Secondary gliomatosis cerebri is characterized by diffuse extension of the tumour sometimes to the opposite hemisphere and it often remains low-grade. Malignant transformation involves progression to a high-grade tumour with characteristics of anaplastic astrocytoma, anaplastic oligodendroglioma or glioblastoma. Imaging shows new areas of irregular contrast enhancement in a previously non-contrast enhancing tumour.

Surgery

The role of surgery in grade 2 tumours is unclear. When safe complete or near complete resection

271

is feasible, it may be attempted. A recent retrospective study showed that gross total resection (complete resection of preoperative FLAIR abnormality) improved survival (10-year OS 76%) compared with near total resection (<3 mm thin residual FLAIR abnormality around resection cavity) (10-year OS 57%) and subtotal resection (residual nodular FLAIR abnormality) (10-year OS 49%; p = 0.017). Incomplete resection is only indicated to control specific symptoms such as seizures or intracranial pressure which may be relieved with removal of the appropriate region of tumour. The majority of patients are followed up or treated with non-surgical treatment after biopsy.

Radiotherapy

Immediate radiotherapy is as effective as delayed radiotherapy (i.e. delayed until progressive symptoms). In a symptomatic patient, radiotherapy reduces the tumour size and leads to symptomatic improvement in 50–75%. However, in patients with well-controlled seizures early radiotherapy does not improve overall survival compared with radiotherapy deferred until clinical progression, but improves the progression-free interval. A randomized study of early vs. delayed radiotherapy showed a 5-year overall survival of 63% with early radiotherapy compared with 66% with delayed radiotherapy. The 5-year disease free survival was better (44% vs. 37% p = 0.02) with early radiotherapy. There is no clinical benefit beyond a radiotherapy dose of 45–50 Gy, and higher doses cause significant side effects of fatigue and poor emotional functioning.

Chemotherapy

Chemotherapy can improve symptoms and lead to a radiologic response. The role of chemotherapy in newly diagnosed disease is however undefined. Chemotherapy is used in malignant transformation. Oligodendroglioma with allelic loss of chromosome 1p/19q usually responds to chemotherapy with alkylating agents (Box 16.3).

Outcome

The median survival of low-grade glioma is 5–8 years. Oligodendroglioma has a better prognosis of 12–16 years.

Management of recurrence or progression after first definitive treatment

Management of recurrence or progression depends on previous treatment. Radiotherapy can be considered for those who have not previously received radiation treatment. Chemotherapy is the option in patients who progress after previous radiotherapy.

Gliomatosis cerebri

Gliomatosis is characterized by diffuse infiltration of the brain with malignant glial cells. It usually presents with headaches, personality changes or seizure. MRI with FLAIR is more sensitive in detecting the lesion which shows diffuse isointense to hypointense lesions on T1W and hyperintense lesions involving at least two lobes of the brain on T2W & FLAIR. Surgery is of little benefit but radiotherapy (principles same as low grade glioma) can stabilize or improve the disease. Chemotherapy can be attempted when radiotherapy is technically difficult. Median survival is around 12 months.

Treatment of high-grade (malignant) glioma (WHO grade 3 and 4)

High-grade gliomas account for around 50% of brain tumours. These can be either anaplastic glioma (grade 3) or GBM. These tumours are highly aggressive and the aim of treatment is to improve neurological deficit, quality of life and to increase survival. Optimal medical management includes steroids to improve oedema, anticonvulsants in patients who have had seizures and rehabilitation.

GBM

GBM accounts for 75% of malignant gliomas. The median survival is around 1 year. There is no randomized data showing superior survival with surgical resection compared with biopsy alone. Maximal resection will improve time to progression as well as tolerability to subsequent radiotherapy and hence, maximal safe resection is recommended.

Adjuvant radiotherapy improves median survival of GBM from 14 weeks to 40 weeks and is given as a dose of 58–60 Gy in 1.8 to 2 Gy per fraction. Hence patients aged <70 years with good performance status (0–1) are considered for radical radiotherapy, whereas patients aged >70 years and performance status of 0–2 may be considered for short course radiotherapy. Patients with poor PS and significant neurological deficit are treated with supportive measures (Box 16.4).

A meta-analysis of adjuvant chemotherapy trials showed a slight improvement in median survival of 2 months. Recently a randomized study reported a significant survival benefit with concurrent and adjuvant temozolomide. In this study of newly diagnosed GBM patients, temozolomide (75 mg/m^2) given concurrently with radiation followed by adjuvant monthly treatment (200 mg/m^2 days 1–5) up to 6 months produced a survival advantage at 2 years of 16% which was sustained at 4 years compared to radiation alone (10–26%). Hence this is the treatment of choice for GBM. However, the benefit of temozolomide is only seen in patients with methylation of the O^6-methylguanine-DNA methyltransferase (MGMT) gene promoter. The overall survival was increased in patients with methylated MGMT promoter regions compared to those with unmethylated MGMT promoter regions (18.2 months and 12.2 months, $p < 0.001$). However test for methylation of the MGMT gene promoter is not routinely used, to select patients for concurrent chemoradiotherapy.

Anaplastic glioma (AG)

AG constitutes 25% of high-grade glioma. Patients with anaplastic astrocytoma have a median survival of 3 years and those with anaplastic oligodendroglioma have a better prognosis, particularly those with loss of heterozygosity of 1p and 19q (median survival 5–7 years). Current standard treatment of AG is maximal cytoreduction with postoperative radiotherapy.

The value of temozolomide in grade 3 astrocytoma and oligodendroglioma is not proven. Patients with anaplastic oligodendroglioma demonstrating LOH on 1p/19q have 60–80% response rates with alkylating chemotherapy. Despite that, early administration of adjuvant chemotherapy before or after radiotherapy does not impact on overall survival and there is no difference in efficacy between PCV and temozolomide chemotherapy.

Management of recurrence and progression

In the majority of patients (>80%) with high-grade glioma, tumours recur within a 2–3 margin of the original tumour (Figure 16.4). Repeat surgery is an option for those with favourable prognostic features such as age <50 years, good performance status, progression free survival of >6 months and well circumscribed tumour, which offers a median survival of 6–8 months with 20% 1-year survival. In this group of patients polymer-based carmustine chemotherapy in a wafer (Gliadel) is proven to be useful. A randomized study showed an increased 6-month survival from 44% to 64% ($p = 0.02$) and median survival from 23 to 31 weeks with Gliadel wafers.

An alternative treatment option is radiosurgery if the recurrent tumour is small. In patients who are not suitable for the above options palliative chemotherapy should be considered. PCV results in 20–50% response with 4–8 months survival.

Brainstem glioma

Brainstem gliomas are rare in adults. Diffuse intrinsic pontine gliomas are generally high grade whereas exophytic tumours are low grade. These tumours usually present as multiple cranial nerve paralysis, ataxia and hemiparesis. MRI shows diffuse enlargement of the pons on T1W images and enhancement is seen in high-grade glioma. Surgery is an appropriate treatment for exophytic low-grade lesions whereas inoperable low-grade lesions and intrinsic lesions are treated with involved field radiotherapy. The median survival of non-enhancing lesions is in the region of 7

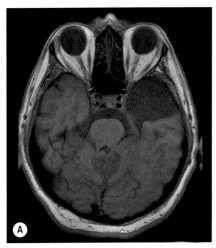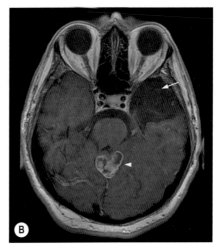

Figure 16.4
GBM recurrence. GBM can spread along the white matter track and manifest with recurrence away from the original lesion. This patient, who had left temporal lobectomy (B-long arrow) for GBM (A), presents with a non-homogenous contrast enhancing recurrent lesion (B-arrow head), which indicates spread along the white matter track.

years and of enhancing lesions is approximately 11 months.

Ependymoma

Ependymomas (grade 2) are slow growing tumours arising from the ependymal or sub-ependymal cells surrounding the ventricles, spinal canal or filum terminale. These are typically low-grade but exhibit a high risk of recurrence and can spread through the CSF. They are rarely infiltrative and seldom metastasize outside CNS. Subependymoma, which occur in the cerebral ventricles and myxopapillary ependymoma, which occurs in the filum terminale are grade 1 variants of ependymoma. Histologically these tumours consist of uniform round cells with widespread pseudorosette formation. Maximal surgical resection followed by postoperative radiotherapy is the treatment of choice in adults (Table 16.2). Local radiotherapy is recommended if spinal MRI and CSF cytology are clear. Craniospinal RT is recommended only in cases of neuraxis spread. There is no recommended role for chemotherapy, except in recurrence after radiotherapy. Postoperative radiotherapy increases 5-year survival from 18% to 68%.

Choroid plexus tumour

Choroid plexus papilloma (grade 1) usually presents as an intraventricular mass in children.

These are cured with excision. Choroid plexus carcinomas (grade 3) are also common in children and behave aggressively with extensive ventricular and subarachnoid space spread. Choroid plexus carcinoma is treated with a combination of surgery and radiotherapy, with or without chemotherapy.

Medulloblastoma and PNET

Medulloblastoma (grade 4) commonly occurs in children, but can also occur in adolescents and adults. It usually affects the cerebellum and can spread locally, through CSF and outside the CNS. Histologically the tumour consists of small primitive round or spindle cells which might express neuron specific enolase, synaptophysin, Leu-7 and protein gene product 9.5.

PNET (grade 4) are aggressive supratentorial tumours in children and young adults. Histology shows highly cellular diffuse sheets of cell with extensive necrosis. The prognosis is worse than medulloblastoma.

Treatment of medulloblastoma and PNET

In medulloblastoma, the extent of surgical resection correlates with survival and hence, maximal surgical resection is attempted in localized disease. All patients are treated with postoperative craniospinal radiotherapy followed by additional radiotherapy to the posterior cranial fossa. Radiotherapy with concurrent vincristine followed by adjuvant chemotherapy with cisplatin, CCNU and vincristine (Packer regime) is an effective regime (Box 16.3); but it is very toxic in adults (especially neurotoxicity) and hence sometimes radiotherapy alone may be used.

Acoustic neuroma (vestibular schwannoma)

Acoustic neuromas are tumours arising from the Schwann cell of the myelin sheath of the eight cranial nerves. These can occur sporadically (4–5th decade of life) or as part of NF2 (2nd–3rd decade of life). These are expansile slow growing tumours. Clinical presentation is usually with progressive sensorineural hearing loss (up to 95%). Large cerebello-pontine angle tumours can lead to trigeminal involvement and pressure effect on the cerebellum and brainstem can give rise to ataxia and lower cranial nerve (IX–XII) involvement.

Imaging shows a homogenously enhancing lesion close to internal auditory canal. Follow-up with regular imaging may be adequate for some patients. When treatment is indicated, for progressive tumours or large tumours with pressure symptoms, the treatment options are surgery and radiotherapy (either radiosurgery or fractionated radiotherapy). Surgery achieves a complete excision of 97% at the expense of complete hearing loss and transient facial palsy. Radiosurgery is appropriate for lesions of <3 cm size. Fractionated radiotherapy may preserve hearing in patients with good control rates; but long-term follow-up is needed.

Pineal tumours

Pineal tumours are common in children. Pineocytoma (grade 2) are slow growing tumours which are treated with surgery and radiotherapy. Pineoblastomas (grade 4) are aggressive tumours treated with surgery, radiotherapy and chemotherapy. Pineal parenchymal tumours of intermediate differentiation have an unpredictable clinical behaviour. Treatment recommendation varies from surgery alone to surgery followed by craniospinal radiotherapy. Management of pineal germ cell tumours is discussed below.

Germ cell tumours

Germ cell tumours occur in the midline structures, pineal, sellar, hypothalamic and third ventricular regions. The majority of patients are diagnosed between 11–20 years. Histological appearance is similar to their gonadal counterpart. Immunohistochemically germinomas may stain for placental alkaline phosphatase (PLAP) and hCG and non-germinoma may stain for hCG and AFP.

Presentation depends on the tumour type and location. These tumours usually arise from the pineal region and present with features of CSF obstruction and Parinaud's syndrome (dorsal midbrain compression leading to failure of up gaze, nystagmus and light-near dissociation of pupil). Suprasellar tumours present with neuro-endocrine deficits.

On imaging germinomas appear as a homogenously enhancing mass and non-germinomas as a heterogeneous mass with cysts, calcification and/or haemorrhage. Spinal imaging with MRI may show leptomeningeal disease in 10–15% of cases.

The role of surgery is mainly to obtain a tissue biopsy. In tumour marker positive disease (AFP above 25 IU/L or serum or CSF hCG of >50 IU/L in Europe and >100 IU/L in USA), imaging alone is sufficient prior to non-surgical treatment. Surgery may have a role in symptomatic residual masses after non-surgical management.

Germinoma is treated with craniospinal radiotherapy, which results in a 5-year survival of 90–95% and 10-year survival of 91%. Chemotherapy is being evaluated to avoid the need for craniospinal radiotherapy and to reduce the dose of radiotherapy in paediatric germinoma. Non-germinoma is treated with platinum based chemotherapy followed by radiotherapy. In non-germinoma, with radiotherapy alone the overall survival is only 10–30%, whereas combined modality treatment results in a 5-year survival of 45%.

Meningeal tumours

Meningiomas (Figure 16.5) account for 30% of primary intracranial neoplasms and occur predominantly in women. Grade 1 meningiomas

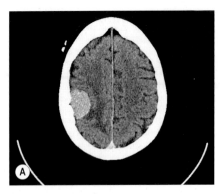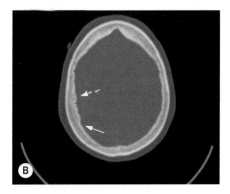

Figure 16.5
CT scan of meningioma. A, A homogenously contrast enhancing lesion arising from the dura. B, Bone window showing increase in thickness of skull bone (hyperostosis) at the site of the tumour (arrows), a feature of meningioma.

(90% of meningiomas) are benign with a low risk of recurrence, atypical (grade 2) meningiomas (5–7%) have a high risk of local recurrence after complete excision and grade 3 meningiomas (3–5%) are aggressive. Papillary meningioma (grade 3) is seen in young patients, shows aggressive behaviour with frequent recurrences, brain invasion and metastasis. Anaplastic (malignant) meningioma is also aggressive.

An incidental finding on CT/MRI is one of the common modes of diagnosis. Presentation depends on the location of tumour. Base of skull tumours usually present with cranial nerve involvement whereas tumours over the convexity of the cerebrum present with headache or seizure.

Treatment of meningioma

Meningiomas can be observed if they are small and asymptomatic. Treatments of choice for progressive or symptomatic meningioma are either complete surgical resection if in an operable location or radical radiotherapy or radiosurgery, if in an inoperable site. Complete resection is usually difficult for skull base (Figure 16.6A), cavernous sinus and cerebellopontine angle meningiomas. After incomplete resection, either a policy of imaging surveillance with delayed radiotherapy on progression or immediate postoperative radiotherapy is adopted. The policy of image surveillance with delayed radiotherapy depends on:

1. Location of tumour – tumour near critical structures may cause neurological damage when it progresses and hence early radiotherapy is indicated (e.g. tumour near optic chiasma).
2. Grade of tumour – grade 2 and 3 tumours have a 5-year recurrence rate of 40–100% even after complete resection whereas that of grade I tumour is 7–12%. Hence all patients with grade 2/3 tumours are treated with immediate postoperative radiotherapy.

Data suggest that postoperative radiotherapy improves local control compared with no radiotherapy after subtotal resection (15-year local control 81% vs. 49%; p = 0.0001).

Primary CNS lymphoma (PCNSL)

PCNSL has a higher incidence in immunocompromised individuals than in the normal population. It commonly presents in the third and fourth decades in immunocompromised individuals whereas it occurs three decades later in those who have a competent immune system. The usual presentations include focal symptoms, raised intracranial pressure, behaviour and personality changes and confusion. Biopsy shows diffuse large cell B cell lymphoma in 80–90%. Up to 20–40% patients have CSF involvement. Less than 5% people have systemic involvement. Tissue diagnosis is made from an open or stereotactic biopsy. Staging investigations include HIV testing, chest X-ray, CSF examination and slit lamp examination (10–20% have uveitis). Systemic staging is only indicated if B symptoms are present (see p. 306).

The role of surgery is limited to biopsy. Steroids may cause complete disappearance of

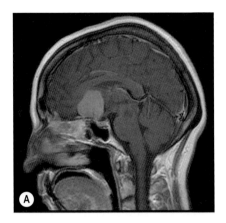

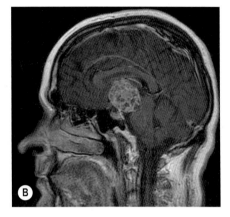

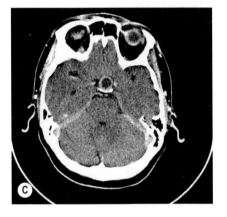

Figure 16.6
Tumours of the base of the brain.
A, Homogeneously enhancing
meningioma. B, Heterogeneously
enhancing craniopharyngioma. C, Cystic
enhancing pituitary adenoma.

tumour (ghost tumours) and hence should be avoided until tissue diagnosis. Current standard treatment is high-dose intravenous methotrexate with whole brain radiotherapy (40–50 Gy) which results in a 2-year survival of 43–73%. However this treatment is extremely toxic particularly in the elderly when 60–80% patients older than 60 years develop progressive leucoencephalopathy and cognitive dysfunction. Hence in the elderly chemotherapy alone with delayed radiotherapy is an alternative. In immunocompromised patients reduction of radiotherapy dose may be necessary to reduce toxicity.

Craniopharyngioma

Craniopharyngioma (Figure 16.6B) arises from the epithelial remnants of Rathke's pouch. These are slow growing tumours often with a solid and cystic component, the latter filled with a fluid having a 'motor oil' appearance.

The clinical presentation is with pituitary hormonal abnormalities, pressure symptoms on the optic pathway (visual field defects) and neurological symptoms.

Surgical resection is the recommended treatment if feasible. Following incomplete resection or cyst decompression and biopsy, postoperative radiotherapy is indicated which results in a 5-year survival of 89% and 10-year survival of 77%.

Pituitary adenoma and carcinoma

Pituitary adenoma

Pituitary adenoma (Figure 16.6C) usually presents between the ages of 30–50 years. These are slow growing tumours with an insidious onset of symptoms. The usual presentation is hormonal dysfunction or symptoms resulting from pressure effects such as visual field defects.

Medical management is important in secretory tumours. Transphenoidal surgery is the standard surgery for secretory tumours other than prolactinoma and macroadenoma producing pressure symptoms. The indication for radiotherapy is relative and usually indicated in tumour progression after surgery, uncontrolled hormone production, extensive residual tumour and invasion of the cavernous sinus. Radiotherapy is usually given as stereotactic fractionated radiotherapy or radiosurgery. Radiotherapy controls hypersecretion in 80% patients with acromegaly, 50–80% with Cushing's disease and 33% with hyperprolactinaemia. In non-secretory tumours, surgery followed by radiotherapy results in a 20-year progression free interval of >90%. The long-term side effects of radiotherapy are hypopituitarism, increased risk of a second cancer (20-year risk of 2.4%), and increased risk of cerebrovascular death (relative risk 4.1).

Pituitary carcinoma

Pituitary carcinomas are rare (0.2% of pituitary tumours). They often present with secretory features (Cushing's or hyperprolactinaemia). There is limited literature, but the prognosis is poor with multiple local recurrences and metastatic spread.

Metastatic tumours of brain

Metastatic brain tumours are four times commoner than primary brain tumours and one quarter of all cancer patients develop brain metastases during their illness. The incidence of brain metastases is increasing because of the improved systemic control of many cancers. The commonest primaries are lung in whom 30–80% develop brain metastases, breast (20–30%) and gastrointestinal cancer. Other cancers include renal cell carcinoma (5–10%) and malignant melanoma (10–20%).

Presentation

Eighty percent of brain metastases are diagnosed after development of the primary cancer and 20% present with brain metastases prior to and simultaneously with the diagnosis of primary. Headache is the commonest symptom. Up to 20% can have seizures and lateralizing signs. 5–10% can present with an acute neurological deficit due to bleeding into the tumour or cerebral infarction.

Diagnosis

Contrast enhanced CT scan is usually diagnostic with more than half of the patients showing multiple metastases (Figure 16.7). The lesions are typically contrast enhancing and located in the junction between grey and white matter. MRI scan is useful in lesions in the posterior fossa, those with negative CT scans, those with suspected leptomeningeal disease and to confirm a solitary lesion if planning for surgical resection.

Prognosis

Untreated symptomatic patients have a median survival of 4–8 weeks. With steroids the survival is 8–12 weeks. A prognostic classification is shown in Table 16.3.

Treatment

Initial management includes high-dose steroids which reduce the symptoms of cerebral oedema, pain management and anti-epileptics for seizures.

Multiple brain metastases

Whole brain radiotherapy (WBRT) is the treatment of choice for the majority of class 1 patients. Most of the Class 2 patients are not suitable for WBRT. Class 3 patients are treated with supportive care only. The standard radiotherapy regime is either 20 Gy in five fractions or 30 Gy in 10 fractions. Around 10% of patients are alive after 12 months.

Table 16.3: Prognostic groups in brain metastases

Prognostic group*	Definition	Median survival (months)
Class 1	Age less than 65 years, KPS ≥70, controlled primary disease and no extracranial metastases.	7.1
Class 2	Neither class 1 nor 2	4.2
Class 3	KPS <70	2.3

*Based on RTOG RPA prognostic group. This is not applicable to chemosensitive tumours such as germ cell tumours, choriocarcinoma etc.

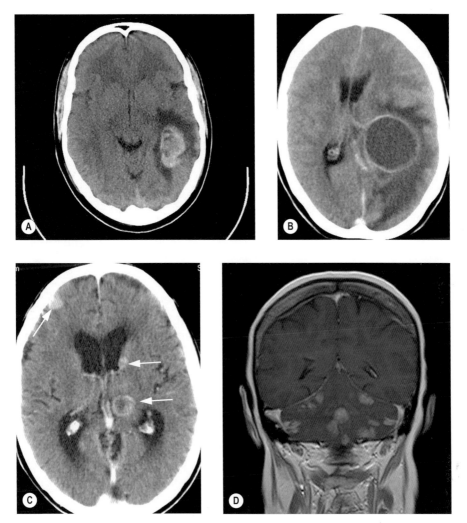

Figure 16.7
Various appearances of brain metastases. A, Bleeding metastasis (melanoma). B, Single cystic metastasis (mucinous carcinoma, breast). C, Multiple metastasis (lung cancer). D, Predominant posterior fossa metastases (HER2+ breast cancer).

There is no role for surgery in multiple metastases, except to relieve hydrocephalus. Patients with highly chemosensitive tumours (e.g. germ cell tumours, choriocarcinoma) are treated with initial chemotherapy followed by consolidation whole brain radiotherapy in some cases.

Single or solitary metastasis (on MRI) (Box 16.5)
In a group of patients with operable single or solitary metastasis, surgical excision followed by WBRT improve survival compared with WBRT alone (40 weeks vs. 15 weeks; p < 0.01). Most benefit is seen in patients <65 years with KPS of ≥70 and no extracranial progression in the

> **Box 16.5: Single or solitary metastasis**
>
> - Single metastasis – one lesion within the brain irrespective of status of systemic disease
> - Solitary metastasis – the one lesion in the brain is the only metastatic disease in the body
> - Oligometastases – solitary or small number (<4) metastases which can be treated aggressively

previous 3 months. Complete excision followed by close imaging follow-up may be appropriate for some patients with good prognosis.

Patients with inoperable tumours due to inaccessible locations may be considered for stereotactic radiosurgery followed by WBRT if they have a PS of 0–1, >1year disease-free interval and controlled systemic disease.

Brain metastasis after prophylactic cranial radiotherapy and previous treatment

Patients with isolated metastasis can be considered for radiosurgery in a selected group of patients. If a patient had previously benefited from WBRT for at least 4 months and the general condition is good (PS 0–1), re-irradiation, either partial brain or whole brain may be considered.

Leptomeningeal carcinomatosis

Infiltration of the leptomeninges by cancer commonly occurs with breast and lung cancer, melanoma, lymphoma and leukaemias. Clinical presentation can be with features of increased intracranial pressure, cranial nerve palsies or impaired higher function. Diagnosis is based on MRI scan (CT has a reduced sensitivity of 30% compared with 70% for MRI) and CSF examination. Typical findings on MRI are subarachnoid or parenchymal nodule (Figure 16.8) and sulcal/dural enhancement. Patients with good prognosis (limited disease, PS0–1, chemo-sensitive tumour and minimal neurologic deficit) are treated with intrathecal chemotherapy with radiotherapy to symptomatic sites and systemic chemotherapy. Median survival in untreated patients is 4–6

weeks, with prompt treatment median survival is around 6–8 months.

Spinal cord tumours

Spinal cord tumours can be either primary or secondary. Primary spinal cord tumours consist of 2–4% of all primary CNS tumours. Common spinal cord tumours are shown in Box 16.6.

Pain is the commonest presenting symptom. There will be varying degrees of spinal cord compression depending on the location of tumour. Evaluation includes a full neurological examination to assess the extent and level of neurological deficit. MRI is the imaging of choice. Intramedullary tumours may expand the cord and other imaging features are similar to that of corresponding tumours in the brain (Table 16.1).

Management

General management includes pain control, steroids which reduce both pain and the neurological deficit and rehabilitative measures.

The definitive treatment is surgery. Early surgery is advocated to avoid further neurological damage. Maximal safe removal with the help of operative microscope and tools such as intraoperative ultrasound and cavitating ultrasonic aspirator is the norm. Indication for and dose of radiotherapy is as in Box 16.7. Radiotherapy is indicated for all intramedullary tumours except the following situations:

1. Pilocytic tumours (grade 1) after complete and incomplete resection (5-year survival 90%).
2. Myxopapillary ependymoma (grade 1) after complete (10-year survival 98%) or incomplete resection (10-year survival 70%).

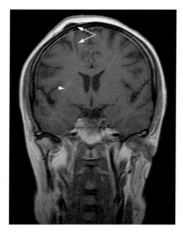

Figure 16.8
Ommaya reservoir (arrows) in situ for intrathecal chemotherapy, and there is an enhancing parenchymal lesion (arrow head).

Box 16.6: Spinal cord tumours

Intramedullary (within spinal cord)
- Glioma – ependymoma or astrocytoma
- Metastasis (rare)

Extramedullary – intradural (outside the cord but within the dura)
- Meningioma – usually grade 1
- Nerve sheath tumours – usually grade 1

Extradural
- Metastasis – lung, breast, prostate etc.
- Primary tumours of spine

Box 16.7: Radiotherapy for intramedullary tumours

Position – depends on the site of tumour
- Cervical – prone
- Thoracic – supine
- Lumbar – supine or prone

Target volume
- CTV – spinal canal in axial direction and 2–3 cm superioinferior margin
- PTV – 1 cm

Dose 50 Gy in 30 fractions

3. Grade 2 astrocytoma after complete resection.

Extramedullary tumours are treated with surgical excision followed by imaging follow-up. Incompletely excised grade 2–3 meningiomas are considered for postoperative radiotherapy.

Extradural tumours treated according to the histologic type of the tumour.

Chemotherapy has a limited role in spinal cord tumours except in high-grade glioma. When necessary, agents used in brain tumours can be used.

Prognosis

Prognosis depends on histologic type and grade, age (younger the better), functional status at presentation, size of the tumour (dictates operability) and extent of resection.

Management of recurrence

A second surgery if feasible is the treatment option in low-grade tumour recurrences. Radiotherapy may be considered if surgery is not possible and radiotherapy has not previously been given. Chemotherapy is an option for high-grade recurrences (Box 16.3).

Further reading

Nieder C, Mehta MP, Jalali R. Combined radio- and chemotherapy of brain tumours in adult patients. Clin Oncol. 2009;21:515–524.

van den Bent MJ, Hegi ME, Stupp R. Recent developments in the use of chemotherapy in brain tumours. Eur J Cancer. 2006;42:582–588.

Noda SE, El-Jawahri A, Patel D, Lautenschlaeger T, Siedow M, Chakravarti A. Molecular advances of brain tumors in radiation oncology. Semin Radiat Oncol. 2009;19:171–178.

Van Meir EG, Hadjipanayis CG, Norden AD, Shu HK, Wen PY, Olson JJ. Exciting new advances in neuro-oncology: the avenue to a cure for malignant glioma. CA Cancer J Clin. 2010;60:166–193.

Soffietti R, Rudà R, Trevisan E. Brain metastases: current management and new developments. Curr Opin Oncol. 2008;20:676–684.

Khuntia D, Brown P, Li J, Mehta MP. Whole-brain radiotherapy in the management of brain metastasis. J Clin Oncol. 2006;24:1295–1304.

Traul DE, Shaffrey ME, Schiff D. Part I: spinal-cord neoplasms-intradural neoplasms. Lancet Oncol. 2007; 8:35–45.

Endocrine tumours

TV Ajithkumar

Thyroid cancer

Thyroid malignancies are the commonest endocrine malignancy. Common types of thyroid cancers are papillary and follicular carcinomas (well-differentiated cancers) arising from epithelial cell, medullary carcinomas from the parafollicular C cells, anaplastic carcinoma and NHL. Well-differentiated cancers typically affect women in their 40s. The median age of presentation of medullary carcinoma is 50–60 years and older for anaplastic carcinoma.

Aetiology

The majority of thyroid cancers are sporadic. Other risk factors include radiation exposure (papillary carcinoma), genetic (e.g. MEN2 with medullary carcinoma, FAP with papillary carcinoma) and endemic goitre (follicular carcinoma).

Presentation

Common presentation is with an enlarging solitary nodule. Cervical lymphadenopathy is common with medullary, papillary and anaplastic carcinoma. Local invasion can lead to symptoms of hoarseness of the voice and dysphagia. Anaplastic carcinoma has an aggressive growth with local invasion and rapid growth which can lead to stridor.

Evaluation

Evaluation includes clinical examination and assessment for thyrotoxicosis which is rare in cancer. Initial investigations include thyroid function tests and FNA of the lesion. Biopsy may be indicated for lymphoma and anaplastic carcinoma and hemithyroidectomy is indicated for all follicular lesions. MRI is the preferred imaging to assess local invasion (Figure 17.1) as the use of iodine containing contrast can cause thyroid stunning which may prevent effective use of radioiodine for at least three months subsequently.

Staging

Box 17.1 shows the TNM staging system. The TNM and MACIS (Box 17.2) have been shown to be the best predictors of outcome in differentiated thyroid cancer.

Management

Well-differentiated cancer

Surgery is the definitive treatment of all malignancies except lymphoma. The majority of patients need total or near total thyroidectomy. In low-risk patients (<1 cm papillary cancer with no nodes, <2 cm follicular cancer in women aged less than 45 years and <1 cm follicular cancer with minimal capsular invasion) lobectomy is adequate. Patients with high-risk disease (male >45 years, tumour >4 cm and extracapsular spread) are at risk of level VI nodal involvement and hence elective central node dissection is indicated. Patients with proven neck node metastases are treated with modified radical neck dissection. All patients should have serum calcium postoperatively to rule out transient hypocalcaemia. Serum thyroglobulin (TG), the tumour marker, is estimated 6 weeks postoperatively which should be undetectable in patients who had total thyroidectomy and have no residual disease. Patients after total thyroidectomy are started on triiodothyronine (T3) 20 mg thrice daily which is subsequently changed to T4. T4 is started

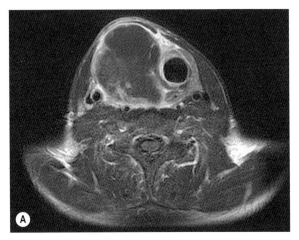
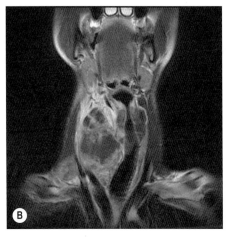

Figure 17.1
Axial (A) and coronal (B) view of MRI scan in anaplastic carcinoma of thyroid.

Box 17.1: TNM staging in thyroid cancer

T stage

pT1	Tumour ≤2 cm in greatest dimension
pT2	Intrathyroidal tumour >2–4 cm in greatest dimension
pT3	Intrathyroidal tumour >4 cm in greatest dimension
pT4	Tumour beyond the thyroid capsule

N stage (cervical and upper mediastinal)

N0	No nodes involved
N1	Regional nodal involvement
	N1a Ipsilateral cervical nodes
	N1b Bilateral, midline or contralateral cervical nodes, or mediastinal nodes

Distant metastases

M0	No distant metastases
M1	Distant metastases
MX	Distant metastases cannot be assessed

Staging of epithelial thyroid carcinomas

Stage I
  Aged 45 or younger with any pT, any N M0
  Aged 45 or older with pT1N0M0

Stage II
  Aged 45 or younger with any pT any N M1
  Aged 45 or older with pT2N0M0 or pT3N0M0

Stage III
  Aged 45 or older with pT4N0M0 or any pT, N1M0

Stage IV
  Aged 45 or older with any pT, any N, M1
  Anaplastic thyroid carcinoma any age or stage

Box 17.2: MACIS (Metastasis, Age, Completeness of resection, Invasion, Size). Scoring system to assess 20-year survival probability of papillary

Scores
Metastasis – Present: score 3
Age – <40 years: score 3.1
     >40 years: score = 0.08 × age
Completeness of resection – incomplete: score 1
Invasion – present: score 1
Tumour size: score = 0.3 × size in cm

Total score and 20-year survival

<6	99%
6–6.99	89%
7–7.99	56%
>8	24%

---

with a dose of 100 mcg daily and increased by 25 mcg every 6 weeks until TSH levels are below 0.1 MiU/L.

Radioablation
Postoperative radioiodine ablation is recommended for all patients except for those who had total thyroidectomy for a well-differentiated unifocal tumour of <1 cm with no vascular or extracapsular invasion. Informed consent should be obtained and instruct female patients not to get pregnant prior to and up to 12 months after treatment (Box 17.3). T4 is substituted with T3 4–6 weeks before radioablation and T3 is withdrawn 2 weeks before ablation. 3–3.7 GBq of radioiodine is administered orally. In patients with a history of myxoedema psychosis, severe

Box 17.3: Side effects of radioablation

Early effects
- Sialoadenitis and taste changes
- Nausea
- Neck pain and swelling
- Radiation cystitis, gastritis
- Symptoms of hypothyroidism for 4–6 weeks

Late effects
- Dry mouth and taste changes
- Dry eyes due to lachrymal gland dysfunction
- Increase in miscarriage rate in first year after treatment
- Pulmonary fibrosis
- Male infertility
- Risk of 2nd malignancy

cardiac disease and high volume disease, T3 withdrawal can be dangerous and hence recombinant human TSH (0.9 mg IM daily for 48 hours before radioablation) is used. Patients are admitted to and remain in a specialist facility with appropriate shielding and sanitation. Isolation is continued until safe levels of radiation are measured by a medical physicist. Patients are advised to keep well-hydrated, empty the bladder frequently and to take prescribed laxatives to avoid constipation and these measures are aimed at minimizing the absorbed dose of radiation. An uptake scan is done 3–10 days after radioiodine to assess residual thyroid tissue. In patients with elevated TG and positive uptake scans, either further surgery or repeat dose of radioiodine (5.5 MBq) is indicated. Further management afterwards is shown in Figure 17.2.

Some patients do not have a take-up of radioiodine when external beam radiotherapy to the entire thyroid bed has been carried out, and level III–VI nodes (60 Gy in 30 fractions) is indicated if there is gross residual disease, extranodal disease and in patients >60 years with T4 disease.

Medullary carcinoma

All patients with medullary carcinoma should have screening for phaeochromocytoma with 24-hour urinary catecholamines and serum calcium to exclude hyperparathyroidism (MEN2 syndrome).

Total thyroidectomy with elective central nodal dissection is the treatment of choice even

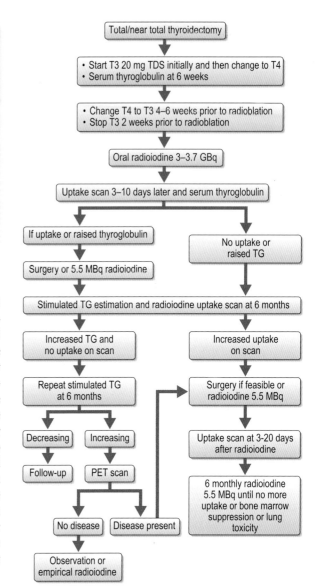

Figure 17.2
Management of well-differentiated thyroid cancer.

if metastatic disease is present. In metastatic disease this helps with optimal local symptom control and control of calcium levels. In patients with level II–V nodal involvement modified radical neck dissection is done. All patients need a suppressive dose of thyroxine.

There is no role for radioiodine ablation. In patients with incomplete resection, postoperative radiotherapy to the thyroid bed, bilateral cervical and upper mediastinal nodes (50–60 Gy in 2 Gy per fraction) may be given to improve relapse-free survival.

Follow-up is life-long with clinical examination, serum calcitonin estimation and ensuring adequate thyroid suppression.

Patients presenting with recurrence may be treated with surgical excision if feasible. Radiotherapy is useful in inoperable local recurrence. Patients with symptomatic metastatic disease may be considered for ^{131}I-MIBG or radiolabelled somatostatin analogues if there is uptake with the corresponding scans.

All patients with medullary carcinoma thyroid require genetic screening for mutations in the RET gene at exon 10, 11, 13 and 16. Prophylactic surgery is indicated in gene carrier mutated relatives (before 1 year in MEN 2B and 5–10 years in MEN 2A).

Anaplastic carcinoma thyroid

Surgery is an option only in a small proportion of patients and the majority of patients present with locally advanced and metastatic disease. Radiotherapy is the principal treatment which is essentially to improve local control. It is given either as 50–60 Gy in 2 Gy per fraction or in combination with chemotherapy (adriamycin).

Prognosis

The long-term survival of well-differentiated thyroid cancer is >90%. 10-year survival of medullary carcinoma thyroid is 50–70% and median survival of anaplastic carcinoma is less than 6 months (5-year survival <10%).

Adrenocortical carcinoma

Introduction

Adrenocortical carcinoma (ACC) is a rare malignancy with heterogeneous manifestations and a poor prognosis. In adults it peaks at 57 years of age. There are no proven aetiological factors. ACC is rarely reported in multiple endocrine neoplasia I (MEN I), Li–Fraumeni and Wiedemann–Beckwith syndromes.

Presentation

Approximately 60% patients present with features of adrenal steroid hypersecretion. Rapidly progressing Cushing's syndrome with or without virilization is the most common presentation. Other presenting symptoms include virilization in women and gynaecomastia and testicular atrophy in men, hypertension and hypokalaemia.

Non-secreting tumours present with abdominal discomfort or back pain due to mass effect. Rarely patients can present with fever, weight loss and anorexia.

Diagnosis

Initial investigations include hormonal workup and imaging with CT chest and abdomen (Figure 17.3). MRI is also useful in identifying invasion of adjacent organs and the inferior vena cava, and hence in planning surgery. Biopsy of an adrenal tumour is controversial because of the theoretical risk of needle tract metastases. However, it may be acceptable if primary surgical management is not feasible and diagnosis cannot be established with non-invasive measures.

Staging

WHO (2004) staging for adrenocortical carcinoma is as follows:

Stage I: localized tumour of ≤5 cm.
Stage II: localized tumour of >5 cm.

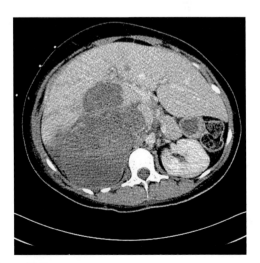

Figure 17.3
CT scan in adrenocortical carcinoma. On CT scan adrenocortical carcinoma is typically more than 4 cm with central necrosis with heterogeneous enhancement and may show calcification (30%) and invasion into adjacent structures.

Stage III: locally invasive or tumours with regional lymph node metastases.

Stage IV: tumour invading adjacent organs or distant metastases.

Management

Complete removal of tumour offers best chance for cure in patients with stage I–III tumours. Radiotherapy has an established role in the palliation of bone and brain metastases. Mitotane (o,p'-DDD) is a specific drug for the treatment of adrenocortical cancer which leads to an objective response of 25% of cases. The main side effects are vomiting, diarrhoea, lethargy, somnolence, depression, and adrenal insufficiency. All patients need high-dose gluococorticoid replacement (e.g. 50 mg hydrocortisone daily) which helps to minimize mitotane-induced side effects.

Combination chemotherapy with mitotane with streptozocin has yielded a response rate (partial and complete) of 36%.

The commonly used combination regimes used are cisplatin, etoposide and doxorubicin (EDP) with mitotane (Berruti Regime) and EDP with streptozocin (Khan Regime). The ongoing FIRM-ACT trial is comparing efficacy of these two combination regimes in patients with inoperable stage III–IV disease.

Outcome

The reported 5-year survival is 60% for stage I, 58% for stage II, 24% for stage III and 0% for stage IV. Median survival of stage IV patients is less than 12 months. Cortisol secreting tumours are associated with worse prognosis, partially attributable to morbidity associated with Cushing's syndrome.

Further reading

British Thyroid Association – Guidelines from the management of thyroid cancer 2nd Edition. 2007. Available from: http://www.british-thyroid-association.org/

Ganti AK, Cohen EE. Iodine-refractory thyroid carcinoma. Rev Recent Clin Trials. 2006;1:133–141.

Tuttle RM, Ball DW, Byrd D et al. Medullary carcinoma. J Natl Compr Canc Netw. 2010;8:512–530.

Sherman SI. Molecularly targeted therapies for thyroid cancers. Endocr Pract. 2009;15:605–611.

Neff RL, Farrar WB, Kloos RT, Burman KD. Anaplastic thyroid cancer. Endocrinol Metab Clin North Am. 2008;37:525–538.

Wandoloski M, Bussey KJ, Demeure MJ. Adrenocortical cancer. Surg Clin North Am. 2009;89(5):1255–1267.

Fassnacht M, Allolio B. Clinical management of adrenocortical carcinoma. Best Pract Res Clin Endocrinol Metab. 2009;23:273–289.

Cancers of unknown primary

18

TV Ajithkumar and HM Hatcher

Introduction

Cancers of unknown primary (CUP) constitute 3–5% of all cancers. The criteria for diagnosis of CUP includes patients who have a biopsy proven metastatic cancer in whom a detailed history, physical examination, blood tests, immunohisto-chemistry of biopsy, chest X-ray, CT scan of the abdomen and pelvis and in certain cases, mammography or FDG-PET fail to detect a primary tumour.

Evaluation

Clinicopathological evaluation aims to identify a primary site, a clinicopathological subset and to rule out non-epithelial tumours. The first step includes clinical history to establish risk factors, clinical examination, investigations and patho-logical evaluation. Initial investigations include blood tests, urinalysis, faecal occult blood test and CT scan of the chest, abdomen and thorax. Endo-scopic evaluation is guided by symptoms and/or signs. In patients suspected to have extragonadal germ cell tumours a serum beta-hCG and AFP should be estimated. Other tumour markers depending on the clinical context include PSA, CEA, CA-125 and CA19-9. Pathological evalua-tion includes light microscopy and expedient use of immunohistochemical techniques. Immunohis-tochemistry is useful in differentiating epithelial from non-epithelial tumours, such as sarcoma and lymphoma (Table 18.1). The majority of epithe-lial tumours are adenocarcinoma (65–80%) fol-lowed by squamous cell carcinoma (10–15%) and undifferentiated carcinoma (5–10%).

The outcome of first step evaluation is identification of a specific clinicopathological entity which may be a favourable (15% patients) or unfavourable (85% patients) (Box 18.1).

All patients should have an assessment of performance status and co-morbidities, which will guide treatment decisions.

Management

The decision to treat depends on the clinico-pathological entity and performance status. Patients with poor performance status (>2) are generally treated symptomatically. Treatment of various subsets is as described below.

Women with isolated axillary lymphadenopathy

Women presenting like this are treated like stage II breast cancer. Previous studies showed an occult primary in 50–60% of cases after mastec-tomy. However, if MRI of the breast failed to show any primary, breast surgery or radiother-apy may not be warranted. Axillary lymphaden-opathy is treated with lymph-node dissection followed by regional radiotherapy based on breast cancer radiotherapy principles (p. 124). Adjuvant systemic treatment is similar to stage II breast cancer. The reported 5-year survival for patients with 1–3 nodes are 87% and those with >3 nodes are 42%.

Women with peritoneal carcinomatosis

Women with peritoneal carcinomatosis are treated like stage III ovarian cancer with initial cytoreduction followed by combination chemo-therapy or vice versa depending on performance status and co-morbidities (p. 201). CA-125 may be used as a tumour marker if elevated and the reported long-term survival is 15%.

© 2011, Elsevier Ltd
DOI: 10.1016/B978-0-7234-3458-0.00023-3

Table 18.1: Immunohistochemistry in cancers of unknown primary

	CK7	CK20	TTF-1	Other markers
Colorectal	–	+	–	CDX-2
Pancreas	+	+		
Stomach	Variable	Variable		CDX-2 (intestinal-type cancers)
Lung	+	–	+*	
Ovary	+	+		
Breast	+	–		ER/PR/HER2
Prostate	–	–		PSA/PSAP
Melanoma	–	–	–	S100+ (except signet ring) HMB-45 and Melan-A
Lymphoma	–	–	–	CD45 CD79a/CD20 (B cell)
Small cell	dot +	dot +	+/–	CD56/chromogranin/synaptophysin

*Adenocarcinoma in lung – TTF-1 is highly specific for lung and thyroid adenocarcinoma, lung small cell, and may stain extra-pulmonary small cell carcinoma.

Box 18.1: Clinicopathological subsets of cancer of unknown primary

Subset

Favourable subset

Adenocarcinoma
- Women with isolated axillary lymph node
- Women with peritoneal papillary serous adenocarcinoma
- Men with sclerotic metastases
- Single metastatic lesion

Squamous cell cancer
- Patients with cervical lymphadenopathy
- Patients with inguinal lymphadenopathy

Poorly differentiated or undifferentiated
- Undifferentiated neuroendocrine carcinoma
- Poorly differentiated carcinoma of the midline in the young

Unfavourable subset
- Metastasis to liver or multiple sites
- Malignant ascites with non-papillary serous carcinoma
- Multiple brain metastases
- Multiple bone metastases

Men with sclerotic metastasis

Men with sclerotic metastasis and with either raised serum PSA or immunohistochemical stain for PSA are treated with hormonal treatment for prostate cancer.

Single metastatic disease

Patients with single metastatic disease are treated with surgical excision or radical radiotherapy or combination. Role of systemic treatment is not known.

Cervical lymphadenopathy

Upper or mid-cervical lymphadenopathy can be due to a head and neck primary whereas lower cervical lymphadenopathy or supraclavicular lymphadenopathy can be due to either a head and neck cancer or lung tumour. Investigations using panendoscopy with CT/MR imaging will help to identify the primary site of the tumour in 85–90% of cases. If a lesion is not identified, unilateral tonsillectomy is done to rule out a tonsillar primary. PET scan may also be useful in identifying the primary. If a primary is detected it is treated accordingly with combined modality treatment with surgery and radiotherapy or chemo-radiotherapy. If no primary is detected, lymphadenopathy is treated with neck dissection followed by radiotherapy or radical radiotherapy. The reported 5-year survival ranges between 20–70%.

Patients presenting with inguinal lymphadenopathy

In this group of patients investigations are to rule out a primary site in the perineal area. If no primary tumour is detected, treatment is node dissection with or without postoperative radiotherapy.

Poorly differentiated carcinoma with midline distribution in young

These patients are usually male under 50 years of age, with mediastinal and/or retroperitoneal tumours. Serum beta-hCG and AFP estimation (raised in 20%), CT scan of chest, abdomen and pelvis and ultrasound of testis are needed. These patients are treated as poor prognostic germ cell tumours with four courses of BEP chemotherapy followed by surgical resection of any residual disease.

Poorly differentiated neuroendocrine carcinomas

These are treated with a combination of chemotherapy with cisplatin and etoposide which yields a response rate of over 70% with 16% durable remission based on a small series of 51 patients.

Poorly differentiated carcinoma without features of neuroendocrine or germ cell tumour

Patients with these tumours are in the good prognosis group and hence treated with a cisplatin regime like that used for germ cell tumours. In a study of 220 patients with median age of 39 years, the overall response rate was 64% with 27% complete response and median survival of 20 months.

Patients with unfavourable disease

Patients in the unfavourable subset are treated with symptomatic and palliative care. Those with good performance status are treated with chemotherapy with cisplatin-based or taxane/platinum combination which yields a response rate between 10–40% and median survival of 5–9 months.

Further reading

Pavlidis N, Fizazi K. Carcinoma of unknown primary (CUP). Crit Rev Oncol Hematol. 2009;69:271–278.

Greco FA, Erlander MG. Molecular classification of cancers of unknown primary site. Mol Diagn Ther. 2009;13:367–373.

Morris GJ, Greco FA, Hainsworth JD et al. Cancer of unknown primary site. Semin Oncol. 2010;37:71–79.

Varadhachary GR, Abbruzzese JL, Lenzi R. Diagnostic strategies for unknown primary cancer. Cancer. 2004;100:1776–1785.

Pavlidis N, Briasoulis E and Pentheroudakis. Cancer of unknown primary site: ESMO clinical practice guidelines for diagnosis, treatment and follow-up. Ann Oncol. 2010;21(suppl 5):v228–v231.

Cancer in pregnancy

TV Ajithkumar and HM Hatcher

Cancer during pregnancy poses a very challenging situation. Cancer complicates 0.02–0.1% of pregnancies. The oncologist faces the difficult situation of optimizing the care of the mother without causing harm to the foetus. The common tumours diagnosed during pregnancy are malignant melanoma, breast cancer and cervical cancer.

Diagnostic work-up

All patients require a complete physical examination. Although histological diagnosis with fine needle aspiration cytology and core biopsies are safe, general anaesthesia during the first trimester carries a 1–2% risk of spontaneous abortion. Endoscopic biopsies as well as lumbar puncture and bone marrow examinations are safe. Radiological investigations should be restricted to minimize the foetal exposure to ionizing radiation. A foetal exposure dose of 1 mGy is considered safe. Box 19.1 shows various imaging procedures and uterine/foetal exposure dose. A dose of less than 100 mGy (10 cGy) is associated with less than 1% risk of foetal malformation and carcinogenesis and hence, in the event of inadvertent exposure of pregnant women to radiation, termination of pregnancy is not recommended if the foetal dose does not exceed this limit.

During the first trimester of pregnancy, radiological investigations are indicated only if absolutely necessary. Chest X-ray with lead apron is considered safe and hence can be used with ultrasound sonogram for initial evaluation. MRI without gadolinium (which crosses the placenta) can be used to rule out metastatic disease in the brain, liver and bone when indicated. Avoidance of MRI in the first trimester of pregnancy has

been suggested due to the risk of foetal heating/cavitation. Abdominal X-rays, CT scans and isotope scans should be avoided during pregnancy. However, a final decision to perform these investigations is based on the risk benefit for the mother (your patient), their expected survival and the gestation of the foetus.

Principles of management

Termination of pregnancy

Termination of pregnancy is an option when pregnancy itself is an obstacle to aggressive management of cancer and is associated with unacceptable risks for the health of mother and foetus. Termination of pregnancy in the first trimester is indicated only when treatment cannot be delayed and should take into consideration the curability of cancer, drugs to be used and wishes of the patient. The indications for termination generally are:

- Abdominal/pelvic tumour necessitating immediate treatment, especially if radiotherapy is needed.
- Aggressive disease course.
- Poor general condition of the patient.
- Inadvertent foetal exposure to more than 100 mGy during the first trimester.

Surgery

Surgery can be performed without major risk to the patient during the first two trimesters, but with a 1–2% risk of foetal loss, small risk of low birth weight (RR 1.5–2.0) and premature delivery. Foetal harm during surgery is due to various factors including placental transfer of drugs, intraoperative complications such as hypoxia,

Box 19.1: Uterine/foetal radiation dose during various radiological investigations

Investigation	Uterine/foetal dose
Chest X-ray	0.000005 Gy
Abdominal X-ray	0.022 Gy
Mammogram	0.04 Gy
Chest CT scan	0.002 Gy
Abdominal CT scan	0.02 Gy
Pelvic CT	0.07 Gy
Barium enema	0.036 Gy
IVU	0.045 Gy
Bone scan	0.018–0.045 Gy

1 Gy = 100 cGy = 1000 mGy

Box 19.2: Foetal radiation dose during radiotherapy

Radiotherapy	Foetal dose
Cervical cancer	45–50 Gy
Mantle field	0.014–0.13 Gy
Breast cancer	0.14–0.18 Gy
Brain tumour and head and neck cancer	0.0015–0.08 Gy

hypotension, and long-term supine positioning of mother during surgery causing placental underperfusion.

In the third trimester surgery after foetal maturation and delayed surgery until post-partum if appropriate are the options.

Intra-abdominal surgery is more likely to interfere with pregnancy. During major abdominal and pelvic surgery, continuous monitoring of the foetus is necessary. Measures to suppress premature labour and prophylactic treatment to improve foetal lung maturity should be undertaken if the surgery carries a risk of premature labour.

Timing of delivery and breast feeding

Delivery is generally planned after weeks 32–35 (earlier in modern neonatal units with better outcome for the baby) and 3 weeks after the last chemotherapy. Breast feeding is not recommended during chemotherapy, up to 2–4 weeks after completion of chemotherapy and during hormonal treatment.

Radiotherapy

The developing embryo or foetus is extremely sensitive to ionizing radiation, which can cause foetal loss, malformations, growth retardation and defects in intelligence. Radiotherapy is therefore contraindicated for abdominal and pelvic malignancies during pregnancy. Several studies support the use of radiotherapy for head and neck cancer, breast cancer and brain tumours. Radical radiotherapy to the head and neck and brain can be achieved with a foetal dose of less than 100 mGy (Box 19.2). During radiotherapy to the breast and chest wall, the dose to the foetus increases with gestational age. The foetal dose depends on the radiation field, dose, the distance between the edge of radiation field and foetus, and the machine and its shielding measures.

Radiotherapy should be delayed until postpartum if possible. If radiotherapy cannot be postponed the second trimester is the preferable time to deliver with appropriate precautions to keep foetal dose below 5–10 cGy.

Systemic treatment

Most cytotoxic drugs have a low molecular weight of less than 600 kDa and can cross the placenta. The concern is that these agents can cause various mutagenic, teratogenic and carcinogenic effects in the foetus. Physiological changes due to pregnancy such as change in haemodynamics and renal clearance will also alter the metabolism, distribution and elimination of cytotoxic agents leading to unpredictable effects. Chemotherapy interferes with organogenesis in the first trimester, leading to a high risk of teratogenesis (10% with single agent and 20% with combination) and hence is not advised. After the first trimester organogenesis is complete except for the brain and gonads. Chemotherapy during this period can cause foetal growth retardation (2-fold risk), stillbirths (5%), premature delivery (5%), low birth weight (7%) and myelosuppression (4%). However, the risk of teratogenesis is almost similar to the general population (2–3%); but there is concern about risk of sterility, defects in intellectual function and other organ dysfunction due to in utero exposure of chemotherapy.

Alkylators and anti-metabolites are the most teratogenic and have high abortive potential.

Vinca alkaloids, anthracyclines, 5-fluorouracil, cytarabine, taxanes and platinums appear to be relatively safe.

Chemotherapy during pregnancy needs to be modified according to the toxicity data of individual drugs. Chemotherapy is not given after 35 weeks and stopped 3 weeks prior to a planned delivery of the baby to allow for recovery of bone marrow function of the mother and foetus and for placental drug excretion from the foetus.

Postpartum care

The placenta should be send for histopathologic examination as there is risk of placental metastasis. Metastases can also occur in the foetus. In the absence of placental metastasis, optimal follow-up of a healthy baby is not known.

Future pregnancies

Most oncologists would recommend women not to become pregnant during follow-up for a period of 2–3 years depending on the type of cancer, risk of recurrence and patient's age and wishes. There is no evidence to suggest that future pregnancies compromise survival.

Care of the baby

Anthracycline exposure in utero may affect heart development so this should be assessed as the child grows. With platinum-based chemotherapy during pregnancy, there is a concern that any non-renally excreted dose will be retained within the tissue which may affect later development, e.g. neural, although there is little evidence of this.

Management of specific cancers

Cervical cancer

The majority of cervical cancers in pregnancy are asymptomatic, diagnosed by abnormal cytology. Though atypical cytology is not uncommon in pregnancy, dysplastic changes are suspicious. Colposcopic biopsy is needed for suspected malignancy. Cone biopsy is associated with increased risk of vaginal bleeding, abortion, infection and premature delivery and hence used only for patients with suspicion of microinvasion

or invasive disease. When indicated conization is done at 14–20 weeks of pregnancy. The majority of cervical cancer in pregnancy is squamous cell carcinoma (80–90%) and 80% present with stage IA–IIA disease. Staging includes physical examination, chest X-ray and MRI of abdomen and pelvis.

Cervical carcinoma-in-situ (CIN) can be managed with close follow-up with cytology and colposcopy. When invasive cancer is diagnosed the choice is between termination of pregnancy followed by treatment or postponing treatment until delivery. Cervical cancer with less than 3 mm invasion can be followed and delivered vaginally, whereas those with 3–5 mm invasion and/or lymphovascular invasion are delivered by caesarean section at 32–36 weeks.

Management of stage IA disease during the first trimester is debatable. Some advise radical hysterectomy for margin positive IA1 disease and IA2 disease. Patients with IA disease diagnosed during the second or third trimester can be followed up and treated only after delivery.

Patients with stage IB–IVA disease during the first and second trimesters of pregnancy are managed by termination of pregnancy and immediate treatment, whereas those diagnosed during the third trimester may be followed up until delivery after 32–38 weeks. Some patients diagnosed with cervical cancer in later second trimester and early third trimester can be treated with neoadjuvant chemotherapy until delivery of the baby. Radical treatment involves radical hysterectomy with lymphadenectomy or chemoradiotherapy.

There is no evidence to suggest that cervical cancer diagnosed during pregnancy has a worse outcome than those diagnosed when not pregnant, stage for stage.

Breast cancer

Breast cancer in pregnancy can occur at any time during pregnancy and within 12 months postpartum. The median age at diagnosis is 33 years and the commonest presentation is a painless palpable lump (80–95%). Presentation is similar to non-pregnant breast cancer. Diagnosis may be delayed accounting for a 2.5-fold increased risk of advanced cancers (40%) at presentation. Diagnosis is by mammogram, ultrasonography and non-enhanced MRI. Cytology may be difficult to interpret due to pregnancy associated changes and hence needle biopsy or open biopsy is diagnostic. The most common histological type is invasive ductal carcinoma (80–90%) followed by lobular carcinoma. The majority of tumours are high grade with axillary involvement (60–90%). Hormone receptors are negative in 40–70% and HER2 positive in 28–58%.

Staging investigations include chest X-ray, USS of abdomen and axilla and MRI if indicated. Serum alkaline phosphatase is doubled during pregnancy, but serum transaminases and CA 15-3 are unaffected.

In patients with non-metastatic disease, mastectomy and breast conserving surgery followed by radiotherapy (post partum) are accepted surgical treatments. Sentinel node biopsy using blue dye (risk of allergic reaction) and radioisotope are not advised (though the exposure is <5–15 mGy). Patients who need adjuvant chemotherapy can be safely treated after 12 weeks of gestation (1.3% risk of malformation) using anthracycline containing regime. Hormonal treatment and transtuzumab are not advised during pregnancy.

Patients with metastasis can be treated with chemotherapy after the first trimester. However, the issue of termination of pregnancy should be discussed in the appropriate context.

Most series suggest that pregnancy does not affect the natural course of illness or prognosis.

Melanoma

Common presenting symptoms are change in size and colour and bleeding or ulceration of pre-existing melanotic lesion as with melanomas diagnosed outside pregnancy (p. 234). Patients can present with lymphadenopathy and features of metastatic disease. Evaluation includes full clinical examination and skin examination followed by excisional biopsy, in limited disease. The commonest type is superficial spreading (74%) followed by nodular melanoma (16%). In the absence of clinical features of metastases, chest X-ray and USS abdomen are sufficient for staging.

The surgical excision margin is based on thickness of primary (p. 234). Treatment of metastatic melanoma is essentially palliative. Pregnancy termination should be discussed with the patient. Chemotherapy using dacarbazine or cisplatin can

be given after the first trimester if the patient decides to continue with the pregnancy.

Studies suggest that the survival following a diagnosis of melanoma in pregnancy is the same as an equivalent stage of melanoma diagnosed in a non-pregnant woman.

Lymphomas

Lymphomas present with lymphadenopathy (70–80%) and B symptoms (20%). A small series suggested that in NHL there is a higher chance of presentation with extranodal manifestation (breast, GI, cervix and ovary). 70% of Hodgkin's disease (HD) presents with stage I–II disease, whilst 70–80% of NHL present with stage III–IV disease.

Investigations include full blood count including ESR (raised in pregnancy), biochemistry, lymph node excision biopsy, bone marrow examination, USS of abdomen and pelvis. ENT examination, endoscopy and nervous system staging are done whenever indicated.

The most common type of HD is nodular sclerosis and 90% of pregnancy associated NHL are high grade.

When the diagnosis is made in the first trimester, termination of pregnancy is considered particularly in those with B-symptoms, bulky stage I–II, stage III–IV and high-grade lymphoma. If the patient refuses termination, single agent vinblastine may be given until the second trimester. The preferred regime for HD is ABVD and for NHL is CHOP (p. 298). Treatment may be delayed until delivery in low volume low-grade NHL. If treatment is needed for low-grade NHL, single agent chemotherapy or limited field radiotherapy is used.

When the diagnosis is made in the third trimester, treatment may be delayed until delivery at 32–35 weeks. Radiotherapy whenever indicated is generally delayed until delivery.

Prognosis of pregnancy associated lymphomas is similar to that of non-pregnant patients. The long term remission is 88% for HD and 45% for NHL.

Ovarian cancer

Ovarian cancer is diagnosed rarely in pregnancy with 35% adenocarcinoma, 30% borderline ovarian tumour and 35% germ-cell/sex cord

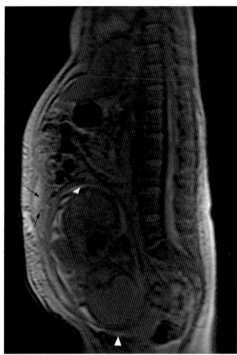

Figure 19.1
Pregnancy associated ovarian cancer – MRI shows uterus with foetus (white arrow heads) and omental thickening (arrow). Biopsy of the omental thickening confirmed serous papillary adenocarcinoma consistent with a primary peritoneal cancer.

stromal tumour (most common dysgerminoma). Most of the borderline and germ cell tumours are diagnosed at an early stage.

Staging includes chest X-ray, abdominal and pelvic ultrasound and MRI if indicated (Figure 19.1). CA-125, beta-hCG and AFP are raised in pregnancy.

Laparotomy or laparoscopy is indicated when there is suspicion of an ovarian lesion (persistent solid or complex mass lesion of >6 cm with asso-

ciated ascites). Surgical principles follow that of ovarian cancer in non-pregnant women (p. 197). Maximum feasible cytoreduction is attempted and bilateral salpingo-oophorectomy after week 7 is feasible as the hormonal function will be taken up by placenta. Other option is neoadjuvant chemotherapy depending on the stage of gestation. In high-grade bulky tumours hysterectomy is also advisable. Chemotherapy may be administered after the first trimester.

Psychosocial support

A diagnosis of cancer during pregnancy is an extremely distressing situation for the patient and family, as they may have to decide about future plans which may not include both of them. This necessitates provision of adequate psychosocial support for both the parents (and probably grandparents!). Needless to say that there will be anxiety about the baby, though evidence shows little harm to date (but is minimal). The risks of a genetically associated cancer in the child should be evaluated by clinical genetics criteria (p. 45) but are not affected by being diagnosed in pregnancy.

Further reading

Azim HA Jr, Peccatori FA, Pavlidis N. Treatment of the pregnant mother with cancer: a systematic review on the use of cytotoxic, endocrine, targeted agents and immunotherapy during pregnancy. Part I: Solid tumors. Cancer Treat Rev. 2010;36:101–109.

Azim HA Jr, Pavlidis N, Peccatori FA. Treatment of the pregnant mother with cancer: a systematic review on the use of cytotoxic, endocrine, targeted agents and immunotherapy during pregnancy. Part II: Hematological tumors. Cancer Treat Rev. 2010;36:110–121.

Kal HB, Struikmans H. Radiotherapy during pregnancy: fact and fiction. Lancet Oncol. 2005;6:328–333.

Pentheroudakis G, Pavlidis N. Cancer and pregnancy: poena magna, not anymore. Eur J Cancer. 2006;42: 126–140.

Human immunodeficiency virus (HIV) related malignancies

20

TV Ajithkumar

Introduction

Malignancies have a significant impact on the morbidity and mortality of people with human immunodeficiency virus (HIV) infection. 30–40% of HIV-infected patients develop malignancies during the course of their illness. Some of the malignancies are AIDS-defining conditions whereas others appear to be more common in HIV patients (Box 20.1). Although AIDS-defining malignancies may be caused mainly by progressive immunosuppression, the exact relationship between immunosuppression and non-AIDS-defining malignancies is yet to be established. The most common cancers in the general population such as breast, prostate and colon do not appear to increase in HIV infection.

Introduction of highly active antiretroviral therapy (HAART) has brought significant changes to the natural history of HIV-infection. The incidence of Kaposi's sarcoma and NHL has generally declined whilst the incidence of Hodgkin's lymphoma and non-AIDS-defining cancers has not changed. With the introduction of antiretroviral therapy, 28% of deaths in HIV infection are due to cancer compared with 10% before HAART.

Pathogenesis

Development of cancers in HIV-infected individuals may be similar to that occurring in patients with immunosuppression and immune-deficiency disorders. The possible mechanisms for increased incidence of various malignancies in HIV-infected people include:

- Immunosuppression – organ transplant recipients have an almost 100-fold increased risk compared with the general population.
- Though HIV is not generally considered as oncogenic, a possible direct role has been suggested recently.
- Increased risk of other viral infections – such as Epstein–Barr virus (Hodgkin's disease), human papilloma virus (cervical cancer, anal cancer), human herpes virus (Kaposi's sarcoma) and hepatitis virus (hepatocellular carcinoma).

AIDS-defining malignancies

Kaposi's sarcoma

KS is one of the most common neoplasms in HIV-infected patients, associated with human herpes virus-8 (HHV-8). With the introduction of highly active anti-retroviral therapy (HAART), the risk of both visceral and cutaneous KS has decreased dramatically.

The clinical manifestation of KS varies from a mild to a fulminant course. Skin lesions appear mainly on the lower extremities, face and genitalia. Skin lesions are typically multifocal and papular (Figure 20.1), but can appear plaque-like or as a fungating mass. Extracutaneous lesions appear in the oral cavity (most commonly palate followed by gingiva), larynx, gastrointestinal tract and lung. Gastrointestinal lesions can be asymptomatic or can cause weight loss, abdominal pain, nausea, vomiting and bleeding. Pulmonary KS may be symptomatic with cough,

DOI: 10.1016/B978-0-7234-3458-0.00025-7

Box 20.1: Cancers in HIV patients

AIDS-defining cancers

- Kaposi's sarcoma
- Invasive cervical cancer
- Non-Hodgkin's lymphoma
  - Burkitt's
  - Immunoblastic
  - Primary cerebral

Non-AIDS-defining cancers

- Anal cancer
- Liver cancer
- Hodgkin's disease
- Penile cancer
- Vulva and vagina cancer
- Oral cavity and pharynx
- Larynx
- Lung
- Myeloma
- Acute myeloid and monocytic leukaemia

Box 20.2: Staging of Kaposi's sarcoma

	Good risk (all of the following)	Poor risk (any of the following)
Tumour (T)	Confined to skin and/or lymph nodes and/or non-nodular disease in palate	• Associated oedema or ulceration • Oral disease other than non-nodular disease in palate • Gastrointestinal KS • Non-nodal visceral KS
Systemic illness	No history of opportunistic infection or thrush No B symptoms* ≥70 KPS	History of opportunistic infection or thrush B symptoms present <70 KPS Other HIV-related illness

*B symptoms – unexplained fever, night sweats, >10% involuntary weight loss or diarrhoea persisting more than 2 weeks

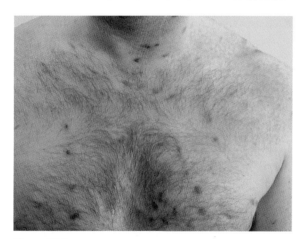

Figure 20.1
Kaposi's sarcoma. From Clutterbuck: Specialist Training in Sexually Transmitted Infections and HIV, with permission.

dyspnoea, haemoptysis etc. or present with asymptomatic radiological features of infiltrates, isolated nodules, pleural effusion and hilar or mediastinal lymphadenopathy.

In the post HAART era, tumour burden and systemic illness are useful to categorize patients into two prognostic groups (Box 20.2). Diagnosis of KS is confirmed by biopsy.

Treatment is aimed at symptom relief, preventing progression, cosmetic improvement, relief of oedema and avoiding organ compromise. For patients with limited cutaneous lesions and HIV viraemia, effective combination HAART is the initial management. Local therapy is indicated for bulky lesions and for cosmetic reasons. Local treatment options include external beam radiotherapy, laser therapy, cryosurgery, photodynamic therapy and intralesional vinblastine.

Indications for systemic chemotherapy (Box 20.3) include:

- widespread skin involvement (>25 lesions)
- extensive oral KS
- symptomatic oedema
- rapid progression
- symptomatic visceral KS
- KS flare.

Cervical cancer

Cervical cancer in HIV-infected women is associated with advanced disease at diagnosis, high recurrence rate and frequent cytotoxicity. Oncological management is similar to seronegative patients with cervical cancer; however special consideration should be given for interaction between cytotoxics and antiretroviral agents

Non-Hodgkin's lymphoma

Almost all of the HIV associated lymphomas are diffuse B cell (immunoblastic) or Burkitt's like. Approximately two-thirds of the patients present with extranodal disease and up to 20% will have meningeal disease, necessitating CSF examination in all.

- Liposomal doxorubicin 20 mg/m² three-weekly
- Liposomal daunorubicin 40 mg/m² two-weekly
- Paclitaxel 100 mg/m² two to three-weekly
- Others: vinorelbine, alpha-interferon, thalidomide and imatinib

Optimal treatment of HIV-related lymphoma is not known. Patients are generally treated similarly to those who are seronegative (p. 302). The overall prognosis is poor with a less than 1 year median survival.

Primary CNS lymphoma is 15 times more common than in the general population. The histology is large cell or immunoblastic type of B cell origin. Treatment involves radiotherapy combined with steroids, which extend the median survival from 2–3 months to 6–8 months (p. 306).

Non-AIDS-defining malignancies

These account for the increased mortality in the HAART era. HIV-infected people have an increased risk of these cancers (RR 1.9), and these tumours occur at a relatively younger age. Apart from duration of immunosuppression, other contributing risk factors include HAART interruption, smoking, sun exposure, oncogenic viruses and family history. The diagnosis needs to be confirmed by biopsy and staging will be affected by the presence of reactive lymphadenopathy as well as unrelated imaging abnormalities. Treatment is based on performance status, co-morbidity and potential for surgery. Non-medical management is also challenging due to chemotherapy-enhanced immunosuppression, added cytotoxicity, drug interaction with HAART and severe radiation reactions. Patients need regular monitoring of their CD4 count. Continuation of HAART, prophylaxis of opportunistic infections and supportive medications such as G-CSF are important.

Anal cancer

The high-risk group includes patients who practice receptive anal intercourse, men who have sex with men and anal co-infection with HPV or syphilis. The clinical presentation and treatment is similar to that of the seronegative population (p. 170). Patients with high-grade anal intra-epithelial neoplasia (AIN), invasive anal margin cancer and those with severe drug reactions require surgical management. Although the response to treatment is equivalent to seronegative patients with anal cancer, there is a high risk of severe radiation toxicity.

Liver cancer

Hepatocellular cancer is increased by 8-fold in the HIV population. Tumours tend to be more symptomatic, advanced at presentation and have an aggressive course. Resection or transplantation is an option for early stage whereas systemic chemotherapy is used in advanced cancer (p. 147). Survival is not influenced by CD4 count.

Hodgkin's disease

Patients present early in HIV infection with unfavourable histologic subtypes (mixed cellularity, lymphocyte depleted). There is a 5–15 fold increase in risk with a high rate of EBV co-infection (75–100%). Clinical presentation with B symptoms and extranodal disease are common. They are treated as seronegative patients (p. 298) and the median survival is 12–18 months.

Other cancers

Other cancers are treated similarly to seronegative patients.

Interactions between chemotherapy and HAART

There are interactions between some cytotoxic agents and antivirals due to cytochrome p450 enzymes and p-glycoprotein. These interactions may account for the better response rate and higher rates of survival seen with combinations of cytotoxics and antivirals compared with cytotoxics alone in patients with HIV associated malignancies. These interactions can also result in higher toxicities with treatment.

Further reading

Spano JP, Costagliola D, Katlama C et al. AIDS-related malignancies: state of the art and therapeutic challenges. J Clin Oncol. 2008;26:4834–4842.

Deeken JF, Pantanowitz L, Dezube BJ. Targeted therapies to treat non-AIDS-defining cancers in patients with HIV on HAART therapy: treatment considerations and research outlook. Curr Opin Oncol. 2009;21:445–454.

Cancers of the haematopoietic system

21

TV Ajithkumar and HM Hatcher

Hodgkin's disease

Epidemiology

Around 1500 cases of Hodgkin's disease are diagnosed every year in the UK and approximately 350 people die of this disease every year. Males are predominantly affected (male:female 1.8:1). There is bimodal peak of incidence with the first peak in those between 15 and 30 and the second peak between 50 and 60 years.

Aetiology

- EBV increases the risk of HD by two- to threefold. In up to 50–90% of classical HD, RS cells stain for EBV DNA.
- Family members of patients affected by HL are at a three to nine fold increased risk of developing the same disease. Same sex siblings have 10 times higher risk of HD.

Pathology

The WHO classification of HD is shown in Table 21.1. Nodular sclerosis is the common subtype in young adults (more common in females), which presents with early stage supradiaphragmatic disease whereas mixed cellularity presents with generalized lymphadenopathy or extranodal disease with B symptoms. Lymphocyte depletion type presents with advanced stage disease with extranodal involvement and aggressive clinical course.

LRCHL usually presents in young males with localized cervical node involvement with no B symptoms.

Histologically HD is characterized by the presence of Hodgkin and Reed–Sternberg (H-RS)
cells in a background of non-neoplastic cells such as lymphocytes, histiocytes, neutrophils, eosinophils and monocytes. Classical HD is characterized by CD30 positive H-RS cells and the nodular lymphocyte predominant form of HL (LPHL) with CD20 positive lymphocytic and histiocytic (L and H) cells. In classical HD, RS cells stain positive for CD15 (80%) and CD30 (90%).

Clinical features

The most common presentation is lymphadenopathy in the cervical or supraclavicular region (60–70%). Almost two-thirds of patients with classical HL have mediastinal nodal disease producing symptoms: tight chest, cough, venous congestion, or dyspnoea. About 40% of patients present with 'B-symptoms' of fever >38°C, drenching night sweats, or weight loss >10% within the previous 6 months (not from other causes). Bone marrow involvement at presentation occurs in less than 10% of cases. Extranodal involvement commonly occurs in the lung.

Investigations and staging

- Blood – full blood count and ESR, biochemistry including LDH.
- Tissue diagnosis – An excision biopsy of a lymph node is required for accurate diagnosis and subtyping. All patients need bone marrow examination.

Imaging

- Chest X-ray may show mediastinal widening (Figure 21.1), pleural effusion or pericardial effusion.
- CT of the neck, thorax, abdomen and pelvis will delineate lymphadenopathy as well as visceral involvement.

© 2011, Elsevier Ltd
DOI: 10.1016/B978-0-7234-3458-0.00026-9

Table 21.1: WHO classification of Hodgkin's lymphoma

Classical Hodgkin's lymphoma	Frequency
Nodular sclerosis Hodgkin's lymphoma (grades 1 and 2)	60–70%
Mixed cellularity Hodgkin's lymphoma	20–30%
Lymphocyte-rich classical Hodgkin's lymphoma (LRCHL)	3–5%
Lymphocyte-depleted Hodgkin's lymphoma (LDHL)	0.8–1%
Nodular lymphocyte-predominant Hodgkin's lymphoma (LPHL)	3–5%

Table 21.2: The Cotswolds modification of Ann Arbor staging for lymphoma

Stage I	Involvement of a single lymph node region or lymphoid structure or involvement of a single extralymphatic site (IE)
Stage II	Involvement of two or more lymph node regions on the same side of the diaphragm; localized contiguous involvement of only one extranodal organ or site and lymph node region(s) on the same side of the diaphragm (IIE)
Stage III	Involvement of lymph node regions on both sides of the diaphragm (III),which may also be accompanied by involvement of the spleen (IIIS) or by localized contiguous involvement of only one extranodal organ site (IIIE) or both (IIISE)
Stage IV	Diffuse or disseminated involvement of one or more extranodal organs or tissues, with or without associated lymph node involvement

Designations applicable to any disease stage

A:	No B symptoms
B:	Presence of B symptoms
X:	Bulky disease (a widening of the mediastinum by more than one third of the chest or presence of a nodal mass with a maximal dimension greater than 10 cm)

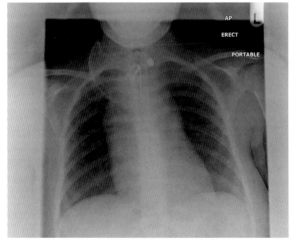

Figure 21.1
Mediastinal widening in Hodgkin's disease.

- Lung function tests, especially for those who may receive bleomycin as part of their treatment.
- PET scan – the role of FDG-PET is increasing. It is useful to define the extent of lymphadenopathy at diagnosis, as well in assessing post-treatment residual disease.
- MRI is useful to delineate disease in bone and the nervous system.

Staging

Cotswolds modification of the Ann Arbor Classification is used for staging (Table 21.2).

Management

HD is a highly curable disease with long-term disease-free survival (DFS) exceeding 80%. Current efforts are to improve the chances of cure with the least long-term toxicity. Measures to preserve fertility should be discussed with all young patients prior to starting chemotherapy.

Patients with early stage disease (clinical stage I/II) are categorized as favourable and unfavourable group based on risk factors (Table 21.3). Prognosis of patients with advanced-stage (stage III and IV) disease is defined using the International Prognostic Score (IPS) (Box 21.1).

Table 21.3: EORTC risk grouping of early stage HD

Treatment group	Definition
Favourable	CS I–II without risk factors
Unfavourable	CS I–II with ≥ 1 risk factors
Risk factors	A large mediastinal mass (>10 cm/> ⅓ thorax)
	B age ≥50 years
	C B symptoms or elevated ESR*
	D ≥4 involved regions

* Erythrocyte sedimentation rate (≥50 mm/h without or ≥30 mm/h with B-symptoms).

Box 21.1: International prognostic score of Hasenclever

- Serum albumin <4 g/dl
- Haemoglobin <10.5 g/dl
- Male sex
- Age >45 years
- Stage IV disease
- White cell count >15,000/mm^3
- Lymphocyte count <600/mm^3 and/or <8% of white-cells

Presence of each prognostic factor reduces the 5-year rates of freedom from progression of disease by 8%. i.e. those without any risk factors have a 5-year rate of 80% which is reduced to 45% by the presence of all 7 factors.

Box 21.2: Radiotherapy techniques in lymphoma

Definitions (see Figure 21.2 showing nodal regions)
- Involved field radiotherapy – involved lymph nodes with or without first echelon nodes.
- Extended field radiotherapy – involved lymph nodes with 1st and 2nd echelon nodes.
- Total nodal radiotherapy – all nodal regions.

Localization – based on CT scan or conventional definition of nodal regions.

Target volume definition – CTV depends on possible microscopic disease and PTV depends on site of treatment.

Dose
Hodgkin's lymphoma
- Macroscopic disease: 30–36 Gy in 20 fractions.
- Prophylactic nodal areas: 30 Gy in 15–20 fractions.
- Postchemotherapy: 30–35 Gy in 15–20 fractions.

NHL
- RT alone: 40 Gy in 20 fractions.
- Postchemotherapy: 30–35 Gy in 15–20 fractions.

Total body electrons
- Whole skin to a depth of 3–5 mm (6 MeV).
- Dose 24 Gy in 8 fractions, 3 fractions per week.

Box 21.3: ABVD regime
- Doxorubicin 25 mg/m^2 IV D1 and D15
- Bleomycin 10 units/m^2 IV D1 and D15
- Vinblastine 6 mg/m^2 (max 10 mg) IV D1 and D15
- Dacarbazine 375 mg/m^2 IV D1 and D15

Cycles repeated every 4 weeks

Nodular lymphocyte predominant (NLP)

Patients with localized NLP HD are treated with involved field radiotherapy (30–35 Gy in 15–20 fractions) which results in a 96% response rate and >90% 8-year survival (99% for stage I and 94% for stage II). Advanced stage and relapsed NLP disease is treated similar to classical HD.

Since this subtype usually expresses CD20, the anti-CD20 antibody, rituximab may have a future role in the management of these patients.

Classical HD

Early-stage favourable

The current standard treatment is combined modality treatment, consisting of two to four cycles of ABVD chemotherapy (Boxes 21.2 and 21.3), followed by 30–35 Gy in 15–20 fractions of involved field radiotherapy (IF-RT).

Early-stage unfavourable

These patients are also treated with combined modality treatment; however, the optimal chemotherapy regime and radiotherapy fractionation are yet be determined. The current treatment is four courses of ABVD followed by involved field radiotherapy of 30–35 Gy in 15–20 fractions (Boxes 21.2 and 21.3). With this treatment 5% patients progress during or immediately after treatment and 15% relapse within 5 years.

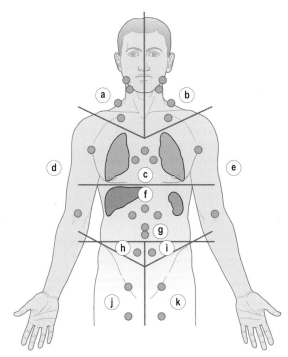

Figure 21.2
Nodal regions: cervical (a-b), mediastinal (c), axillary (d-e), mesenteric (f), paraaortic (g), iliac (h-i) and inguinal (j-k).

Advanced stage

Combination chemotherapy with 6–8 cycles of ABVD is the current treatment of choice; although this regime is not as successful as in earlier stage disease. Various attempts are being made to modify the ABVD regime by adding newer drugs and increasing dose intensity.

The role of consolidation radiotherapy in advanced stage HD is also not clear. A meta-analysis of combined modality treatment showed equal tumour control but inferior overall survival compared with chemotherapy alone. An EORTC study suggested that involved field radiotherapy did not result in better outcomes in patients who achieve complete response after chemotherapy, but may be beneficial in patients with a partial response. Hence consolidation radiotherapy is considered in those with initial bulky disease and those who fail to achieve a complete response to chemotherapy.

Recurrence

Combination chemotherapy is usually the treatment of choice for patients who relapse after previous radiotherapy alone. Treatment options for relapse after prior chemotherapy include salvage radiotherapy for localized relapse in previously non irradiated areas, salvage chemotherapy, or high-dose chemotherapy followed by autologous stem cell transplantation (SCT).

Patients who relapse after autologous stem cell transplantation may be candidates for allogeneic transplantation. Patients who cannot have intensive chemotherapy may be treated with palliative intent with drugs such as gemcitabine, vinca alkaloids, idarubicin etc.

Survival

With combined modality treatment patients in the early-favourable group achieve a disease free survival (DFS) of more than 90% and an overall survival of about 95% at five years. Patients in the early unfavourable group have a DFS of about 84% and an OS of 91%. In advanced stage combination chemotherapy results in 5-year failure free survival of 78% and overall survival of 90%. High-dose therapy and autologous stem cell transplantation results in DFS of 55% and the overall survival 71% at 5 years.

Follow-up

Two-thirds of relapses occur within 3 years of initial treatment and more than 90% occur within 5 years. Since a significant proportion of patients who relapse can be successfully salvaged, all patients need regular follow-up (Box 21.4). Follow-up is also helpful in identifying and managing long term side effects such as endocrine dysfunction.

Survivorship issues

The major causes of excess death in survivors of HD are second malignancies and ischaemic heart disease (p. 58).

One of the most common second malignancies is lung cancer which is attributed to mediastinal radiotherapy, chemotherapy and smoking. Patients who had thoracic radiotherapy are encouraged not to smoke. There is 20–50% risk of second breast cancer after mediastinal/axillary radiotherapy in young females and these patients should be screened for breast cancer. Common haematological neoplasms include acute myeloid leukaemia, myelodysplastic syndrome (develops

301

> **Box 21.4: Follow-up and screening after treatment for HD**
>
> - History and physical examination, FBC, ESR, LDH, electrolytes, liver function tests and chest X-ray at each visit if chest CT is not done: 3–4-monthly for first 2 years, 6-monthly for years 3–5 and then annually.
> - CT scan chest: 6–8 monthly for first 2 years, yearly for years 3–5 and then only if any abnormality on CXR.
> - CT abdomen and pelvis: in stage I–II annually for 5 years; in stage III–IV, 6-monthly for first 2 years, annually for years 3–5.
> - Others:
>   - Serum TSH estimation 6-monthly if radiotherapy to neck.
>   - Mammogram: annually beginning at age 40; if received radiotherapy above the diaphragm start at age ≥30 years.
>   - MRI breast: consider for those who received radiation above the diaphragm before age 30 years.

within 3–5 years) and non-Hodgkin's lymphoma (develops after 5–15 years).

Future perspectives

Future studies will address the issues of improving survival whilst minimizing the risk of long-term side effects. Newer imaging modalities such as functional imaging are already being incorporated into risk stratification to determine future treatments.

Non-Hodgkin's lymphoma

Introduction

Non-Hodgkin's lymphomas are a group of lymphoid malignancies of varying subtypes with a range of clinical behaviours and treatment strategies. Around 8450 new cases are diagnosed per year in the UK and 65,980 cases in the USA. The median age is 65, although aggressive B-cell lymphomas are the predominant NHL in younger adults. Male:female ratio is 1.5:1. Almost ⅔ of cases are due to two specific subtypes: diffuse large B-cell lymphoma and follicular lymphoma.

Pathology

The cell of origin is different for each subtype of lymphoma. Classification is by the updated WHO modification of the REAL (revised European and American lymphoma) classification system which is broadly divided into B-cell, T-cell/natural killer cell and Hodgkin's disease (Table 21.4). Table 21.5 shows cytogenetic and molecular characteristics of NHL.

Clinical features

The most common presenting symptom is painless lymphadenopathy. B symptoms (weight loss >10% within the previous 6 months, fever, night sweats) occur in up to half of the patients, predominantly in those with high-grade disease. Symptoms can be due to involvement of specific organs such as dyspnoea due to mediastinal nodes or effusion, abdominal symptoms and neurological symptoms such as cord compression.

Evaluation and staging

Initial evaluation includes detailed history, full clinical examination and assessment of performance status. Blood tests include FBC with peripheral smear, serum biochemistry, serum LDH and serological tests for HIV and hepatitis.

Biopsy – Excisional biopsy of an enlarged lymph node or generous incision biopsy is required to make an accurate diagnosis. Immunohistochemistry and genetic analyses are important in making an accurate diagnosis. All patients need bone marrow biopsy with aspiration.

Imaging

CT scans of the neck, chest, abdomen and pelvis are carried out to assess lymphadenopathy and organ involvement (Figure 21.3).

Other investigations

- Lumbar puncture-CSF studies are needed for patients with neurological symptoms or those with paranasal sinus or testicular involvement.
- Endoscopy depends on the clinical situation and type of lymphoma.

Staging

Staging is similar to Hodgkin's disease (p. 299).

Prognostic factors

Stage, age, LDH and performance status have prognostic value. The Follicular Lymphoma International Prognostic Index (FLIP) score is used for indolent lymphomas (Box 21.5). The interna-

Table 21.4: Abridged WHO/REAL classification of NHL

B-cell neoplasms

- Precursor B-cell neoplasm
- Peripheral B-cell neoplasms
  - B-cell chronic lymphocytic leukaemia/small lymphocytic lymphoma
  - Mantle cell lymphoma
  - Follicular lymphoma
  - Extranodal marginal zone B-cell lymphoma of mucosa-associated lymphatic tissue (MALT) type
  - Hairy cell leukaemia
  - Plasmacytoma/plasma cell myeloma
  - Diffuse large B-cell lymphoma
  - Burkitt lymphoma

T-cell and putative NK-cell neoplasms

- Precursor T-cell neoplasm
- Peripheral T-cell and NK-cell neoplasms
1. T-cell chronic lymphocytic leukaemia/prolymphocytic leukaemia
2. T-cell granular lymphocytic leukaemia
3. Mycosis fungoides/Sézary syndrome
4. Peripheral T-cell lymphoma, not otherwise characterized
5. Enteropathy-type intestinal T-cell lymphoma
6. Adult T-cell lymphoma/leukaemia (human T-lymphotrophic virus [HTLV] 1+)
7. Anaplastic large cell lymphoma

Table 21.5: Cytogenetic and molecular characteristics of NHL

Lymphoma	Cytogenetics	Genes
Burkitt's	t(8;14)(q24q32) Or t(2;8) or t(8;22)	c-MYC (8q24) Immunoglobulins (other chromosome)
Follicular lymphoma	t(14:18)(q32;q21)	BCL-2 (18q) Ig heavy chain (14q)
Diffuse large B-cell lymphoma	t(14:18)(q32;q21)+others such as p53, p16, p15	
Mantle cell lymphoma	t(11;14)(q13;q32)	BCL-1 or PRAD1 (11q) Ig heavy chain (14q)
Anaplastic lymphoma	t(2;5)(p23:q35)	TCR-ALK T cell receptor

tional prognostic index (IPI) is used for patients with diffuse large B-cell lymphoma (Box 21.6).

Treatment

Follicular lymphoma

Follicular lymphoma accounts for approximately 20% of all lymphomas and has a variable clinical course. The median age at presentation is 50 years. Most patients present with advanced disease and median survival is 10–15 years from diagnosis. Spontaneous regression can occur and 40% of patients transform to an aggressive histologic type. Over 90% have rearrangement of the bcl-2 gene which inhibits apoptosis.

Early stage

Only about one-third of patients with follicular lymphoma present with stages I and II or limited stage III (with up to five involved lymph nodes

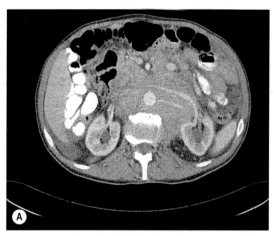
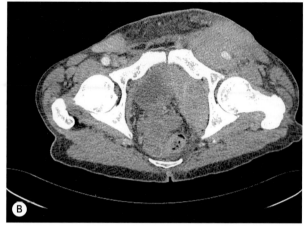

Figure 21.3
CT scan in NHL. Figure shows massive para-aortic lymphadenopathy (A) and iliac and inguinal lymphadenopathy (B).

Box 21.5: Follicular Lymphoma International Prognostic Index

1. Age (≤60 years vs. >60 years).
2. Serum LDH (normal vs. elevated).
3. Stage (stage I or stage II vs. stage III or stage IV).
4. Haemoglobin level (≥12 g/dL vs. <12 g/dL).
5. Number of nodal areas (≤4 vs. >4).

Patients with 0 to 1 risk factors have an 85% 10-year survival rate. Those with three or more risk factors have a 40% 10-year survival rate.

Box 21.6: The International Prognostic Index (IPI) for aggressive NHL (diffuse large cell lymphoma)

1. Age (≤60 years of age vs. >60 years of age).
2. Serum LDH (normal vs. elevated).
3. Performance status (0 or 1 vs. 2–4).
4. Stage (stage I or stage II vs. stage III or stage IV).
5. Extranodal site involvement (0 or 1 vs. 2–4).

Patients with two or more risk factors have a less than 50% chance of relapse-free survival and overall survival at 5 years.

---

areas) disease. Treatment options include watchful waiting, or radiotherapy (Box 21.2).

Advanced stage

The optimal treatment for patients with bulky stage II, III and stage IV disease is yet to be defined. There is no proven role for early chemotherapy in asymptomatic patients. A watch and wait policy is appropriate for these patients. Alternatives include the anti CD20 antibody (rituximab), alkylating agents or experimental therapies. Indications for systemic treatment are:

- Symptomatic bulky disease
- Massive hepato-splenomegaly
- Bone marrow suppression
- B symptoms
- Transformed lymphoma

The commonly used regime is either single agent chlorambucil or fludarabine. Chlorambucil results in 50–75% response rate with no complete response, whereas fludarabine can result in a complete response (15%). Combination chemotherapy (e.g. CVP and CHOP) (Table 21.6) have no overall survival benefit. The role of chemotherapy with rituximab is being investigated. Elderly patients may be treated with rituximab or single agent chemotherapy.

Relapse

Two trials report prolonged event-free survival and overall survival with a combination of rituximab with chemotherapy (CHOP).

High-grade lymphoma

High-grade lymphomas include a number of lymphoma subtypes including:

- Diffuse large B cell (DLBCL)
- Burkitt's
- Mantle cell

Table 21.6: Chemotherapy regimes in NHL

- CHOP – cyclophosphamide, adriamycin, vincristine and prednisolone
- CVP – cyclophosphamide, vincristine and prednisolone
- ESHAP – etoposide, methylprednisolone, cytarabine and cisplatin
- BEAM – BCNU, etoposide, cytarabine, melphalan
- CODOX-M – cyclophosphamide, vincristine, doxorubicin, araC, methotrexate

---

- Lymphoblastic lymphoma/leukaemia (precursor T/B lymphoma/leukaemia) (p. 310, leukaemias).
- HIV associated (p. 296).

DLBCL

Diffuse-large cell lymphoma (DLBCL) comprises 30% of NHL and is characterized by an aggressive clinical behaviour with rapidly enlarging lymphadenopathy frequently associated with extra-nodal disease.

In early-stage disease without adverse factors (see Box 21.6), treatment is with 3–4 cycles of CHOP in combination with rituximab (R-CHOP) followed by involved-field radiation therapy (30–35 Gy in 1.75–3 Gy per fraction) or 6–8 cycles of R-CHOP.

Patients with early stage disease with adverse factors and advanced disease are treated similarly. CHOP chemotherapy with rituximab shows a significant improvement in response rate, event-free and overall survival in younger and older patients. Patients with bulky disease seemed to benefit the most from rituximab. The role of additional locoregional radiotherapy in patients with bulky sites or extra-nodal disease is of no proven benefit. With this approach, the 5-year survival of early stage disease is 80–90% and that of advanced disease is around 50%.

In diffuse-large cell lymphoma, risk factors for CNS relapse are involvement of the skull, more than one extra-nodal manifestation (especially testis), IPI >1 and bone marrow infiltration and hence need to be considered for CNS prophylaxis.

Burkitt's lymphoma

Burkitt's lymphoma is a rare (2–3%) aggressive B cell NHL There are two main forms: the endemic form observed in Africa and associated with EBV and the sporadic form which accounts for up to 30% childhood lymphomas (p. 323, children's cancers). The endemic form classically presents with enlargement of the jaw. The sporadic form presents rapidly increasing disease with intra-abdominal masses often involving the gastrointestinal tract (especially ileocaecal), ovaries or kidneys. Bone marrow and CNS involvement is frequent. These patients are at a high risk of developing tumour lysis syndrome due to an almost 100% cell turnover (p. 342). Survival rates vary from 30% to 70% and have improved with intensive regimes and risk group. Low-risk patients include those with a low LDH and those with a completely resected abdominal/single lesion. All others should be considered high risk.

Treatment with intensive multiagent chemotherapy (e.g. CODOX-M) is started rapidly with tumour lysis prophylaxis. There is no evidence to support high-dose treatment with transplantation as first line treatment. CNS involvement is extremely common and hence CNS prophylaxis is essential for all cases.

Relapse should be treated with further intensive chemotherapy and young fit patients should then be considered for autologous or allogeneic stem cell transplantation.

Mantle cell lymphoma

Mantle cell lymphoma (MCL) comprises less than 4% of NHL. The median age at presentation is 62 years. It usually presents with advanced disease involving the bone marrow and/or spleen. Overall long term survival is poor at less than 20% but with recent improvement in median survival from 2.7 to 4.8 years.

Optimal initial treatment in MCL is yet to be established. The commonly used first line chemotherapy regime is CHOP. Other first line options include fludarabine-containing regimens, single agent cladribine and a combination of high-dose methotrexate with cytarabine. Consolidating autologous stem cell transplantation in first remission improves progression free survival in eligible younger patients. Rituximab maintenance therapy seems to be a therapeutic alternative particularly in elderly patients. In relapsed patients, fludarabin-containing regimens, bendamustine and bortezomib seem to be effective. In the absence of allogenic stem cell transplantation, a potentially curative but investigative treatment option, the median survival is 4–6 years.

Primary extra-nodal NHL

Primary extra-nodal NHLs are defined as lymphomas which present with a predominantly extra-nodal tumour mass which represent approximately 25 to 30% of NHL.

Histologically, nearly 50% of all extra-nodal lymphomas are diffuse, large B-cell lymphomas. It is the most common histological subtype in the testis, brain, bone, thyroid and sinus.

The vast majority of the remaining group arise from the mucosa-associated lymphoid tissue (MALT) and represents 5–10% of all NHL. The most common involved sites are the stomach, small intestine, orbit, salivary glands and the lung.

Primary CNS lymphoma

Primary CNS lymphoma occurs are a median age of 60 years in immunocompetent patients and 30 years in HIV patients. Primary CNS lymphoma often has a rapidly progressive course. Systemic dissemination is rare. The finding of characteristic features on CT (Figure 21.4) and MRI imaging should prompt a stereotactic biopsy. Management of primary CNS lymphoma is discussed on p. 276.

The prognosis of HIV-associated primary CNS lymphoma is generally worse and depends on the CD4+ cell count. Whereas patients with a CD4+ cell count >200/μl can achieve a long-term remission, those with a CD4+ cell count less than 200/μl do not respond to chemotherapy. These patients may respond to highly active antiretroviral therapy.

Bone lymphoma

In most cases, involvement of the bone is secondary in patients with advanced-stage lymphoma whereas primary bone lymphoma is rare. The presenting symptom is mainly localized bone pain. DLBCL is the most common histological diagnosis.

The median age is 63 years. 10-year overall survival is approximately 41%. Three different prognostic groups (patients <60 years with IPI 1–3, patients ≥60 years with IPI 0–3, and patients ≥60 with IPI 4–5) with significantly different overall survival at 5 years of 90%, 61% and 25%, respectively, have been identified. The treatment involves combination of rituximab and CHOP with or without radiotherapy. Radical surgery does not improve outcome.

Testicular lymphoma

Primary testicular lymphoma represents 1–2% of all NHL. It is the most common malignancy of the testis in men older than 60 years and the most common presentation is unilateral painless

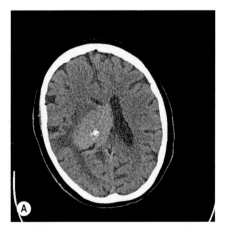 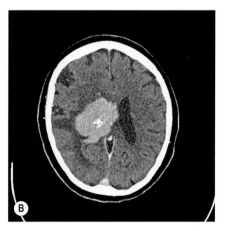

Figure 21.4
CT scan in primary CNS lymphoma. Non-contrast enhancing CT scan shows a periventricular hyperdense lesion (A) which uniformly enhances on contrast administration (B).

scrotal swelling. DLBCL is the most common histology and diagnosis is usually established by initial orchidectomy. Approximately 80% of cases are stage I or II at presentation. A low IPI, no B-symptoms, the use of anthracyclines, and prophylactic contralateral scrotal radiotherapy are significantly associated with longer survival. Systemic chemotherapy alone seems not to be effective in preventing relapses in the contralateral testis because the testis is a sanctuary site (p. 35). Treatment consists of 6–8 courses of R-CHOP followed by prophylactic irradiation of the contralateral testis. Although data are not convincing, prophylactic intrathecal therapy should be considered. This approach results in a 3-year overall survival of 86% and 3-year progression-free survival 77%.

Cutaneous NHL

Primary cutaneous lymphomas differ considerably in their clinical course and outcome from systemic lymphomas. Primary cutaneous lymphomas are generally divided into lymphomas with an indolent or an aggressive clinical course. Approximately 75% of primary cutaneous lymphomas are T-cell lymphomas which include mycosis fungoides (MF) and Sezary syndrome (SS) and 25% are primary cutaneous B-cell lymphomas.

Clinical features

Mycosis fungoides typically presents with erythematous patches, plaques and tumours usually in areas not often exposed to sunlight (Figure 21.5). Most patients have multiple lesions and ulcerations can occur. The course of the disease is indolent.

The lesions of mycosis fungoides can be classified into four groups: Patches, papules and/or plaques affecting less (T1) or more (T2) than 10% of body surface, T3 with tumours >1 cm and T4 with erythroderma affecting more than 80% of body surface. In T1 disease outcome is excellent and also patients with T2 disease have a median overall survival of more than 10 years.

Patients with erythrodermic mycosis fungoides have a median survival of 5 years and those with visceral involvement have an even worse survival with only one or two years.

Sezary syndrome is defined as an erythrodermic cutaneous T-cell lymphoma with haemato-

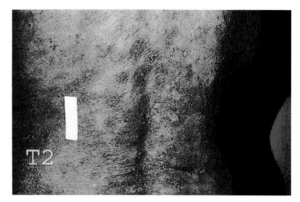

Figure 21.5
Cutaneous lymphoma. From Darell Rigel: Cancer of the Skin (Saunders), with permission.

logic evidence of leukaemic involvement and can be preceded by mycosis fungoides. The clinical behaviour of the disease is aggressive.

Primary cutaneous marginal zone B-cell lymphoma and primary cutaneous follicle centre B-cell lymphoma usually show an indolent clinical behaviour.

Spontaneous resolution may occur. Primary cutaneous follicle centre B-cell lymphoma preferentially involves the head and trunk with solitary or grouped plaques and tumours. The 5-year survival is excellent with more than 95% in both entities.

In contrast, primary cutaneous diffuse-large B-cell lymphoma, leg-type, behaves aggressively and affects predominantly elderly patients. This entity typically presents as red solitary or multiple nodule on the leg but can also rarely be found at other sites. Both cutaneous relapses and extracutaneous dissemination are frequent. With a 5-year survival of only 50%, prognosis is significantly worse than in the other two entities.

Management of cutaneous T-cell lymphoma

In patients with early stages of MF topical therapy with mechlorethamine or bexarotene, superficial radiotherapy and phototherapy (PUVA) are appropriate treatment options.

Patients with more advanced disease will require systemic treatment. Total skin electron beam therapy (TSEBT) is appropriate in patients with generalized thickened plaques due to its depth of penetration. The rate of complete responses is greater than 80% but the long-term outcome is not affected. TSEBT should be followed by an adjuvant therapy such as mechlorethamine or PUVA.

Systemic therapy with the orally administered retinoid bexarotene can achieve response rates of 50%. MF and SS are relatively chemoresistant diseases. The most frequently used combination chemotherapy regimens include cyclophosphamide, vincristine and prednisone (CVP) with or without doxorubicin. High-dose chemotherapy followed by autologous stem cell transplantation in patients with advanced disease has been shown to induce high response rates in most patients but the responses were predominantly of short duration. In contrast, allogeneic transplantation seems to induce long-term durable remissions of more than 3 years.

Management of cutaneous B-cell lymphoma
Due to their indolent course and excellent outcome in primary cutaneous marginal zone and follicle centre B-cell lymphoma a watch-and-wait strategy is the adequate management in most cases. In patients with limited symptomatic skin lesions, local excision or radiotherapy (20–36 Gy) are the first treatments of choice. Cutaneous relapses can be treated in the same way as the initial lesion and do not worsen prognosis.

In patients with extensive skin lesions rituximab is the treatment of choice. Oral chlorambucil is a treatment option often used in Europe. A multiagent chemotherapy is rarely indicated in these types of cutaneous lymphomas with the exception of patients developing extracutaneous disease.

The role of stem cell transplantation in aggressive lymphoma
Autologous stem cell transplantation has become the standard treatment in younger patients with a first chemosensitive relapse of aggressive lymphoma. The role of autologous stem cell transplantation in relapse after rituximab-containing front-line treatment has not been determined.

The role of allogeneic transplantation in the management of patients with aggressive lymphoma remains controversial.

Recent advances
The use of FDG-PET imaging in lymphomas is evolving. It is useful to define the extent of disease as well as allow cessation of treatment when a previously metabolically active area becomes inactive after treatment.

Several new monoclonal antibodies are under investigation including atumumab (a human monoclonal IgG1 antibody against a small loop epitope on the CD20 molecule) and epratuzumab (anti-CD22). Radioimmunotherapy (RIT) is an innovative treatment modality that combines the tumour cell targeting ability of monoclonal antibodies with the cytotoxic effect of radiation by linking a radioisotope to the antibody. This is under investigation for NHL with ^{90}Y-ibritumomab tiuxetan and ^{131}I-tositumumab. Other agents under investigation include bortezomib (30–40% response) and lenalidomide.

Follow-up in NHL
The purpose of follow-up is to detect early relapse and to educate about possible long-term complications. A typical schedule is 3-monthly follow up for 1 year, 4-monthly during the 2nd year, 6 monthly for the 3rd year, annually up to 10 years and then on alternate years. At each visit detailed history is taken and clinical examination is done with routine bloods including LDH and ESR. Chest X-ray is done in patients with chest disease at presentation. Further investigations are needed depending on any new symptoms or signs or other abnormal tests.

Acute leukaemias

Introduction
Acute lymphoblastic leukaemia (ALL) occurs most frequently either between the ages of 15–25 (p. 321) or over the age of 75. In the UK there are 200 new adult cases per year and the male : female ratio is roughly equal. Acute myeloid leukaemia (AML) occurs more frequently and the median age at presentation is 65. In the UK, around 2000 new cases are diagnosed per annum.

Aetiology
The majority of acute leukaemias are sporadic, although some genetic syndromes and other factors can predispose to acute leukaemia.

- Genetic syndromes
  - Down's syndrome
  - Fanconi anaemia
  - Neurofibromatosis

- Chemicals:
  - benzene
  - pesticides
- Previous chemotherapy (AML):
  - alkylating agents
  - topoisomerase II inhibitors

Pathology

AML and ALL are characterized by circulating blasts cells which may be seen in the peripheral blood. Bone marrow examination with immuno-phenotypic analysis is needed for establishing a diagnosis. Both myeloblasts and lymphoblasts are characterized by a high nuclear:cytoplasmic ratio and prominent nuclei. Azurophilic Auer rods are pathognomonic of AML (Figure 21.6).

The French–American–British (FAB) classification recognizes three subtypes of ALL: L1 (30%), L2 (60%) and L3 (10%), whereas the current WHO classification incorporates immunopheno-typing and cytogenetics. By immunophenotyp-ing, 75% ALL arise from B-cell progenitors and 25% from T-cells.

The FAB classification recognizes eight sub-types of AML: M0 minimal myeloid differentia-tion (3%), M1 poorly differentiated myeloblasts (15–20%), M2 myeloblastic with differentiation (25–30%), M3 promyelocytic (5–10%), M4 myelo-monoblastic (20%), M5 monoblastic (2–9%), M6 erythroblastic (3–5%), and M7 megakaryoblastic (3–12%). The recent WHO classification incorporates cytogenetics and classifies AML as:

- AML with recurrent cytogenetic abnormalities.
- AML with multilineage dysplasia.
- AML and MDS, therapy related.
- AML not otherwise categorized.

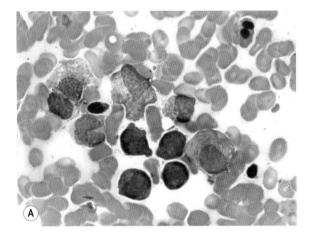

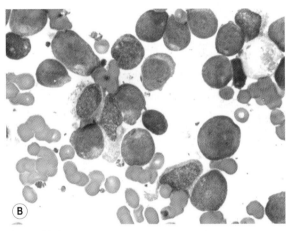

Figure 21.6
AML M3 shows promyelocytes with multiple/stacked Auer rods (A) and AML with a blast in the centre showing an Auer rod (B). Courtesy of Dr. Priyanka Mehta, Bristol Oncology Centre.

Clinical features

The majority of patients present with features of bone marrow failure, which include anaemia, neutropenia and thrombocytopenia, clinically manifesting as fatigue, and pallor, fever and pate-chiae, easy bruising or bleeding. ALL can produce weight loss, bone pain, symptoms of CNS disease and features of extramedullary infiltration (in 50%) such as lymphadenopathy, splenomegaly or a mediastinal mass. AML can present with gum infiltrates (M4/M5) and disseminated intra-vascular coagulation (M3). A small proportion of acute leukaemia can present with features of hyperleucocytosis (WBC >100 × 10^9/L) such as dyspnoea and CNS symptoms.

Clinical examination may show lymphaden-opathy, bruising, patechiae, gum hypertrophy, hepato-splenomegaly, chest signs of effusion, and mediastinal mass.

Diagnosis

Blood tests include FBC and peripheral smear with cytogenetics and immunohistochemistry and biochemistry, including uric acid. Bone marrow examination is essential for definitive diagnosis of acute leukaemia and subtyping.

Prognostic factors and risk classification

The most important predictor of outcome in both AML and ALL are presentation, karyotype, age and response to initial treatment.

ALL

Clinical features (age >50 years, WBC count), immunophenotyping (pro-B, early-T, mature-T), cytogenetics and molecular biology [t (9;22), t (4;11)], and response to treatment (late achievement of response, minimal residual disease [MRD] positivity) have prognostic importance and are used to define standard risk (those without any risk factors) and high risk (those with one or more risk factors) ALL. Philadelphia chromosome positive (Ph+) ALL (t (9; 22)/BCR-ABL) predicts a high relapse rate and <10% chance of overall survival with chemotherapy alone. This group of patients is eligible for treatment with tyrosine kinase inhibitors such as imatinib.

AML

Based on cytogenetics there are three prognostic groups in AML:

- Favourable group with core binding factor (CBF) leukaemias [inv (16), t (16; 16), or t (8;21)], and t (15;17). This group represents 10% of patients and involves mainly patients <60 years of age. With intensive treatment survival rates are around 60%.
- Unfavourable group with monosomies or partial deletions of chromosome 5 and/or 7, or with abnormalities involving chromosome 3. This group constitutes about 30–40% of all patients, on average older (>50–60 years) often with an antecedent haematological disorder or AML related to therapy. The survival rates are around 20%.
- Intermediate group – the remaining 50–60% of patients with normal cytogenetics falls into this group whose outcome is intermediate.

Treatment

The principle of management of acute leukaemia is to achieve a morphological complete remission (<5% blast cells in bone marrow) with induction chemotherapy followed by further chemotherapy as consolidation chemotherapy. CNS directed treatment and maintenance treatment (up to 2 years) are part of the ALL treatment. It is being increasingly recognized that an early allogeneic transplantation is beneficial in high-risk ALL patients.

ALL

Current treatment of adult ALL leads to long-term survival of 30–40%. Initial chemotherapy utilizes vincristine, corticosteroids and daunorubicin (induction). Such intensive combination chemotherapy results in a complete remission (CR defined as <5% blast cells with return of marrow cellularity and function and disappearance of extramedullary manifestations) in 80–90% cases. Once CR is achieved consolidation therapy is started with a combination of chemotherapy. In patients with Ph+ disease, concurrent tyrosine inhibitor imatinib (a tyrosine kinase inhibitor [p. 312]) may improve survival. CNS directed treatment with intrathecal methotrexate and high-dose methotrexate and/or cranial radiation to treat the central nervous system is required for patients who are not planned to have undergo bone marrow transplantation.

After consolidation, maintenance therapy given over 1.5 to 2 years is still standard in ALL. Omission of maintenance therapy has been associated with shorter DFS rates. Daily doses of mercaptopurine and weekly doses of methotrexate are the backbone of maintenance, and are combined with monthly pulses of vincristine and corticosteroids. Intrathecal treatment is also continued but the frequency decreases in the maintenance phase. Patients with mature B-ALL do not require maintenance. In T-ALL, the benefit of maintenance chemotherapy has been questioned.

Transplantation

Unrelated donor transplant is generally advised in Ph+ ALL and high-risk ALL, which gives a survival of 50%. For patients under the age of 45 years with an available HLA identical sibling, allogenic transplant may be considered.

Salvage therapy

The outcome of salvage therapy remains unsatisfactory. CR rates range from 10–50% and long-term DFS is poor. Various combinations of chemotherapy are used. Although stem cell transplantation (SCT) is superior to chemotherapy with long-term DFS rates of 20–40% in salvage therapy, only 30–40% of patients who achieved a second complete remission are eligible for SCT and fewer than 50% have enough time before disease recurrence to undergo SCT.

AML

Induction

70–90% patients achieve a CR with two courses of induction chemotherapy with cytarabine and an anthracycline (usually idarubicin). Complete remission is defined as <5% blasts cells in the bone narrow, absence of cells with Auer rods and resolution of peripheral blood cytopenia.

Post-induction

Patients with favourable cytogenetics receive two further courses of consolidation chemotherapy with cytarabine, an anthracycline and etoposide. Patients with intermediate and unfavourable cytogenetics, those under 40 years with a HLA identical sibling are considered for allogeneic transplantation. The role of post-consolidation maintenance therapy is not clearly defined and hence not recommended.

There is some suggestion that in younger patients with primary refractory AML, allogeneic transplant may improve survival and hence may be considered for those who fail to achieve CR after two courses of induction chemotherapy.

Allogeneic stem cell transplantation is also indicated after a second CR with salvage chemotherapy in relapsed patients.

Acute promyelocytic leukaemia (APML)

APML has a high risk of disseminated intravascular coagulation (DIC). Patients with DIC should be treated with supportive measures (frozen plasma, fibrinogen and platelet support) and all-trans retinoic acid (ATRA) to reverse the coagulopathy. ATRA acts by stimulating differentiation of the leukaemic blasts. In addition to treating DIC, when administered with idarubicin it reduces the risk of disease relapse (DFS >80%). In patients achieving a CR, two further courses of anthracycline based chemotherapy are given

as consolidation. ATRA syndrome is the major toxicity of this treatment characterized by fever and leakage of fluid into the extravascular space producing fluid retention, dyspnoea, effusions, and hypotension. It is treated with high doses of methylprednisolone or dexamethasone.

In patients relapsing after initial CR, arsenic trioxide achieves a CR of 80%. Some studies show that in patients with APML and t (8;21) and inversion (10), a second CR autologous transplantation can result in high rates of DFS.

New agents

Monoclonal antibodies are an attractive treatment option in ALL, especially in the setting of MRD. The agents studied include rituximab (anti-CD20 antibody) and alemtuzumab (anti-CD52).

New drugs being studied for AML include drugs that specifically bind to the surface of the AML blasts such as Mylotarg (gemtuzumab ozogamicin), agents that inhibit the multidrug-resistant (MDR) protein (PSC-833, Zosuquidar) etc.

Chronic myeloid leukaemia

Chronic myeloid leukaemia (CML) accounts for 20% of leukaemia. The median age at diagnosis is 55 years. Males are affected more frequently than females (male:female ratio of 1.3:1). There are 750 new cases per year in the UK. Only recognized risk factor is prior radiation.

Cytogenetics

About 90–95% patients with CML exhibit a chromosomal translocation that results in one shortened chromosome 22 (22q– called the Philadelphia [Ph] chromosome) and one elongated chromosome 9 (9q+). The resulting fusion oncoprotein from the BCR-ABL1 fusion gene has deregulated tyrosine kinase activity which probably is thought to be the initiating event in the chronic phase of CML.

Patients with CML but without Ph chromosome may still have *BCR-ABL* rearrangement which will behave similar to Ph+ disease. Patients without Ph chromosome and *BCR-ABL* molecular abnormalities are classed as atypical CML and they often need a different approach to treatment approach.

Natural history

The three phases of disease are:

- Chronic phase (CP) – 90% of patients present at this stage. Without treatment median survival is 3–4 years.
- Accelerated phase (AP) – characterized by increasing blast count and organomegaly. Median survival is 1–2 years and most progress to blastic phase in 4–6 months.
- Blast phase (BP) – resembles acute leukaemia with >20% blasts in peripheral blood or marrow. 20–30% of BP is lymphoid, 50% myeloid and 25% undifferentiated. Median survival is 3–6 months.

AP and BP are combined as advanced phase disease.

Clinical features

50% patients are asymptomatic and are diagnosed following an abnormal blood count. The remainder presents with non-specific symptoms of weight loss, excessive sweating, spontaneous bleeding and pain due to splenic enlargement and hyperviscosity. Some patients with hyperuricaemia present with a gout-like arthritis. Symptoms of advanced stage include general cachexia, fever, bone marrow failure and bone pain.

Investigations

Full blood count and peripheral smear

- Chronic phase – WBC count is usually around 20–30×10^9/L. Peripheral smear shows myelocytes and myeloblasts.
- Accelerated phase – raised WBC count, anaemia, thrombocytosis or thrombocytopenia.
- Blastic phase – shows blasts or blasts and promyelocytes in the blood.

Bone marrow

Bone marrow shows hypercellular marrow with complete loss of fat spaces. Metaphase cytogenetics or FISH is useful to identify Ph chromosome. The presence of the *BCR-ABL1* fusion gene may be identified by real time quantitative polymerase chain reaction (RQ-PCR).

Management

Chronic phase

Initial treatment is with the tyrosine kinase inhibitor (TKI), imatinib (400 mg daily). This results in 5-year event free survival of 83%, overall survival of 89% and a cumulative complete cytogenetic response (CCyR) of 87%. Indefinite treatment is recommended. RQ–PCR for the *BCR-ABL* transcript is the cornerstone for monitoring patients for response to treatment. Patients with a suboptimal response or failure to respond to an initial dose are treated either with an increased dose of imatinib (600–800 mg daily) or a second generation TKI such as dasatinib (70 mg twice daily).

Patients who fail treatment with a TKI may be considered for allogenic stem cell transplant. The suitable candidates are aged <60 years and have an HLA-identical sibling or an HLA-matched unrelated donor.

Advanced phase

Newly diagnosed patients with advanced phase disease are treated with imatinib 660–800 mg daily. The median survival of these patients is 7.5 months and hence fit patients who respond to treatment should proceed to allogenic SCT if there is an appropriate donor. Those who have had previous imatinib are treated with dasatinib or allogenic SCT.

Chronic lymphocytic leukaemia

Chronic lymphocytic leukaemia (CLL) is the most frequent (30%) leukaemia in the Western world. The median age at diagnosis is 70 years. There is a 2 : 1 male : female ratio. The aetiology is unknown. No specific risk factors have been identified.

Clinical features

About 50–70% patients are asymptomatic. The most frequent presentation is painless symmetrical lymphadenopathy. Other presenting features include systemic symptoms of weight loss, night sweats, tiredness and features of bone marrow failure. Autoimmune complications especially haemolytic anaemia and immune thrombocytopenia can occur. Infections are common due to hypogammaglobulinaemia.

10% patients can undergo transformation to a more aggressive tumour, most commonly diffuse large B-cell lymphoma, called Richter's syndrome.

Diagnosis

CLL is a proliferative disorder of monoclonal CD5+ B lymphocytes. The diagnostic criteria for CLL are:

- Lymphocytosis >5 × 10⁹/l.
- Typical morphology – small to medium sized lymphocytes with clumped chromatin, absent nucleoli and scanty cytoplasm.
- Typical immunophenotype – SmIg (weak), CD5+, CD19+, CD20 (weak) and CD23+.

A direct Coombs test and serum immunoglobulin estimation is needed. Bone marrow examination helps to establish the extent and pattern of marrow involvement and to evaluate response to treatment.

Staging

Two staging systems exist based on the extent of disease and bone marrow failure and correlate with median survival (Table 21.7).

Treatment

Most patients need only active monitoring. Treatment is indicated only when one of the following features is present:

- Progressive marrow failure.
- Massive (>10 cm) or progressive lymphadenopathy.
- Massive (>6 cm) or progressive splenomegaly.

- Rapidly rising lymphocyte count in peripheral blood (doubling time <6 months or >50% rise in lymphocyte count within 2 months).
- Systemic symptoms:
  - weight loss >10% in six months
  - fever >38°C for >2 weeks
  - extreme fatigue or night sweats
- Autoimmune cytopenias (this may only require treatment of the autoimmune component not necessarily the leukaemia).

The treatment options are chlorambucil, fludarabine with cyclophosphamide and alemtuzumab (if no response or relapse following fludarabine). Most patients are actively monitored after initial treatment. Recently the role of consolidation treatment with monoclonal antibodies and stem cell transplantation are being evaluated.

The choice of salvage treatment depends on the first line treatment and clinical situation at relapse. Patients with previous prolonged remission (>12 months) will respond to the same treatment but with a shorter duration of remission. Patients who are refractory to chlorambucil can be treated with fludarabine or its combination. Treatment options after fludarabine treatment are alemtuzumab, CHOP chemotherapy, and allogeneic transplantation.

Richter's transformation is treated with CHOP chemotherapy which yields 40% response and a poor survival of <6 months.

Supportive treatment

Patients with hypogammaglobulinaemia with recurrent infection need regular intravenous

Table 21.7: Staging systems and survival in CLL					
Risk group	Binet staging		Rai staging		Median survival (years)
Low	A	0–2 areas involved*	0	Lymphocytosis	>10
Intermediate	B	≥3 areas involved	I	Lymphadenopathy	5–7
			II	Splenomegaly and/or hepatomegaly	
High	C	Hb <10 g/dL or platelet <100 × 10⁹/L	III	Hb <11 g/dL	<3–4
			IV	Platelet <100 × 10⁹/L	

* Areas are liver, spleen or lymph nodes (either unilateral or bilateral) in inguinal, axillary and cervical region immunoglobulin (400 mg/kg 3–4 weekly). Patients on intensive treatment with purine analogues and alemtuxumab (Campath) need *Pneumocystis jiroveci* prophylaxis. All patients need influenza vaccine annually.

Splenectomy may be useful for patients with features of hypersplenism and symptomatic splenic enlargement.

New agents

Oblimersen sodium, an antisense molecule to Bcl-2 (Bcl-2 is an anti-apoptotic protein, is highly expressed in CLL cells), in combination with fludarabine and cyclophosphamide has shown to improve CR. Lenolidomide, an anti-angiogeneic agent, and flavopiridol, a cyclin dependent kinases inhibitor, are shown to have activity in CLL.

Hairy cell leukaemia

Hairy cell leukaemia (HCL) constitutes 2% of lymphoid leukaemias. The median age at presentation is 55 years and males are commonly affected. There is no known aetiological factor.

One-quarter of patients are asymptomatic and diagnosis is made after an incidental finding of splenomegaly or cytopenia. One-quarter of patients present with abdominal symptoms due to splenomegaly; one quarter of patients with non-specific symptoms of fatigue, weight loss and fever and the remainder present with features of bleeding or recurrent infections.

Peripheral smear shows cytopenia and the presence of hairy cells, cells twice the size of a normal lymphocyte with cytoplasmic projections and an oval nucleus (Figure 21.7). Bone marrow biopsy is important in definitive diagnosis, which shows an interstitial or focal pattern of infiltration. Immunophenotyping is necessary to distinguish HCL from other B-cell lymphomas.

Asymptomatic patients can be observed until the development of cytopenia or systemic symptoms, when treatment is indicated. The mainstay of treatment is nucleoside analogues, Pentostatin and cladribine, which give a complete remission of >80% with a 10-year overall survival of 95–100%. Since both drugs can cause lymphopenia, patients presenting with cytopenia are treated either with G-CSF support during nucleoside analogue treatment or initial interferon alfa for

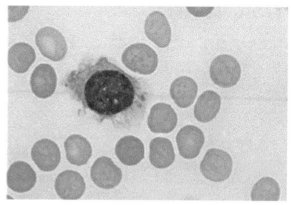

Figure 21.7 Peripheral-blood smear showing characteristic hairy-cell features. From Mey U, Strehl J et al. Advances in the treatment of hairy cell leukaemia, Lancet Oncology 2003;4:86–94.

two months followed by nucleoside analogue treatment.

Patients with a large spleen and with little or moderate bone marrow can be treated with splenectomy with delayed purine analogues until progression.

The majority (70%) of relapsed patients respond to retreatment with pentostatin or cladribine. In patients who fail to respond to nucleoside analogues, rituximab is useful.

Myelodysplastic syndromes

Myelodysplastic syndrome (MDS) is a heterogeneous group of clonal stem cell disease characterized by dysplasia and ineffective haematopoiesis in one or major cell lineages. Although the marrow is producing an excess of cells, these are immature and destroyed before reaching the circulation such that the peripheral blood appears hypocellular. The median age of occurrence is 70 years with over 90% patients over the age of 50 at the time of diagnosis.

There are a number of types including:

- Refractory anaemia
- Refractory anaemia with ring sideroblasts
- Refractory anaemia with excess blasts
- Refractory anaemia with excess blasts in transformation
- Chronic myelomonocytic leukaemia

In the majority of cases, MDS occurs as a de novo disorder; recently secondary MDS/AML as a result of chemotherapy/radiotherapy is increasing. Radiotherapy and alkylating agent related MDS occurs 5–6 years after treatment whereas topoisomerase II inhibitor (e.g. etoposide and teniposide) related MDS develops at a median interval of 33–34 months after exposure.

Presentation depends on the associated cytopenia. Evaluation includes bone marrow biopsy with iron stain and cytogenetic studies, erythropoietin levels and iron studies. The International Prognostic Scoring System (IPSS) defines four risk groups for overall survival and AML evolution, based on the percentage of marrow blasts, specific cytogenetic abnormalities and number of cytopenias. Treatment is complex which depends on the subtype of MDS, IPSS, performance status and co-morbidities which is not dealt with in this text-book. In general the initial treatment is supportive but can later involve chemotherapy or even stem cell transplantation. Median survival is related to IPSS score and ranges from a few months to many years.

Solitary plasmacytoma

The incidence of solitary plasmacytoma is one-tenth of myeloma. Solitary plasmacytomas can occur in bone (solitary bone plasmacytoma – SBP) or in extramedullary sites (extramedullary plasmacytoma – SEP). SBP commonly involves the spine, ribs, femur, humerus, and skull and SEP commonly occurs (80%) in the upper respiratory tract. In >50% cases solitary plasmacytoma is a precursor of myeloma. It is more common in men and the median age at diagnosis is 10 years younger than patients with multiple myeloma.

Clinical features

Pain is the most common clinical symptom of solitary bone plasmacytoma. Spinal plasmacytoma can present with spinal cord compression. Presentation of extramedullary plasmacytoma depends on the site of origin.

Diagnosis

The diagnostic approach is the same as that for myeloma and solitary plasmacytoma is diagnosed when there is no evidence of myeloma. MRI of the spine and pelvis should be performed

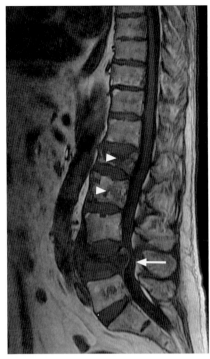

Figure 21.8
MRI scan of the lumbo-sacral spine of a 69-year-old man who presented with cauda equina syndrome due to L4 compression (arrow). Biopsy of L4 vertebra showed plasmacytoma and MRI showed another lesion in L1 and changes in L2 (arrow heads), suggesting myeloma.

in all patients as up to one-third of patients may have additional occult lesions that will be missed on skeletal survey (Figure 21.8). There may be a monoclonal gammopathy, which has prognostic significance, in 24–72% of patients.

Treatment

Radical radiotherapy is the treatment for choice of SPB and SEP (Box 21.7). There is no role for surgery in SPB in the absence of structural instability or neurological compromise. Patients who need surgery receive postoperative radiotherapy. There is no data to recommend adjuvant chemotherapy. Some consider chemotherapy for patients at high risk of failure (e.g. tumour >5 cm).

Surgery is avoided in head and neck SEP. Surgery may be considered for SEP at other sites. After a complete excision, radiotherapy may not be necessary and patients with incomplete excision require radiotherapy. Adjuvant

Clinical target volume
- Solitary bone plasmacytoma:
  - Visible tumour on MRI with a margin of at least 2 cm.
  - For a lesion in the long bones, there is no need to include the entire bone marrow.
  - For vertebral disease, the target volume is the involved bone with one uninvolved vertebra above and below.
- Solitary extramedullary plasmacytoma:
  - Primary tumour with a margin of at least 2 cm.
  - Cervical lymph nodes are included in the target volume if involved.
  - In SEP of Waldeyer's ring, first echelon cervical nodes should be included.

Dose
- Lesion <5 cm – 40 Gy in 20 fractions.
- Lesion >5 cm – 50 Gy in 25 fractions.

Monitoring and further treatment
- 6-weekly for 6 months and then at long interval.
- Patients not responding to radiotherapy should be treated as multiple myeloma.

Patients with apparent SBP with extensive disease on MRI
- Consider as having multiple myeloma.
- Treatment is either with radiotherapy for symptomatic plasmacytoma followed by observation until progression or as multiple myeloma.

chemotherapy may be considered for tumours of >5 cm and high-grade tumours.

Prognostic factors

Increased serum M protein level and an abnormal free light chain ratio are risk factors for progression to myeloma. The 10-year myeloma free survival is 29% in patients with a persistent serum or urinary M protein compared with 91% in those in whom the M protein was not detectable following radiation therapy. Other factors associated with progression to myeloma include axial disease, lesion >5 cm and old age.

Survival

The 10-year overall survival is >50% and DFS is 25–50% for SBP. The 10-year DFS for SEP is 70–80% and has a less risk of distant relapse compared with SBP. Median time to progression of SBP to myeloma is 2–4 years and the overall survival of SBP varies from 7.5–12 years.

Myeloma

Introduction

Myeloma accounts for 1–2% of all malignancies and 10% of all haematological cancers. About 4000 cases are diagnosed in the UK annually. The median age at presentation is 70 years and men are more commonly affected. The aetiology of myeloma is not known.

Myeloma is the result of clonal proliferation of plasma cells. 98% cases have production of paraprotein with IgG being most frequent (60%), followed by IgA (20%), light chain (20%), IgD (9%) and rarely IgE or IgM. 2% of tumours are non-secretory.

Clinical features

The most common presenting symptoms of myeloma are fatigue and bone pain. Pain may be due to bone disease, pathological fracture or nerve compression. Other presenting features include symptoms due to anaemia, renal failure (20–30%), hypercalcaemia and infections.

Investigations and diagnosis

Initial investigations for suspected myeloma include full blood count with ESR, biochemistry including albumin, calcium and uric acid, and electrophoresis of serum and concentrated urine.

Further investigations include serum and urine immunofixation to confirm and type monoclonal protein. Patients with heavy chain myeloma, serum electrophoresis (82%) or serum immunofixation (93%) can detect immunoglobulins. Up to 20% of patients have light chain myeloma which requires detection by urine electrophoresis, immunofixation or serum free light chain test. 1–2% patients have non-secretory myeloma. Serum beta2 microglobulin estimation is important in staging.

Imaging

A skeletal survey reveals lytic bone lesions in myeloma (Figure 21.9). CT and/or MRI studies are indicated when symptomatic areas show no abnormality on routine radiographs.

Bone marrow

A unilateral bone marrow aspirate and trephine is indicated in all patients with myeloma which

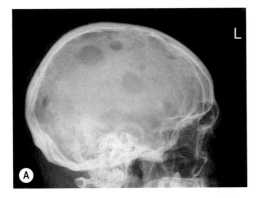

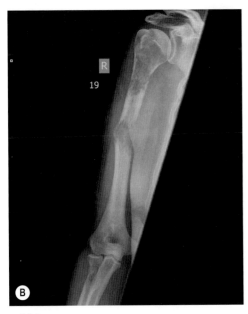

Figure 21.9
Skeletal survey in myeloma.

Box 21.8: Diagnostic criteria of myeloma

Myeloma is diagnosed by the following three criteria:

- Bone marrow plasma cells ≥10%, and
- Presence of serum and/or urinary monoclonal protein (except in patients with true non-secretory multiple myeloma), and
- Any myeloma-related organ or tissue impairment:
  - Bone lesions: lytic lesions, osteoporosis or pathologic fractures.
  - Anaemia: haemoglobin value of >2 g/dL below the lower limit of normal or a haemoglobin value <10 g/dL.
  - Hypercalcaemia: corrected serum calcium >0.25 mmol/L above the upper limit of normal or >2.75 mmol/L), or
  - Renal failure: serum creatinine >195 mg/L.
  - Others: symptomatic hyperviscosity, amyloidosis, >2 episodes of bacterial infection in 12 months.

Table 21.8: International Staging System for Myeloma

Stage (% of patients)	Criteria	Median survival (months)
I (29)	Serum beta2-microglobulin <3.5 mg/L Serum albumin ≥3.5 g/dL	62
II (38)	Not stage I or III*	44
III (34)	Serum beta2-microglobulin ≥5.5 mg/L	29

Categories of stage II:

- Serum beta2-microglobulin <3.5 mg/L but serum albumin <3.5 g/dL
- Serum beta2-microglobulin 3.5 – <5.5 mg/L irrespective of serum albumin level

will show ≥10% clonal bone marrow plasma cells.

The diagnostic criteria of myeloma is shown in Box 21.8.

Staging

An International Staging System (ISS) has replaced the Durie–Salmon staging (Table 21.8).

Prognostic factors

Performance status is one of the important predictors of outcome and is a key determinant of transplant eligibility. Other prognostic factors include age, ISS stage, creatinine, calcium, albumin, immunoglobulin subtype, extent of bone marrow involvement, plasmablastic morphology and lactate dehydrogenase and cytogenetic changes.

Treatment

Myeloma is rarely curable and a minority of patients achieve long-term remission following allogenic stem cell transplantation. Chemotherapy is indicated for symptomatic myeloma and asymptomatic myeloma with myeloma-related organ damage. The median time to progression from asymptomatic to symptomatic myeloma is

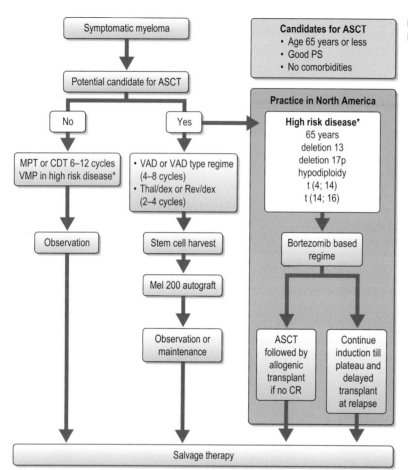

Figure 21.10
Management of myeloma.

12–32 months. Monitoring of asymptomatic myeloma includes 3-monthly clinical assessment and measurement of paraprotein.

Treatment of newly diagnosed multiple myeloma is rapidly evolving. The North American approach involves risk categorization of patients based on molecular cytogenetics and upfront use of novel agents such as bortezomib (a proteasome inhibitor) and lenalidomide (an analogue of thalidomide) whereas such an approach is yet to be adopted in the UK (Figure 21.10). Table 21.9 shows regimes in newly diagnosed myeloma. Treatment response is assessed by the International Myeloma Working Group definitions of response criteria.

In patients eligible for autologous stem cell transplantation (ASCT) prolonged melphalan based chemotherapy can interfere with adequate stem cell mobilization and is therefore avoided.

Patients not eligible for ASCT are treated with melphalan-based regimes (Figure 21.2 and Table 21.9). MPT is the preferred regimen for standard-risk patients who are not candidates for transplantation. ASCT prolongs the median overall survival in myeloma by approximately 12 months.

Refractory and relapsing myeloma

Almost all patients with myeloma eventually relapse. If relapse occurs more than 6 months after stopping therapy, the initial chemotherapy regimen should be re-instituted. Patients who have cryopreserved stem cells early in the disease course can derive significant benefit from ASCT as salvage therapy. In general, patients who have indolent relapse can often be treated with single agents whereas those with more aggressive relapse often require a combination of agents.

Table 21.9: Regimes in newly diagnosed myeloma

Regimen	Response rate
Regime for patients not eligible for ASCT	
Melphalan–prednisolone–thalidomide (MPT)	75%
Bortezomib–melphalan–prednisone (VMP)	70%
Cyclophosphamide–dexamethasone–thalidomide (CDT)	72%
Regime for patients eligible for ASCT	
Vincristine–Adriamycin–dexamethasone (VAD)	52%
Thalidomide–dexamethasone (Thal/Dex)	65%
Lenalidomide–low dose dexamethasone (Rev/Dex)	70%
Bortezomib–dexamethasone (Vel/Dex)	80%
Bortezomib–thalidomide–dexamethasone (VTD)	90%

Supportive care

- Bone disease – all patients with symptomatic myeloma receive regular bisphosphonate for at least one year from diagnosis.
- Pain control is by analgesics and palliative radiotherapy. Percutaneous vertebroplasty and kyphoplasty are useful for vertebral compression fractures that do not respond to standard measures within 6 weeks.
- Hypercalcaemia is treated with bisphosphonates.
- Renal impairment: managed with adequate hydration, avoidance of nephrotoxic drugs and prompt treatment of infection and hypercalcaemia.
- Anaemia – transfusions, erythropoietin or darbepoietin are useful.
- Infections – all symptomatic patients need vaccination against influenza, pneumococci, meningococci and *Haemophilus influenza*. Prompt treatment of infection is required.
- Hyperviscosity syndrome needs plasmapheresis.

Monoclonal gammopathy of unknown significance (MGUS) and smouldering myeloma

MGUS is defined by a serum M-protein concentration of <3 g/dL, <10% plasma cells in the bone marrow and absent myeloma-related organ or tissue impairment (ROTI). Around 1% per year will transform to myeloma or another plasma cell disorder. It does not require any treatment but needs life-long monitoring (6–12 monthly) with clinical assessment and quantification of paraprotein.

Smouldering myeloma is the stage between MGUS and myeloma characterized by serum M protein of ≥3 g/dL and/or ≥10% plasma cell in the bone marrow and no ROTI. Transformation to myeloma or other plasma cell disorders occur at a rate of 10% per year. Management is 3–4 monthly observation until evidence of progression to myeloma.

Further reading

Evens AM, Hutchings M, Diehl V. Treatment of Hodgkin lymphoma: the past, present, and future. Nat Clin Pract Oncol. 2008;5:543–556.

Peggs KS, Anderlini P, Sureda A. Allogeneic transplantation for Hodgkin lymphoma. Br J Haematol. 2008;143:468–480.

Diehl V, Fuchs M. Early, intermediate and advanced Hodgkin's lymphoma: modern treatment strategies. Ann Oncol. 2007;18 Suppl 9:ix71–79.

Lenz G, Staudt LM. Aggressive lymphomas. N Engl J Med. 2010;362:1417–1429.

Zucca E. Extranodal lymphoma: a reappraisal. Ann Oncol. 2008;19 Suppl 4:iv77–80.

Estey E, Döhner H. Acute myeloid leukaemia. Lancet. 2006;368:1894–1907.

Hehlmann R, Hochhaus A, Baccarani M. Chronic myeloid leukaemia. Lancet. 2007;370:342–350.

Shanafelt TD, Kay NE. Combination therapies for previously untreated CLL. Lancet. 2007;21;370:197–198.

Rajkumar SV. Multiple myeloma. Curr Probl Cancer. 2009;33:7–64.

Paediatric, teenage and young adult cancers

HM Hatcher

Introduction

Cancers in this group of patients present specific challenges in diagnosis, treatment, recruitment to clinical trials and survival. Childhood cancers have seen a significant improvement in survival in the last 30 years from less than 30% to greater than 70% long-term survival. Unfortunately the same is not the case in the teenage and young adult cancers (TYA) with very little improvement seen over the same time period.

In addition they have particular social, educational, developmental and psychological needs which, if not addressed, have long-term consequences for the patient and their family. Those who survive cancer at a young age may also be left with significant medical late effects which need to be recognized and managed (p. 58).

Incidence/epidemiology

The incidence of malignancy in the UK is:

- 12.4 per 100,000 up to 15 years.
- 14.4 per 100,000 in those 15–19.
- 22.6 per 100,000 in those 20–24.

Those aged 14–24 account for 0.5% of all cancer registrations in the UK. In a study from the north-west of England the incidence was 174 cases per million with a male:female ratio of 1.22:1. In the same study the incidence was found to be increasing, particularly for bone tumours, testicular tumours, thyroid cancer and malignant melanoma.

Cancer is the most frequent natural cause of death in this age group, second only to accidents.

- Male:female ratio is 1.2:1.

Aetiology

The majority of older adult cancers are related to specific risk factors such as smoking, whereas the majority of paediatric malignancies are thought to be developmental in origin. A number of syndromes are associated with childhood cancer (e.g. Down's syndrome associated with leukaemia) but the majority arise without an underlying genetic predisposition (e.g. Li–Fraumeni and sarcomas). TYA malignancies fall between the two age extremes and may represent a late developmental malignancy or an early adult malignancy due to other factors, e.g. familial adenomatous polyposis. In most cases the aetiology is not known.

Types of cancer

The types of cancer vary not only between children and adults but as the age increases in certain age group bandings (Table 22.1).

In children leukaemias represent the most common malignancy with acute lymphoblastic leukaemia (ALL) being most frequent. Brain tumours also make up a significant group, but the incidence falls as a proportion of cases from childhood towards early adulthood. In the 15 to 19-year-olds, the most frequent malignancies are lymphomas, leukaemias and carcinomas (especially thyroid and nasopharyngeal). For the 20 to 24-year-olds, lymphomas remain the most common malignancy but with carcinomas (especially cervix, thyroid and breast) and germ cell tumours as next common. Osteosarcomas and germ cell tumours peak in late teenage and early adulthood.

Table 22.1: Distribution of cancer types according to age

Age 0–14 years	Age 15–19 years	Age 20–24 years
Leukaemia 35%	Lymphoma 27%	Lymphomas 24%
Brain tumours 24%	Sarcomas 16%	Carcinomas 21%
Lymphomas 12%	Leukaemia 15%	Germ cell tumours 17%
Wilms' tumour 7%	Carcinomas 11%	Melanoma 10%
Neuroblastoma 7%	Brain tumours 11%	Sarcomas 8%
Sarcomas 11%	Germ cell tumours 10%	Leukaemia 8%
Retinoblastoma 3%	Melanoma 6%	Brain tumours 8%
Others 1%	Others 4%	Others 4%

Clinical features

The clinical features in children, teenagers and young adults are similar to those seen in other age groups with the same malignancies, but are often not recognized as such due to the rarity of malignancy in these age groups. In addition for children who are unable to explain symptoms clearly, the disease has usually progressed so that symptoms are obvious to their family. Delays in diagnosis are very common in the adolescent and young adult and can contribute to reduced survival at all ages.

In children warning signs may be due to localized disease, or the manifestations of disseminated disease are listed in Box 22.1.

In the older child and young adult, the same warning features apply but also include additional signs specific to the different malignancies.

Diagnosis and delays

Diagnosis of malignancy currently follows the pathways for either paediatric or adult cancers. Paediatric cancers are diagnosed and treated in specialist principal treatment centres with some care shared with local hospitals. For TYA cancers, currently they may be seen in a paediatric or adult setting and treated according to those protocols. In the UK TYA cancer will soon be treated in specialized centres. This may mean referral to a specialist TYA centre or to an adult cancer specialist in a particular site of the body in a designated regional hospital with appropriate TYA facilities (Figure 22.1).

Box 22.1: Warning signs of cancer in children

- Obvious lump or swelling around the head, neck, abdomen or elsewhere.
- Increasing and persistent pain in bone or joints, often leading to less use of the limb or limping.
- Pallor, especially if associated with unexplained bruising or bleeding.
- Worsening headaches, especially if associated with vomiting in the morning.

Delays in diagnosis can occur in children if symptoms are occult, especially in very young children but are more common in the TYA group.

Specific childhood cancers

Some cancers are specific to children and young adults, or their treatment is different to that in adults. These tumours will be highlighted below. For other malignancies, covered by other chapters, only specific changes in management for children and young adults will be made.

Leukaemias

In childhood acute lymphoblastic leukaemia (ALL) is by far the most frequently occurring leukaemia representing over 75% cases. (p. 308).

Presentation is usually with symptoms and signs of bone marrow infiltration and these can appear to occur quite rapidly, although are often preceded by several weeks of general malaise or recurrent infections and fevers. Usual features at the time of diagnosis are pallor, abnormal bruising or bleeding, bone pain (which may manifest

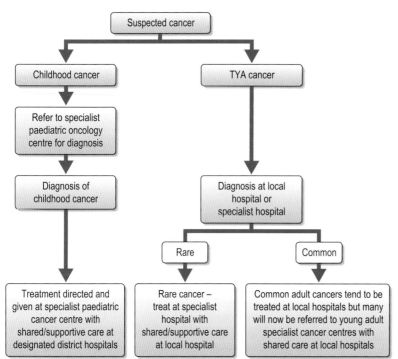

Figure 22.1
Referral for treatment of childhood and TYA malignancy.

Box 22.2: Prognostic features in childhood and adolescent ALL

Patients are stratified according to risk by combining age, initial white count, cytogenetics, immunology and response to initial treatment.

Very high risk (5-year survival <50%).
• Philadelphia chromosome or hypodiploidy or who fail to achieve remission after induction therapy.

High risk (<75% 5-year survival).
• Age greater than 10 years or with unfavourable cytogenetics.

Standard risk (80% 5-year survival).
• Age 1–10, low white count, no unfavourable cytogenetics.

Low risk (90% 5-year survival).
• Age 1–10, low white count, favourable cytogenetics.

Favourable cytogenetics
• Hyperdiploidy, trisomies of 4, 10, 17, t(12;21).

Unfavourable cytogenetics
• Hypodiploidy, tetraploidy, Philadelphia chromosome [t(9;22)], t(1;19), t(4;11).

---

as limping in young children) and on clinical examination lymphadenopathy and hepatomegaly in some children.

Diagnosis is suspected on the differential blood count but bone marrow examination is essential to confirm the diagnosis (p. 308), to perform immunocytochemical stains and cytogenetics which are of diagnostic and prognostic significance (Box 22.2).

Treatment of childhood and young adult ALL is performed according to risk stratification as in Box 22.2. In general treatment involves several phases which is similar to that of adult ALL (p. 308).

Relapsed ALL may still be curable with high-dose chemotherapy and stem cell transplantation, but the chances of long-term cure are much lower with the high-risk subgroups and if relapse is within a year of completing initial treatment.

In addition certain subgroups such as B-cell ALL are often treated on different regimens similar to those used for a Burkitt's lymphoma (p. 305, Burkitt's lymphoma). Both these malignancies are associated with a t(8;14) translocation so may be variations of the same malignancy.

Brain tumours

Brain tumours are the second most common malignancy in children and remain a significant cause of cancer into young adulthood. In children the majority of tumours occur infratentorially but this proportion changes with increasing age.

Presenting features include headaches, often worse in the morning and associated with morning vomiting, papilloedema (sometimes detected by an optician), ataxia, personality change, nerve palsies and nystagmus.

Common subtypes of brain tumour include astrocytoma, medulloblastoma, glioma, craniopharyngioma and ependymoma. In children, particularly in the very young, the emphasis of treatment is to delay, avoid or minimize the need for radiotherapy to avoid long-term side effects. These are covered in more detail on p. 264.

Wilms' tumour

Wilms' tumour or nephroblastoma occurs most frequently in children under 5 years of age and very rarely in older children or young adults. Most tumours are unilateral, but are bilateral in 5% of cases and in a further 5–10% will have more than one tumour in the same kidney. Risk factors include certain genetic syndromes such as Beckwith–Weidemann syndrome. They are often asymptomatic until they present as an abdominal mass, pain and/or anorexia.

Histologically they are divided into a favourable group with well-defined elements and the anaplastic (or unfavourable group) with poorly defined cellular morphology. Less than 25% have a mutation within the WT1 (Wilms' tumour) gene.

Staging is undertaken with imaging and treatment is according to stage (Figure 22.2). Anaplastic tumours are treated with more aggressive chemotherapy except in stage I where their prognosis is similar to favourable histology tumours.

Overall more than 80% are cured of their disease. Treatment for relapse is rarely curative.

Neuroblastoma

Neuroblastoma is a neuroendocrine tumour which originates from any neural crest element of the sympathetic nervous system. It predominantly occurs in those under 3 years of age. The highest incidence is in the first 12 months of life with less than 10% of cases occurring in those over the age of 5 years.

Clinical presentation is varied depending on the location and extent of the tumour. Fatigue, fever and anorexia are the most common initial presenting features with more localizing features dependent on tumour site. Adrenal primaries are often extensive at presentation and may involve the IVC. Paravertebral tumours may lead to spinal cord compression. At least 50% of cases are metastatic at presentation. Elevated catecholamines are found in over 90%. Staging includes a CT, bone scintigram, bone marrow sampling and radiolabelled MIBG (meta-iodobenzylguanidine) scan. MIBG is taken up by 95% of neuroblastomas and acts as a tool for staging and monitoring disease response.

Poor prognostic features are advanced stage, age over 1 year, and over-expression of N-*myc* oncogene.

Treatment may be with surgery alone in early stage disease, but the majority require combination chemotherapy. Trials are examining the role of intensification of treatment in poor prognosis disease. The risk of relapse is high and the long-term survival for those with metastatic disease at presentation is less than 30%.

Lymphomas

Lymphomas occur in childhood and Hodgkin's disease has a peak in incidence in young adulthood (p. 298). In general these tumours are treated similar to their adult counterparts except that radiotherapy is avoided, except in refractory disease, to reduce the risk of its effect on growth and the risk of second malignancy. Chemotherapy regimens are similar to adults but trials are ongoing to assess the role of rituximab in children. The most common subtypes of NHL in children are Burkitt-like lymphomas (p. 305) and diffuse large B-cell lymphomas (Table 22.2).

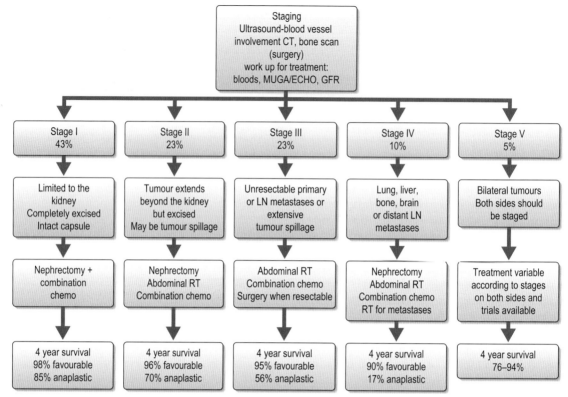

Figure 22.2
Staging and management of Wilms' tumour.

Table 22.2: Major histopathological categories of non-Hodgkin lymphoma in children and adolescents

Category (WHO Classification/ updated REAL)	Immuno-phenotype	Clinical presentation
Burkitt and Burkitt-like lymphomas	Mature B cell	Intra-abdominal (sporadic), head and neck (non-jaw, sporadic), jaw (endemic)
Diffuse large B-cell lymphoma	Mature B cell; may be CD30+	Nodal, abdomen, bone, primary CNS, mediastinal
Lymphoblastic lymphoma, precursor T-cell/leukaemia, or precursor B-cell lymphoma	Pre-T cell	Mediastinal, bone marrow
	Pre-B cell	Skin, bone
Anaplastic large cell lymphoma, systemic	CD30+ (Ki-1+)	Variable, but systemic symptoms often prominent
	T cell or null cell	
Anaplastic large cell lymphoma, cutaneous	CD30+ (Ki-1+usually)	Skin only; single or multiple lesions
	T cell	

Anaplastic large cell tumours are rare as are other adult subtypes such as cutaneous T-cell lymphoma and MALT lymphoma (p. 306). Prognostic factors are similar to adult tumours.

Sarcomas

Both bone and soft tissue sarcomas occur in children and young adults. These are covered in detail in Chapter 15. Some sarcomas, however, peak in this age group. Osteosarcomas peak in early adolescence with Ewing's sarcomas having their peak incidence in older adolescence. Rhabdomyosarcoma (RMS), a tumour of striated muscle, is the only soft tissue sarcoma to peak in children and adolescents. It is divided into two main histological subgroups, embryonal and alveolar. Alveolar rhabdomyosarcoma (ARMS) is characterized by one of two specific translocations, either t(2;13)(q35;q14) resulting in fusion of PAX3-FOXO1 in 60% ARMS or t(1;13)(q36;q14) resulting in PAX7-FOXO1 in 20% ARMS. Embryonal RMS is not associated with a specific translocation, but loss in chromosome 11. Common tumour sites include the head and neck, paratesticular and limb (Figure 22.3). It frequently presents with advanced disease. If localized it can present with a mass or proptosis if retro-orbital. It can give rise to nodal metastases and regional lymph nodes should be examined. Staging involves local MRI, CT of chest (and regional), bone scan, and bone marrow biopsy. Localized disease is treated with surgery, but due to the aggressive nature of these tumours, combination chemotherapy with e.g. IVADo (ifosfamide, vincristine, actinomycin and doxorubicin), is given. Radiotherapy is often given if margins are positive or there has been tumour regrowth after initial surgery. An Italian pilot study suggested that maintenance therapy with cyclophosphamide and vinorelbine may prolong progression free survival. In advanced disease combination chemotherapy is used but the outlook is poor. Poor prognostic factors include increasing age, particularly over age 16, advanced stage and alveolar subtype.

Germ cell tumours

Germ cell tumours of the ovary and testes peak in young adulthood and are described in more detail in Chapters 12 and 13. Similar treatment modalities are used in children and young adults, but there has been a move to reduce long-term side effects from chemotherapy and to try to maintain fertility in ovarian germ cell tumours. Trials are underway to examine the role of carboplatin rather than cisplatin and to reduce the dose of bleomycin in adolescent germ cell tumours to reduce late effects. Fertility sparing surgery is preferred if possible for ovarian germ cell tumours and many women retain their fertility with this type of surgery and BEP chemotherapy (p. 220).

Langerhans cell histiocytosis (LCH)

LCH is a proliferative disorder of histiocytes. Although not strictly a malignancy it may exhibit aggressive behaviour and require combination chemotherapy. Multiple bony lesions can occur at any site, but can occur within the skull leading to hypothalamic infiltration and diabetes insipidus. Systemic LCH tends to present in infancy as a widespread rash with bone marrow and soft tissue involvement. Organ dysfunction is a better indication of poor prognosis than the number of involved sites. Treatment of advanced disease is with chemotherapy.

Hepatoblastomas

Hepatoblastomas are rare but are most common malignancy of liver in children. There is an association with FAP. Hepatocellular carcinoma can also occur rarely but in older age groups. Clinical

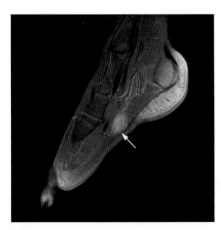

Figure 22.3
MRI of sagittal section through the foot showing a mass deep to the plantar fascia. Histology showed an embryonal rhabdomyosarcoma.

presentation is usually with a mass or abdominal distension. Jaundice is rare. Alpha-foetoprotein (AFP) is elevated in most cases. Unlike adult liver tumours, most hepatoblastomas respond to combination chemotherapy (cisplatin and doxorubicin) with good long-term survival.

Retinoblastoma

Retinoblastomas are very rare childhood tumours. All bilateral tumours and 20% of unilateral tumours are thought to be hereditary. The retinoblastoma tumour suppressor gene is on chromosome 13 with the pattern of inheritance being autosomal dominant with incomplete penetrance (Chapter 5, p. 55). Most cases present before age 3. In children not known to be in a retinoblastoma family presentation is with a squint or white papillary reflex. Those related to retinoblastoma families should be part of a screening programme. Surgery may be necessary for some but most cases are treated with radiotherapy. Long-term survival is over 95%, but second malignancy is common (osteosarcomas in radiotherapy field) and in those with hereditary retinoblastoma other malignancies, especially sarcomas can occur elsewhere in the body in young adulthood up to middle age.

Clinical trials

Traditionally children have a high recruitment to clinical trials (>80%) and there are often available trials in the most frequent childhood cancers. However, trial recruitment is lowest in the adolescent and young adult population when compared with either children or older adults. This is partially due to the rarity of cancers concerned, but also to the fact that these patients are treated in a wide range of settings. Many fall between different groups of physicians who may not be able to provide available trials. It is hoped this will be changed with the evolving changes in the organization of TYA cancer management.

Psychological support

Children and their families frequently need support to help them manage the consequences of a diagnosis of cancer at such a young age, and the consequences it will have on the family over an often protracted treatment period. The fact that many children are now cured of their disease but with long-term effects from their treatment also has a psychological impact on them and their family. Adolescents and young adults are at a vulnerable stage of development and treatment for cancer has been shown to have a detrimental long-term psychological impact in many patients. Appropriate support should be offered to patients and their families to try to prevent some of these conditions occurring later on.

Risk-taking behaviour is also at its greatest in the TYA age group and can affect drug compliance as well as coping mechanisms.

Body image and fertility

Sexual identity and future fertility are important considerations for the adolescent or young adult. Loss of hair or a limb will significantly affect body image at an age when this is especially vulnerable. The type of cancer or its treatment may also affect future fertility, but this is not universal so specific knowledge is required for each patient (p. 59, late effects).

Education

The majority of children and young adult patients will be in full-time education at the time of diagnosis. If treatment is lengthy or affects the ability to study in the longer term, this can also result in difficulties reintegrating into school or obtaining a job. Continuing education should be supported throughout treatment.

Late effects

Late effects are an important factor in the treatment of children and young adults (p. 58, late effects). Late effects are dependent upon the original cancer, its treatment, the family genetics and the developmental stage of the individual when treated for cancer. Every organ system can be affected, but the most significant include the risk of second malignancy, neurocognitive impairment, growth problems, and cardiac and endocrine abnormalities. Many centres run late effects clinics to monitor for these and other sequelae of cancer treatment.

Transition

Patients in the adolescent age group are at a critical stage of development between childhood and independent adulthood. Their ongoing care necessitates an understanding of the transition between these stages. There must be clear communication between different medical teams and an agreement to the future care and follow-up of an individual. This can be facilitated by multidisciplinary teams from paediatric, TYA and adult services as well as joint clinics to facilitate knowledge and experience.

Terminal care and bereavement

Unfortunately many young adults and some children with cancer will not survive and this will have an enormous impact on their families and friends. Family support at this time, as with the rest of the child or young adult's treatment, is essential. Liaison with community services and children's hospices is an important part of this process.

Further reading

Albritton K, Bleyer WA. The management of cancer in the older adolescent. Eur J Cancer 2003;39:2584–2599.

Birch JM, Alston R, Quinn M, Kelsey A. Incidence of malignant disease by morphological type in young persons aged 12–24 years in England, 1979–1997. Eur J Cancer 2003;39:2622–2631.

Martin S, Ulrich C, Munsell M, et al. Delays in cancer diagnosis in underinsured young adults and older adolescents. The Oncologist 2007;12:816–824.

Ramanujachar R, Richards S, Hann I, et al. Adolescents with ALL: outcome on UK national paediatric and adult trials. Pediatr Blood Cancer 2007;48:254–261.

Guidance on Cancer Services – Improving outcomes in children and young people with cancer. August 2005. Available from www.nice.org.uk

Oncologic emergencies

23

J Wrigley and TV Ajithkumar

Metastatic spinal cord compression

Introduction

Metastatic spinal cord compression (MSCC) occurs in 3–5% of patients with cancer. Prostate, breast and lung cancer each account for 15–20% of cases; lymphoma, myeloma and renal cell cancer account for 10% and the remainder is due to colorectal cancers, sarcomas and cancers of unknown primary. Although more frequent in patients with known malignancy, MSCC is the presenting feature in up to 20% of patients with no prior diagnosis of cancer, particularly lung cancer.

Aetiology

The mechanisms by which MSCC may develop include:

1. Direct tumour extension into the epidural space from a vertebral or paravertebral mass.
2. Haematogenous spread to the vertebral spine causing collapse and compression.
3. Direct deposition of tumour cells within the cord.

Early stage compression of the cord results in oedema, venous congestion and demyelination, and neurological recovery may still be possible during this phase with prompt decompression. Continued compression causes secondary vascular injury and irreversible infarction. The most common location of compression is thoracic (50–70%) followed by lumbo-sacral (20–30%) and cervical spine (10–20%). Up to 85% patients have multiple vertebral metastases and impor-

tantly, around 17% of patients have two or more levels of compression at presentation.

Spinal cord metastases can be of three types depending on the location of tumour deposit:

- Extradural – occurs in more than 90%, usually due to direct extension of vertebral metastases. 75% of these are caused by soft tissue extension and 25% by bone collapse and compression by bony fragments.
- Intradural extramedullary – occurs in 5% of cases and is due to deposit via CSF spaces.
- Intramedullary (0.5–3.5%) – are commonly associated with brain metastases and lepto-meningeal disease and can occur in lung, breast and renal cell cancers, lymphoma and myeloma.

Clinical features

Back pain is the most frequent (95%) first symptom, which commonly precedes the diagnosis of MSCC by up to 3 months in patients with known cancer and up to 5 months in those without a known malignancy. The pain may be localized or neurogenic and is typically worse when the patient is supine.

Limb weakness is the second most common symptom. Up to 85% of patients will have abnormal power in the limbs at presentation, which depends on the neurologic level of compression.

Sensory deficit may manifest itself as paraesthesia or sensory loss and is present in up to 65% of patients with MSCC. Up to 50% of patients will have a dermatomal sensory level, although this may vary by several dermatomes above or below the true level of compression.

© 2011, Elsevier Ltd
DOI: 10.1016/B978-0-7234-3458-0.00028-2

Autonomic dysfunction is a late complication affecting up to 50% of patients with MSCC. It includes impotence, bladder and bowel dysfunction, with constipation occurring most frequently.

There are two clinical variants of MSCC, which require early recognition:

- Isolated ataxia: thoracic SCC may present with isolated ataxia due to spinocerebellar pathway dysfunction.
- Cauda equina syndrome: epidural extension of metastases below the level of the spinal cord (L1/L2) can present with early sphincter dysfunction, saddle anaesthesia (buttocks and perineal region), flaccid paraparesis of hip extension and abduction, knee flexion and movement of feet and toes, and absent ankle reflexes.

Investigations

MRI of the whole spine is the investigation of choice for suspected MSCC. CT is used only when MRI is contraindicated. A sagittal screening of the whole spine with T1 and short T1 inversion recovery (STIR) images should be done to ensure that multiple levels of compression are not missed and also to identify asymptomatic metastases. T2 weighted images help to detect the degree of compression by a soft tissue component and intramedullary lesions (Figure 23.1).

In patients who have not been previously diagnosed with cancer, a histological diagnosis is required before definitive treatment can be planned. Patients should be investigated like any other patient with cancer of unknown primary and an appropriate area most amenable to biopsy should be established. However, treatment should not be delayed during these investigations and prompt neurosurgical involvement should be established if biopsy is not possible.

Management

The aim of treatment is to preserve or improve neurological function and achieve pain control.

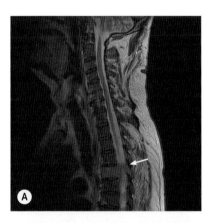

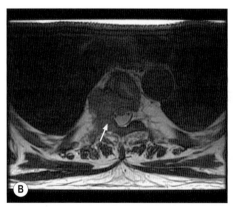

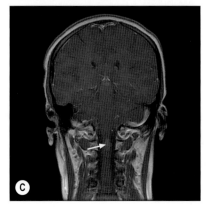

Figure 23.1
Imaging in cord compression. MRI scan shows spinal cord compression due to a collapsed vertebra (A,B) and an intramedullary metastasis from lung cancer (C).

70–100% patients who are ambulant at the beginning of treatment remain ambulant with prompt treatment, whereas only 30–50% patients who are non-ambulant regain the ability to walk and only 5–10% of paraplegic patients become ambulant. Hence it is important to have definitive treatment within 24 hours of presentation with suspected cord compression. Patients with MSCC secondary to a vascular event will not respond to treatment.

Initial measures

All patients with suspected MSCC, except those without known cancer and those who are likely to have lymphoma, are started on oral dexamethasone 16 mg/day after assessment. This dose of steroid is continued until definitive treatment, after which the steroids are weaned down as quickly as neurological symptoms will allow.

Optimal pain control and cervical collar for patients with suspected cervical spine involvement are advised.

Specific measures

Definite treatment of MSCC depends on the histologic type and associated spinal stability. In patients with no prior history of cancer, surgical decompression with histologic confirmation is appropriate. If surgical decompression is not possible, a CT guided biopsy is needed.

Surgery may involve decompression, stabilization and or resection and reconstruction of the spinal canal. The patient's overall prognosis and performance status should be taken into consideration and patients who have had no distal neurological function for >24 h should not be considered for surgery (Boxes 23.1 and 23.2).

Radiotherapy is the treatment most frequently used and is most effective for patients with radiosensitive tumours who are ambulatory at the beginning of treatment. For those without mechanical pain or structural instability, radiotherapy may significantly improve pain control and neurological function. The most commonly used regimes are 20 Gy in five fractions (more appropriate for patients with expected short survival) or 30 Gy in 10 fractions (Box 23.3). Some patients may deteriorate during radiotherapy when the steroid dose may be increased or they may be considered for surgery if appropriate.

Box 23.1: Patients with MSCC according to outcome after surgical intervention

Good surgical candidates	Poor surgical candidates
'Good prognosis tumours' e.g. breast cancer, testicular cancer etc.	'Poor prognosis tumours' e.g. lung cancer, melanoma
Single level of compression with solitary or few vertebral metastases	Multiple levels affected or multiple spinal metastases
Absence of visceral metastases	Presence of visceral metastases
Good neurological function	Poor neurological function
No previous radiotherapy	Recurrence following radiotherapy
Minimal co-morbidity	Medically unfit for surgery
Unknown primary or no histopathological diagnosis	Prognosis <3 months

---

Box 23.2: Indications for surgical treatment*

- Relapse after radiotherapy
- Progression while on radiotherapy
- Radiation resistant tumours
- Unknown primary tumour
- Unstable spine or pathological fractures

*With a single site of cord compression and no total paraplegia for longer than 48 h.

Box 23.3: Radiotherapy in spinal cord compression

- Position – supine or prone
- Treatment volume – one vertebra above and below MRI proven compression
- Ensure that all paravertebral disease is enclosed in the volume if feasible
- Direct posterior beam 6 MV (parallel lateral in cervical region if feasible)
- Prescription point – anterior spinal canal (either measured from MRI or arbitrary, see Figure 23.2)
- Dose – 30 Gy in 10 fractions or 20 Gy in five fractions

Patients with established paraplegia are treated with an 8 Gy single fraction for pain control.

The issue of whether surgery or radiotherapy or a combination of both gives best functional outcome is yet to be resolved. A randomized study compared radiotherapy (30 Gy in 10 frac-

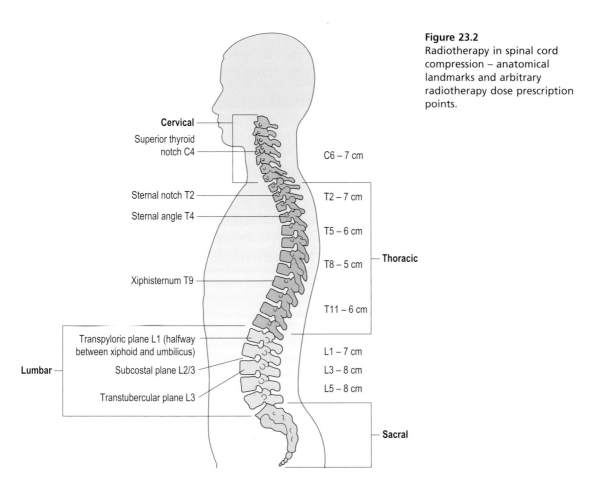

Figure 23.2
Radiotherapy in spinal cord compression – anatomical landmarks and arbitrary radiotherapy dose prescription points.

Cervical

Superior thyroid notch C4

Sternal notch T2

Sternal angle T4

Xiphisternum T9

Transpyloric plane L1 (halfway between xiphoid and umbilicus)

Lumbar

Subcostal plane L2/3

Transtubercular plane L3

C6 – 7 cm

T2 – 7 cm

T5 – 6 cm

T8 – 5 cm — Thoracic

T11 – 6 cm

L1 – 7 cm

L3 – 8 cm

L5 – 8 cm

Sacral

tions) started within 24 hours of onset of MSCC with surgery within 24 hours followed by radiotherapy within 2 weeks of surgery. Results showed that initial surgery followed by radiotherapy offers a longer period with ability to walk compared with those treated with radiotherapy alone (median, 126 days vs. 35 days, p = 0.006). This study showed that surgery permits most patients to remain ambulatory and continent for the remainder of their lives, while patients treated with radiation alone spend approximately two-thirds of their remaining time unable to walk and incontinent. However, results of this study may not be extended to all patients as the study was limited to patients with less radiosensitive tumours and with different tumour types and presentations.

Chemotherapy alone is not an option for treatment even in chemosensitive tumours as the response to treatment is often slow and unpredictable. Hence MSCC in chemosensitive tumours is treated with a combination of radiotherapy and chemotherapy.

Supportive measures

Supportive care requires a multidisciplinary team approach. Analgesia needs to be optimized and venous thromboembolism prophylaxis prescribed. Urinary or supra-pubic catheters should be considered and faecal continence should be controlled with the use of stool softeners and suppositories every 2–3 days. In patients with bone metastases, there is no evidence that bisphosphonates can reduce the risk of cord compression.

Prognosis

The median survival following a diagnosis of MSCC is 3–6 months, with 17% of patients alive at 1 year and 10% alive at 18 months.

Pre-treatment motor function is an important predictor of the ambulatory outcome. Patients who develop motor dysfunction more slowly also may have a better outcome.

Recurrence of spinal cord compression

7–14% of patients can present with recurrence of spinal cord compression after initial decompression. If the second cord compression is in a different area, treatment is the same as that of the original compression. However, if patients present with spinal cord compression at the initial radiation portal, surgical decompression is the initial option, particularly if the recurrence is within three months of initial treatment. If they are not a candidate for surgery, re-irradiation may be considered. It is important to make sure that the total dose to spinal code is kept below 100 Gy_2 (biologically equivalent dose of 100 Gy when delivered as 2 Gy per fraction). Many clinicians use a dose of 20 Gy in 8–10 fractions.

Paediatric spinal cord compression

Paediatric MSCC differs from adult MSCC in that it is often caused by chemosensitive histological types not seen in adults such as neuroblastoma, Wilms' tumour (p. 323). The usual pathogenesis is the direct invasion of tumour through neural foramina. The most common histologic type is neuroblastoma, which responds to chemotherapy. Decompressive surgery is offered when patients present with rapid progression or progress during chemotherapy. Radiotherapy is only offered when there is no response after chemotherapy and/or surgery and for those who require palliation after failure of multiple systemic regimens.

Intramedullary spinal cord metastasis

This is rare (1% incidence) and lung cancer is the most common primary. Sensory deficit (79%), sphincter dysfunction (60%) and weakness (91%) are common manifestations. Up to 40% patients will have brain metastases. Treatment is with corticosteroids and radiotherapy.

Raised intracranial pressure

Approximately 25% of patients with cancer develop brain metastases and can present with features of raised intracranial pressure and focal neurological deficits. Seizures and bleeding into the metastases can result in an acute medical emergency. Malignant melanoma, renal cell carcinoma, thyroid cancer and choriocarcinoma are commonly associated with bleeding into the metastases. Initial treatment is dexamethasone 16 mg daily. Patients who present with seizures require anticonvulsants. Role of prophylactic anticonvulsants is not known; it may be considered in patients with high risk features of seizure such as metastasis to the motor cortex, bleeding metastasis and leptomeningeal metastasis. Further management of brain metastasis is given on p. 278.

Encephalopathy

Introduction

Encephalopathy is an important complication of cancer, which presents with an acute confusional state or delirium subsequent to abnormal brain function resulting from interference with brain metabolism. A number of aetiological factors can contribute to the development of encephalopathy in cancer patients. Generally, these are due to infection, metabolic abnormalities (such as hyponatraemia, hypercalcaemia) and drugs. A number of anti-neoplastic agents such as ifosfamide, methotrexate, cisplatin, vincristine, cytosine arabinoside etc. can cause encephalopathy.

Clinical features

The usual presentation is cognitive and behavioural changes. Patients can present with insomnia followed by acute confusion and delirium. Occasionally focal signs such as ataxia may predominate.

Clinical examination shows an altered level of consciousness, abnormalities of respiration, small reactive pupils and spontaneously roving eye movements. Grading of encephalopathy is as follows:

- G1 – mild transient drowsiness or nightmares. This may not be noticed by the patient at the time of treatment, but nightmares may be reported at the next clinic visit.
- G2 – drowsy <50% time.
- G3 – drowsy >50% time, severe disorientation, tremor, psychosis. Patients will often present with 1 or 2 of these features but not all.
- G4 – coma or seizures.

Management

Investigations include biochemical tests, infection screening, MRI brain, EEG and CSF examination and drug level estimation in selected cases.

In most cases of anti-neoplastic induced encephalopathy, the management is cessation of the drug and continuation supportive measures until recovery, and a re-challenge is seldom attempted. One exception is ifosfamide.

Ifosfamide encephalopathy can occur within minutes or hours of starting ifosfamide, or up to 24 hours after the completion of ifosfamide. The risk factors for ifosfamide encephalopathy are pelvic tumour, low albumin, impaired renal function, previous cisplatin, high dose of ifosfamide and CNS disease. In patients on ifosfamide, encephalopathy can be prevented by prophylactic dose of methylene blue (50 mg IV 4 times daily).

In patients with ifosfamide encephalopathy, treatment is based on the grade of the encephalopathy:

- G1 – no action required.
- G2 – If on antiemetics such as levomepromazine (Nozinan), stop the drug and reassess in 1–2 hours. If there is improvement, replace the anti-emetics. If there is no improvement, give methylene blue (50 mg IV 4 times daily) and continue ifosfamide if the patient is undergoing curative treatment. Ensure regular review so that the patient's condition does not deteriorate.
- G3/4 – stop ifosfamide infusion (even for curative treatment) and give or increase methylene blue (50 mg 6 times daily). Correct any metabolic abnormalities/infection. If there is no improvement, consider thiamine 100 mg, intravenous albumin (in cases of low albumin) or haemodialysis.

Visual loss

Optic neuropathy

Anti-neoplastic drug-induced optic neuropathy (ON) can be acute with rapidly progressive loss of vision. Cisplatin, carboplatin, carmustine, 5-fluorouracil, methotrexate, vinca-alkaloids, paclitaxel, tamoxifen and bisphosphonates are reported to cause optic neuropathy.

Clinical examination reveals reduced visual acuity in the affected eye and there may be associated field defects. Eye pain can also occur secondary to optic nerve sheath oedema. If papilloedema is present this suggests anterior optic neuritis, but this sign will be absent in retrobulbar neuritis.

Investigations may be normal but MRI can exclude intracranial metastases. Visual evoked potentials may display reduced amplitudes and increased latency suggesting optic nerve involvement.

Treatment of drug-induced optic neuritis involves the immediate withdrawal of the drug and exclusion of other causes. Intravenous methylprednisolone has been used but there are no randomized data to support this. Recovery can occur with drug withdrawal. However, the majority of patients have some permanent visual deficit.

Choroidal metastasis

Choroidal metastasis can result in sudden loss of vision. It is most common with breast and lung cancer and up to 20% may be bilateral. Cancer patients presenting with visual symptoms require detailed ophthalmologic assessment including a slit lamp examination. CT scan or MRI of the brain is needed to rule out brain metastasis.

Urgent radiotherapy is needed to avoid further visual deterioration and maintain useful vision. The entire choroid and retina of the affected eye is treated with a dose of 20 Gy in five fractions or 30 Gy in 10 fractions at 2.5 cm depth using a posteriorly angled lateral beam (to avoid opposite lens).

Febrile neutropenia

Introduction

Febrile neutropenia is defined as an oral or tympanic membrane temperature of $\geq 38°C$ on two occasions, at least one hour apart within a 12 h period or a single temperature of $>38.5°C$ with an absolute neutrophil count of $\leq 0.5 \times 10^9/l$ or $\leq 1.0 \times 10^9/l$ with a predictable decline to $\leq 0.5 \times 10^9/l$ in 24–48 h.

Febrile neutropenia is one of the most common complications of cancer treatment. 50–60% of patients with febrile neutropenia have an established or occult infection and 20% of patients with a neutrophil count $\leq 1.0 \times 10^9/l$ have bacteraemia.

Susceptibility to infection increases as the neutrophil count drops below $1.0 \times 10^9/l$. The frequency and severity of infection are inversely proportional to the absolute neutrophil count, with the duration of neutropenia also contributing to overall risk. The timing of the neutrophil nadir depends on the type of chemotherapy and generally, it occurs 5–10 days after the last dose. Usually the neutrophil count recovers 5 days after the nadir.

In the majority of cases, bacterial pathogens are responsible for febrile neutropenic episodes with fungal (Figure 23.3), viral and protozoal infections occurring more commonly as secondary events. Currently, Gram-positive bacteria account for 60–70% of microbiologically detected infections, which may in part be due to the prevalent use of quinolones as prophylactic antibiotics. Other possible causes of this change in trend include widespread use of intravenous catheters, along with more profound and prolonged neutropenia due to intensive and recurrent treatment regimes.

Clinical presentation and assessment

Fever, rigors, hypotension or generalized malaise may be the only presenting features of infection in the neutropenic patient, and even they may be masked by concurrent use of NSAIDs or steroids. Clinical deterioration can be rapid (especially in those aged <45 years) and therefore, prompt assessment is essential. Due to lack of neutrophils, most infections present with atypical manifestations.

It is important to enquire and look for signs of infection at the following sites:

- Head and neck – look at the teeth, gums and pharynx. Ask about ENT problems, especially involving the sinuses and ears.
- Gastrointestinal system – ask about mucositis, diarrhoea and constipation. The perineal/peri-anal area should be inspected and palpated gently; but do not perform a rectal examination.
- Respiratory system – ask about cough, shortness of breath and sputum production.
- Genito-urinary system – ask about symptoms suggestive of infection such as vaginal discharge, abdominal pain, urinary frequency and dysuria.
- Central nervous system – ask about headache. Examine for altered level of consciousness, cranial nerve lesions and meningism.
- Look at vascular access sites and establish whether symptoms are related to flushing of the device.

Antibiotic treatment should not be delayed whilst waiting for results; however, urgent investigations should include:

- FBC and differential, U+E, CRP, LFTs, Ca^{2+}, coagulation screen and group and save.
- Blood cultures should be taken both peripherally and through any central venous line.
- Stool, urine and throat swabs should be sent for microscopy, bacterial culture and sensitivity (viral culture also for throat swab).
- Skin, wound or genital swabs should be collected when appropriate.
- Sputum sample if possible.
- Chest X-ray.

Management (Figure 23.4)

The mainstay of management is the prompt administration of broad-spectrum antibiotics. The Multinational Association for Supportive Care in Cancer (MASCC) scoring system categorizes patients with febrile neutropenia into low and high-risk groups (Box 23.4). Patients with

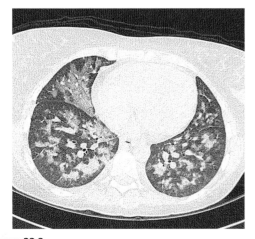

Figure 23.3
CT scan of the chest shows diffuse fungal infection in a neutropenic patient.

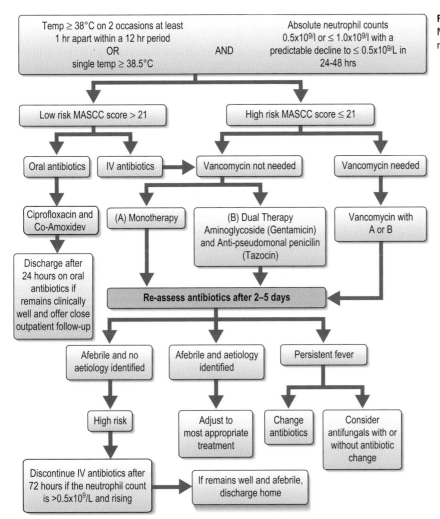

Figure 23.4
Management of febrile neutropenia.

low-risk febrile neutropenia can be managed with oral antibiotics and discharged after 24 hours observation, whereas those with high risk febrile neutropenia require intravenous antibiotics (Figure 23.4).

Although most patients with low-risk febrile neutropenia can be managed in the outpatient setting, close follow-up and unrestricted access to health care are essential for institution of such a policy. Certain social situations such as a previous history of non-compliance, inability to care for oneself, lack of caregivers and lack of unrestricted healthcare access are contraindications to outpatient therapy.

The most commonly used antibiotic regime for high-risk febrile neutropenia is a combination of broad-spectrum, anti-pseudomonal penicillin (e.g. Tazocin) with an aminoglycoside (e.g. Gentamicin). The synergistic effect of combination therapy can be beneficial and dual treatment reduces the risk of drug resistant strains emerging. Alternatively, a carbopenem (e.g. meropenem) can be used as monotherapy in uncomplicated episodes of neutropenic fever when it has been shown to be equally as effective as dual therapy. Vancomycin may be added to mono- or dual-therapy when the patient is felt to be at high risk of Gram-positive bacteraemia (*Staphylococcus aureus* bacteraemia in those with central venous access and severe sepsis with or without hypotension). Gram-positive coverage should also be considered in patients

Box 23.4: The MASCC risk-index score

Characteristic	Score
Extent of illness[a]	
• No symptoms	5
• Mild symptoms	5
• Moderate symptoms	3
No hypotension	5
No chronic obstructive airways disease	4
Solid tumour or no fungal infection	4
No dehydration	3
Outpatient at onset of fever	3
Age <60 years[b]	2

[a]Choose 1 item only.
[b]Does not apply to patients <16 yrs. Initial monocyte count >1.0 × 10^9/l, no co-morbidity and normal chest radiograph findings indicate children at low risk for significant bacterial infections.
Low risk – a score of >21.
High risk – score of ≤21.

with suspected skin infection or severe mucosal damage and when prophylactic antibiotics against Gram-negative bacteria have been used.

Along with reverse-barrier nursing, other supportive measures such as the administration of fluids and blood or blood products are often also required.

Monitoring

Intravenous antibiotics should be reviewed daily and modified depending on organism sensitivities and patient response. The median time to clinical response after the administration of antibiotics to febrile neutropenic patients is 5–7 days and patients who fail to respond to first-line antibiotics should be discussed with a microbiologist who may consider anti-fungal or anti-viral treatments. Antibiotic therapy may be discontinued when no infection is identified after 3 days of treatment, if the neutrophil count is ≥0.5 × 10^9/l for 2 consecutive days and if the patient has been afebrile for ≥48 h. Recovery of the neutrophil count is the single most important determinant of successful antibiotic treatment.

Prophylactic antibiotics

For regimes that are associated with a high risk of febrile neutropenia (stem cell transplantation, acute leukaemias and neutropenia for greater than 10 days), or for patients who have had a previous febrile neutropenic episode, quinolones

are often used prophylactically on days 8–15 of the chemotherapy cycle. Trials have consistently shown that the use of prophylactic antibiotics in the afebrile neutropenic patient reduces the number of febrile episodes; however, data demonstrating beneficial effects on mortality are more variable and less convincing. With the growing problems of antibiotic resistance and antibiotic associated infection, the use of prophylactic antibiotics in all aspects of medicine is being questioned.

Haematopoietic colony stimulating factors

Haematopoietic colony stimulating factors (CSFs) such as granulocyte CSF (G-CSF) and granulocyte-macrophage CSF (GM-CSF) are glycoproteins that stimulate the proliferation and differentiation of haematopoietic cells. A pegylated formulation of G-CSF has the benefit of being given as a one-off dose rather than a daily subcutaneous dose.

CSF use is recommended in both the therapeutic and the prophylactic setting for patients at high risk of developing infection-associated complications or who have prognostic factors predictive of a poor clinical outcome (Box 23.5).

The risk of febrile neutropenia and hospitalization due to febrile neutropenia is substantially reduced by the prophylactic use of CSFs. CSFs may also have a beneficial effect on infection related mortality, although effects on overall mortality remain to be established.

Thrombocytopenia

Thrombocytopenia (a platelet count of <150 × 10^9/l) can occur due to treatment, bone marrow metastasis and in association with disseminated intravascular coagulation. The assessment of patients with thrombocytopenia is to establish presence of bleeding, whether the bleeding is life threatening and contributory factors.

Patients without bleeding, and a platelet count of >10 × 10^9/l (>20 × 10^9/l if with ongoing infection) may be managed conservatively. Patients with a platelet count of <10 × 10^9/l (<20 × 10^9/l in those with infection) or those with bleeding need random donor platelets. The aim of a platelet transfusion is to maintain platelets above 10 × 10^9/l (20 × 10^9/l in those with infection) in the prophylactic setting, to stop bleeding in those with bleeding, and to maintain platelets above $50 \times 10^9/l$ in those with life-threatening bleeding. Each five donor unit or one single donor apheresis pack increases the platelet count by approximately $10 \times 10^9/l$ at 24-hours post-transfusion. In the absence of such an increment, platelet refractoriness should be suspected and managed appropriately.

Chemotherapy dose needs to be reduced for future courses according to the regime and risk of bone marrow toxicity of individual drugs.

Superior vena cava obstruction

Introduction

Superior vena cava obstruction (SVCO) can occur as a result of either extrinsic compression of the superior vena cava or intrinsic obstruction

---

Box 23.5: Indications for G-CSF

Prophylactic
1. Regimes associated with >20% risk of FN

Breast cancer
AC followed by decetaxel

Paclitaxel followed by AC

TAC

Lung cancer
Cisplatin-etoposide

ACE

ICE

Ovarian cancer
Paclitaxel

Docetaxel

NHL

DHAP

ESHAP

CHOP-21

Urothelial
Carboplatin/paclitaxel

BOP-VIP-B

Germ cell tumour
VeIP

2. Regimes with 10–20% risk of FN and with factors that may increase the risk of FN to ≥20%. The risk factors are:
- Age ≥65 years
- Advanced disease
- Prior FN
- No antibiotics prophylaxis
- Multiple co-morbidities
- Bone marrow involvement

Therapeutic use of G-CSF during an episode of febrile neutropenia
Patients with ongoing neutropenia who do not respond to antibiotics

Those with life-threatening infections
- Shock
- Severe sepsis
- Multi-organ dysfunction

---

to blood flow. Lung cancer is responsible for nearly three-quarters of cases of malignant SVCO and SVCO occurs in 2–4% of patients with lung cancer. The remainder of cases is largely due to lymphoma (12%) and metastatic malignancies (most commonly from a breast primary).

Clinical presentation

Malignant SVCO usually presents insidiously over a period of weeks. The most common symptoms are cough and dyspnoea (>50%). Clinical examination shows facial puffiness (80%), distended veins (>60%), and arm oedema (46%). Symptoms are commonly progressive, although there may be some clinical improvement with the formation of a collateral circulation over time. Symptoms tend to be worse first thing in the morning and can be exacerbated by manoeuvres that increase venous pressure, e.g. bending forwards, coughing, sneezing and straining.

Investigations

A plain chest radiograph will often show a right paratracheal mass or widened mediastinum. A CT scan will demonstrate SVC compromise and distinguishes between external compression and thrombus (Figure 23.5). In patients without a histologic diagnosis, a biopsy is required prior to deciding treatment.

Management

The management of SVCO depends on the underlying aetiology and severity of symptoms. In patients with no prior diagnosis of cancer, a histologic diagnosis is essential.

General measures include oxygen, dexamethasone 16 mg daily, and diuretics. Endovascular stent insertion (Figure 23.5) is the gold-standard treatment which relieves obstruction in 95% of cases, usually within 72 h (Box 23.6). Complications of stent placement are in the region of 3–7% and include: transient chest pain, infection, misplaced stent, stent migration and pulmonary emboli. SVCO recurs in approximately 11% of patients (due to stent occlusion secondary to either thrombus or tumour ingrowth). However, secondary patency rates are good and long-term patency is achieved in 92% of patients.

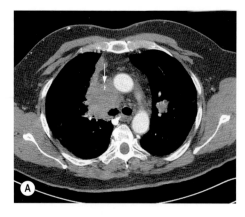

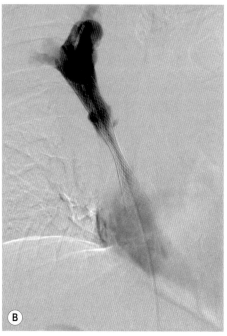

Figure 23.5
Superior vena caval obstruction. CT scan (A) shows significant compression of SVC (arrow) and SVC stent in situ (B).

Radiotherapy was traditionally used first line for the treatment of SVCO prior to endovascular stenting. In radiosensitive tumours, radiotherapy results in symptomatic response rates of up to 78% at 2 weeks. However, complete resolution of obstruction is seen in only 31% on serial venograms with a partial resolution in 23%.

Radiotherapy is given to a dose of 20 Gy in five fractions or 30 Gy in 10 fractions.

Chemotherapy is useful in chemosensitive tumours. Chemotherapy alone relieves SVCO in

> **Box 23.6: Indications for endovascular stent insertion**
>
> - Severe and life-threatening SVCO requiring rapid relief of symptoms
> - Persistent SVCO after radiotherapy or chemotherapy
> - Patients with an underlying disease that is unlikely to respond well to chemotherapy or radiotherapy
> - Patients with symptomatic benign SVCO

80% of patients with non-Hodgkin's lymphoma or small-cell lung cancer and 40% of patients with non-small cell lung cancer.

Prognosis

The median survival for patients with SVCO is generally 6 months; however, this varies widely depending on the aetiology. Prognosis appears to be determined by the underlying malignancy with overall survival being equal between patients of the same tumour type and stage, with or without SVCO.

Life-threatening haemoptysis

Approximately 10% of haemoptysis due to cancers tends to be massive (>500 ml in 24 hours) and <5% of haemoptysis is life-threatening. The reported in-hospital mortality of bleeding at a rate of >1 litre in 24 hours is 80%. It is difficult to predict life-threatening haemoptysis and most patients die suddenly at home.

The immediate management of patients with life-threatening haemoptysis is to maintain a secure airway, adequate ventilation and circulation. Attempts should be made to localize the site of bleeding with bronchoscopy (which can be therapeutic) and/or imaging. Once bleeding is localized the patient is positioned with the bleeding lung in the dependent position.

Specific measures to control bleeding include bronchoscopy with tamponade using a balloon catheter, laser photocoagulation or iced-saline lavage. Bronchial artery embolization is an option in specialist units.

Central airway obstruction and stridor

Malignant central airway obstruction produces progressive symptoms of dyspnoea, stridor and obstructive pneumonia. A central airway narrowing to <25% cross sectional area is usually needed to produce dyspnoea and stridor at rest. Airway obstruction can be produced by either extrinsic or intrinsic compression.

Immediate measures are needed for symptomatic relief, which is monitored with pulse oximetry. These include comfortable positioning, high-dose steroid (if known case of cancer, if not withhold until definitive histologic diagnosis) and supplemental oxygen or heliox (heliox is a mixture of 80% helium with 20% oxygen; lower density of helium helps in the easy flow through areas of turbulence and may decrease the work of breathing). Muscle relaxants and respiratory depressants should be avoided as are attempts to instrument airway without expert help and positive pressure ventilation. CT scan of the neck and chest may reveal the area and type of obstruction.

Further management is shown in Figure 23.6. Stent results in prompt relief of symptoms; with cryotherapy 75% achieve symptomatic relief. Radiotherapy is given either as 20 Gy in five fractions or 30 Gy in 10 fractions. Radiotherapy response usually occurs within 72 hours with 70–95% patients becoming symptom-free by 2 weeks.

Malignancy associated hypercalcaemia

Introduction

Hypercalcaemia (a corrected serum calcium concentration >2.6 mmol/l) occurs in up to 30% of cancer patients during their illness. The mechanisms of hypercalcaemia include secretion of parathyroid-related-protein (80%), osteolytic hypercalcaemia (20%) and rarely due to increased secretion of 1,25-D3 and ectopic secretion of PTH.

Clinical presentation

The symptoms of hypercalcaemia are typically non-specific and their severity depends on the rapidity with which the calcium level rises. When the serum calcium concentration increases above 2.6 mmol/l, symptoms include fatigue, malaise, depression, anorexia, nausea, vomiting, bone pain, polydipsia, polyuria, constipation and mus-

cular weakness. If the concentration continues to rise above 3.6 mol/l, neurological symptoms become more prevalent and patients may become confused, leading to coma and death.

Hypercalcaemia has few examination findings specific to its diagnosis. However, a thorough history and physical examination may help yield the underlying cause.

Investigations

Along with serum corrected calcium, baseline laboratory investigations should include a full blood count, urea, creatinine and electrolytes, liver function tests, serum phosphate, magnesium and PTH concentrations. ECG changes consistent with hypercalcaemia include a shortened QT and prolonged PR interval. At very high levels, a broad QRS complex may develop, T waves may flatten or invert and a variable degree of heart block can occur.

All further investigations are aimed at establishing a cause and are likely to include imaging, particularly of the chest. In a patient without a diagnosis of cancer, a myeloma screen should be considered and in some patients a bone scan may be helpful.

Management (Figure 23.7)

Saline rehydration is an important aspect of the management of hypercalcaemia. Hydration alone may adequately treat mild hypercalcaemia. Hypercalcaemic patients are universally dehydrated as a result of calcium-induced nephrogenic diabetes insipidus and poor oral intake. The speed of administration of normal saline depends on the degree of dehydration and renal impairment, the level of hypercalcaemia and the patient's underlying cardiac function. Fluid balance must be carefully monitored. The aim of saline treatment is two-fold, firstly, to increase the glomerular filtration rate (GFR) and thereby increase the filtered load of calcium into the tubular lumen from the glomerulus. Secondly, calcium reabsorption is inhibited in the proximal nephron because of the calciuretic effects of saline. Once dehydration has been adequately treated, loop diuretics can be used to increase calcium excretion. Any drug that may be contributing to the hypercalcaemia e.g. thiazide diuretics, lithium and calcium supplements should be

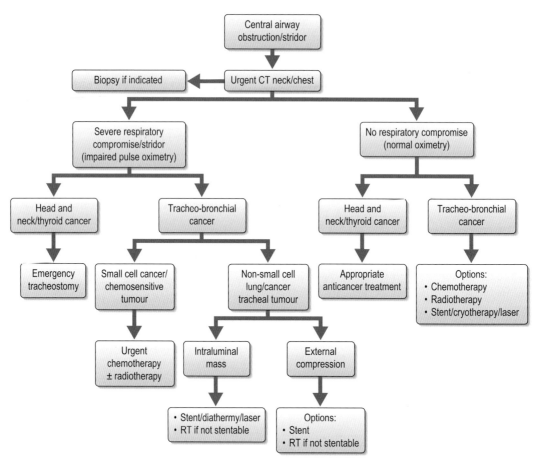

Figure 23.6
Management of central airway obstruction/stridor.

discontinued. Hypophosphataemia is common and phosphate levels should hence be monitored and replaced as appropriate.

Bisphosphonates have been shown to be superior to saline alone in the treatment of malignancy-associated hypercalcaemia. Bisphosphonates inhibit osteoclastic bone resorption by adsorbing to the surface of bone hydroxyapatite. The bisphosphonates of choice for the treatment of malignancy-associated hypercalcaemia are intravenous zoledronate, ibandronate and pamidronate. Pamidronate (60–90 mg IV in 500 ml normal saline over 2 h) or Zoledronate (4 mg IV in 50 ml normal saline over 15 min) are the most widely used bisphosphonates for this indication in the UK. The nadir response to intravenous bisphosphonates is gen-

erally reached at 7–10 days, with the beginnings of a biochemical response evident at 2–4 days. Up to 90% of patients will achieve normocalcaemia after a single dose; however, a second dose can be given after 7–10 days if the calcium remains elevated. Patients with renal impairment may require a dose reduction and this differs between products. Although the administration of bisphosphonates should not be delayed, prior rehydration may reduce the risk of further renal impairment. Another common adverse effect of intravenous bisphosphonates is a transient flu-like syndrome with fever, myalgias and chills. For patients in whom bisphosphonates are unsuccessful, alternative treatments such as glucocorticoids, calcitonin and gallium nitrate can be tried following specialist endocrine advice.

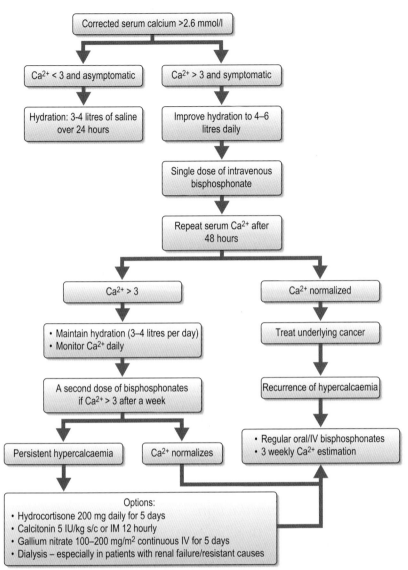

Figure 23.7
Management of hypercalcaemia.

Prognosis

Malignancy related hypercalcaemia carries a very poor prognosis with more than 50% of patients dying within 30 days of treatment. Overall, median survival is less than 12 months.

Acute tumour lysis syndrome

Introduction

Acute tumour lysis syndrome (ATLS) is a group of metabolic abnormalities that occur following the destruction of large quantities of rapidly dividing tumour cells. Typically, it occurs 12–72 h after the initiation of treatment with cytotoxic chemotherapy, cytolytic antibody therapy and/or radiation therapy.

ATLS is most frequent in patients with non-Hodgkin's lymphoma (especially Burkitt's lymphoma), acute lymphoblastic leukaemia (ALL) and acute myeloid leukaemia (AML). It has also been rarely reported following the treatment of ovarian, breast and small-cell lung cancer. Several characteristics inherent to the tumour type predispose to TLS and these include high tumour proliferation rate, large tumour burden, tumour chemosensitivity and increased lactate dehydrogenase (LDH) levels. Pre-existing uraemia or hyperuricaemia, decreased urinary flow, low urinary pH, dehydration, oliguria and renal impairment have also been identified as risk factors for TLS.

Clinical features

ATLS is characterized by hyperuricaemia, hyperphosphataemia, hypocalcaemia and hyperkalaemia. These biochemical abnormalities lead to a range of non-specific symptoms (Table 23.1). When the electrolytes are severely deranged, patients are at risk of seizures, cardiac arrhythmias and sudden death.

Management

Management is essentially aimed at the prevention of ATLS. It is important to identify patients at risk of developing ATLS and to treat them prophylactically with intravenous fluids and allopurinol.

Normal saline re-hydration should aim to produce a urine output of approximately 100 ml/h and diuretics may be required once euvolaemia has been achieved. Improving intravascular volume, renal blood flow and glomerular filtration rate promotes the excretion of uric acid and phosphate. Alkalinization of the urine through the use of sodium bicarbonate is sometimes required.

Allopurinol is a xanthine oxidase analogue, which prevents the conversion of xanthine and hypoxanthine to uric acid. It has proven efficacy in the prevention and treatment of hyperuricaemia in patients with or at risk of ATLS. Allopurinol prevents the formation of uric acid and should be commenced prior to starting treatment with intensive chemotherapy. It has been associated with hypersensitivity reactions and reduces the clearance of other purine-based chemotherapeutic agents such as 6-mercaptopurine and azathioprine.

Rasburicase is a recombinant urate oxidase that promotes the catabolism of uric acid to allantoin. Unlike allopurinol, there is no risk of xanthine nephropathy or calculi. It is licensed for the treatment and prophylaxis of acute hyperuricaemia in patients who have high tumour burden haematological malignancies and are at high risk of ATLS. It is more effective than

Table 23.1: Biochemical and clinical features of tumour lysis syndrome

Biochemical abnormality	Clinical consequence
Hyperuricaemia (serum uric acid >0.5 mmol/L)	Renal impairment
Hyperphosphataemia (serum phosphate >1.4 mmol/l)	Nausea, vomiting, diarrhoea, lethargy, seizures
Hypocalcaemia (serum Ca^{2+} <2.12 mmol/l)	Cardiac arrhythmias, hypotension, tetany, muscular cramps
Hyperkalaemia (serum K^+ >6.5 mmol/l)	Cardiac arrhythmias (VT/VF), muscle cramps, paraesthesia

allopurinol in reducing uric acid levels, but significantly more expensive.

Specific management of established ATLS includes the close monitoring of uric acid, phosphate, potassium, creatinine, calcium and LDH levels. Fluid balance should be measured and electrolyte abnormalities should be corrected (Table 23.2). Haemodialysis and intensive care facilities should be available if required.

Hypersensitivity reactions

Introduction

Nearly all systemic agents used to treat cancer have the potential to cause hypersensitivity reactions; however, severe reactions are rare. Provided patients receive appropriate pre-medication, close monitoring and prompt intervention when required, severe hypersensitivity reactions occur in less than 5% of patients. Platinum compounds, taxanes and monoclonal antibodies are most likely to cause a reaction, although the timing of such reactions may differ, as do their likely underlying aetiology (Table 23.3).

Platinum compounds such as cisplatin, carboplatin and oxaliplatin classically cause reactions following multiple cycles of treatment, typically after 6–8 doses. This is consistent with a type 1 hypersensitivity reaction following repeated exposure to the drug and leads to IgE-mediated release of histamine, leukotrienes and prostag-

Table 23.2: Management of electrolyte abnormalities

Electrolyte abnormality	Management
Hyperphosphataemia	Avoidance of additional phosphate Administration of a phosphate binder e.g. calcium carbonate Haemodialysis/ haemofiltration
Hypocalcaemia	Calcium gluconate (10 ml 10% IV administered slowly with ECG monitoring)
Hyperkalaemia	Avoidance of additional potassium Cardiac monitoring Calcium resonium (15 g po tds) Calcium gluconate (as above) for cardio-protection Insulin–dextrose (10–15 units insulin with 50 ml 50% dextrose) Haemodialysis/ haemofiltration

Table 23.3: Showing the incidence of any grade hypersensitivity in a range of chemotherapy agents

Drug	Incidence
Carboplatin or oxaliplatin	12–19%
Paclitaxel	8–45%
Docetaxel	5–20%
Trastuzumab	40%
Rituximab	Up to 77%
Cetuximab	16–19%

landins from mast cells in the tissues and basophils in the peripheral blood. This causes smooth muscle contraction and peripheral vasodilatation, leading to urticaria, rash, angioedema, bronchospasm and hypotension.

Although a similar clinical picture can be produced following administration of a taxane, 95% of these reactions occur during the first or second exposure to the drug and 80% occur within the first 10 minutes of the infusion. In this scenario, IgE-mediated type-1 hypersensitivity is unlikely, and it is postulated that direct effects on mast cells and basophils lead to release of immunomodulators and an anaphylactoid reaction. The solvent used in paclitaxel, but not docetaxel (Cremophor EL) has been shown to cause histamine release and hypotension and is felt to be partly responsible for the hypersensitivity reactions seen with paclitaxel.

Monoclonal antibody infusions can also produce hypersensitivity reactions, which become less likely with each subsequent infusion. Delayed reactions are still seen in 10–30% however, the underlying aetiology of these reactions is largely unknown.

Clinical features

The National Cancer Institute Common Toxicity Criteria (NCI-CTC) distinguish between hypersensitivity and acute infusion reactions (Table 23.4).

Clinical features of hypersensitivity include pruritis, rash, urticaria, rigors/chills/fevers, headache, arthralgia/myalgia, tumour pain, fatigue, dizziness, sweating, nausea/vomiting, cough, dyspnoea, bronchospasm, hypotension/hypertension and tachycardia.

Management

Prophylaxis with antihistamines and corticosteroids is recommended for infusions that carry a high risk of hypersensitivity reactions and for any patient that shows early signs of a hypersensitivity reaction. Pre-medication for paclitaxel would likely include 20 mg dexamethasone (preferably given several hours before the infusion), chlorpheniramine 10 mg and cimetidine 300 mg. Patients should be closely monitored throughout all infusions.

Treatment of anaphylaxis is outlined in Figure 23.8.

Re-challenging patients following a hypersensitivity reaction depends on the aim of treatment and the severity of the reaction. The majority of patients who have a mild–moderate reaction

Table 23.4: Grading of hypersensitivity reactions according to the NCI-CTC for adverse events

	Grade				
	1	2	3	4	5
Hypersensitivity (allergic reaction)	Transient flushing or rash, fever <38°C	Rash, flushing, urticaria, dyspnoea, fever ≥38°C	Symptomatic bronchospasm, with or without urticaria, parenteral medication indicated, allergy-related oedema/angioedema, hypotension	Anaphylaxis	Death
Acute infusion reaction (cytokine mediated)	Mild reaction, infusion interruption not indicated, intervention not indicated	Requires therapy or infusion interruption but responds promptly to symptomatic treatment, prophylactic medication indicated for ≥24 h	Prolonged recurrence of symptoms following initial improvement, hospitalization indicated for other clinical sequelae (e.g. renal impairment, pulmonary infiltrates)	Life-threatening, pressor or ventilatory support indicated	Death

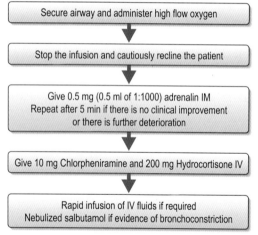

Figure 23.8
Management of anaphylaxis.

during their first drug exposure (often seen with taxanes and monoclonal antibodies) are likely to tolerate re-challenge of the drug if pre-medication is used with a slower rate of infusion. Desensitization protocols have been used with some success in patients who have a reaction to taxanes, however, re-challenge of platinum compounds is usually less successful with approximately 50% of patients experiencing recurrent hypersensitivity reactions.

Extravasation

Introduction

An extravasation injury is any tissue damage that occurs as a result of leakage of cytotoxic drugs into the surrounding tissue.

- An irritant is a chemotherapeutic agent capable of producing venous pain at the venopuncture site or along a vein, with or without an inflammatory reaction.
- A vesicant is an agent capable of blister formation and/or tissue destruction.

Vesicant drugs are more likely to lead to extravasation because of their potential for endothelial damage (Table 23.5). The risk of vesicant extravasation is very low, in the range of 0.01–6% and although the use of implanted ports reduces the risk of extravasation, it can still occur.

Tissue damage occurs due to three main factors:

Table 23.5: Vesicant vs non-vesicant drugs

Vesicant drugs	Non-vesicant/irritant/ exfoliant drugs
Busulfan	Bevacizumab
Carmustine	Bleomycin
Dactinomycin (Actinomycin D)	Carboplatin
Daunorubicin	Cisplatin
Doxorubicin	Cyclophosphamide
Epirubicin	Cytarabine
Mitomycin C	Cetuximab
Treosulfan	Docetaxel
Vinblastine	Etoposide
Vincristine	Fludarabine
Vinorelbine	Fluorouracil
	Gemcitabine
	Ifosfamide
	Irinotecan
	Liposomal doxorubicin
	Methotrexate
	Oxaliplatin
	Paclitaxel
	Rituximab
	Topotecan
	Trastuzumab

1. Direct cellular toxicity of the antineoplastic drug causing cellular necrosis.
2. Differences in osmotic pressures between the infused solution and the tissue environment.
3. Cellular damage due to the alkalinity or acidity of the solution.

Clinical features

Symptoms and signs of extravasation include:

- Pain, discomfort and burning sensations at or around the cannula site.
- Reduced flow rate of the infusion.
- Lack of blood return through the cannula.

- Erythema, blotching, blistering, swelling and tenderness.
- Early firm induration is often an indication of eventual ulceration.
- The skin may become white and cold, later developing into a black eschar.
- Ulceration does not usually occur until at least 48 h, but may be delayed until one or more weeks after the injury.

Management

Prevention is the key. The technique of cannulation and administration of the drug is important. Cannulas should ideally be inserted in the back of the hand where they are readily accessible and extravasation can be easily detected. Use of a central venous access device is preferable; however, vesicant administration should only proceed when there is blood return through the device.

Management of extravasation includes stopping the infusion and aspirating from the intravascular device. Extravasation of anthracyclines is initially managed with cooling of the area, however, heat application is generally used following the extravasation of plant alkaloids. Early review by the plastic surgeons for consideration of surgical debridement is vital when tissue necrosis is possible.

Hyaluronidase increases the permeability of connective tissue and can be injected into the extravasation sites of plant alkaloids. Used in combination with a saline flush out of the area, it aids the dispersion of the vesicant drug.

Dexrazoxane is a derivative of EDTA that chelates iron. It has shown benefit in the treatment of extravasation from intravenous anthracycline therapy; although the exact mechanism of action is unknown. It is a systemic treatment that is infused over 1–2 h each day for three days into a large vein, away from the extravasation site. Side effects include nausea and vomiting, diarrhoea, stomatitis, bone marrow suppression, elevated liver enzymes and infusion site burning.

Bone fractures or impending fractures

Bone metastasis is the third most common site of metastatic disease. Bone metastasis can be lytic,

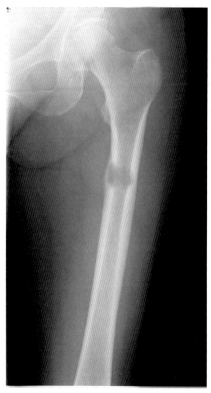

Figure 23.9
A lytic lesion in the femur with high risk features of impending fracture.

sclerotic and mixed. Risk of pathological fracture is highest in lytic lesions. 50% of pathological fractures are due to metastatic breast cancer and the commonest site is femur. A lesion involving 50% of the cortex, 2.5 cm in diameter, or which remains painful after weight-bearing after radiotherapy is at risk of a pathological fracture (Figure 23.9).

The common presentation is bone pain at the site of bone destruction. 10–15% patients present with hypercalcaemia. Pathological fracture of long bones presents with pain and loss of function whereas that of vertebrae presents with pain and neurological deficits.

Plain X-ray will reveal bone metastases in long bones, and it is helpful in deciding Mirel's scoring (Table 23.6).

Surgery is the main treatment for patients with fracture or impending fracture of long bones. All patients with a Mirel score of ≥8 and expected survival of at least 3 months should be referred

Table 23.6: Mirel scoring for impending fracture

Variable	Score		
	1	2	3
Site	Upper limb	Lower limb	Peritrochanteric
Pain	Mild	Moderate	Functional
Lesion	Blastic	Mixed	Lytic
Size*	<1/3	1/3–2/3	>2/3

*Indicates maximal cortical destruction as seen on plain X-ray in any view.
Score and fracture rate:
0–6: 0%
7: 5%
8: 33%
9: 57%
10–12: 100%

for prophylactic surgical fixation. However, surgical fixation of a pathological fracture in a weight-bearing bone may be considered even with a lesser life expectancy to improve pain. In solitary bone metastases, a radical excision may be feasible especially in renal cell carcinoma.

Surgical repair of non-axial pathological fractures can be achieved by a variety of different methods.

Other emergencies

Chemotherapy induced haemorrhagic cystitis

High-dose cyclophosphamide as a marrow ablative regime as well as ifosfamide can produce significant haemorrhagic cystitis. It is produced by a metabolite of these agents, acrolein, by an unknown mechanism. Sodium 2-mercaptoethane sulfonate (mesna) is used as a uroprotective agent along with these agents. Mesna needs to be started prior to the chemotherapy and continued after the last dose of chemotherapy.

- In patients with frank haematuria, urology consultation should be sought as there is a risk of clot retention. A 3-way continuous irrigation may be needed to maintain urine flow. If urine flow cannot be established, cystoscopy with clot wash out is indicated.

- Patients with 1+ blood on urine dipstix can be managed without any intervention.
- Patients with 2+ or 3+ blood on urine dipstix. Ensure that it is current urine void (within last hour) as there will be some haematuria during chemotherapy. If there is uncertainty about dipstix results, repeat the test on a fresh urine sample. If the abnormal treatment is early during mesna treatment, continue monitoring and give the remaining mesna. If there is persistent 2+ reading at the end of mesna treatment, additional mesna is needed and patient should be discharged only after the dipstix is 1+ or less. At discharge patients are given oral mesna 1200 mg/m^2 every 4 hours for three doses and asked to take along with 2 litres water over 12 hours.

Malignant obstructions and bleeding

The management of malignant obstructions and bleeding is dealt in individual chapters.

Further reading

Scott-Brown M, Spence R, Johnston P. Emergencies in Oncology, Oxford University press, 2007.

Samphao S, Eremin JM, Eremin O. Oncological emergencies: clinical importance and principles of management. Eur J Cancer Care. 2009 Dec 17. [Epub]PMID: 20030695.

Walji N, Chan AK, Peake DR. Common acute oncological emergencies: diagnosis, investigation and management. Postgrad Med J. 2008;84:418–427.

Marti FM, Cullen MH, Roila F; ESMO Guidelines Working Group. Management of febrile neutropenia: ESMO clinical recommendations. Ann Oncol. 2009;20 Suppl 4:166–169.

Innes H, Marshall E. Outpatient therapy for febrile neutropenia. Curr Opin Oncol. 2007;19:294–298.

Management of common radiotherapy side effects

24

TV Ajithkumar

General side effects

Skin

Radiation dermatitis generally starts 10–14 days after the first fraction of radiotherapy and peaks at the end or within one week of completion of radical treatment. It progresses from skin erythema, to dry desquamation (dry, itchy, flaky), moist desquamation (raw painful area which may drain serous exudates) and finally necrosis (rare). Skin reaction is intense when skin dose is high (e.g. electrons, bolus over the field), over areas with skin folds (e.g. inframammary fold, groin, perineum etc.), when radiotherapy is given concurrently with chemotherapy (particularly with anthracyclines, methotrexate, and 5-fluorouracil) and over areas of surgical wounds.

Measures to minimize skin reaction include avoiding mechanical, chemical and thermal irritations such as pat drying rather than rubbing, using simple soap, avoiding perfumes, powders, deodorants over the irradiated area, shaving with razor blade, heat, cold and sun and using loose fitting and cotton clothes. 1% hydrocortisone cream is useful for itchy areas.

During dry desquamation, hydrophilic moisturizing ointment with no heavy metals (e.g. aqueous cream) can be applied to the skin after radiation treatment every day. For moist desquamation, dress the moist area with hydrogel, hydrocolloid or alignate dressing and continue applying aqueous cream to other areas. When radiotherapy is stopped, zinc oxide or silver sulfadiazine (flamazine) may be applied to the skin with non-adhesive dressing. Superadded infection may need antibiotics depending on culture and sensitivity.

Radiation reaction heals in 3–4 weeks followed by tanning of the skin which takes a few more days to subside. Patients are asked to protect irradiated skin with sun block when sun exposure is unavoidable.

Late skin reactions include atrophy and fibrosis of skin and telangiectasia. Radiation recall is the phenomenon of skin reaction occurring in the previous radiation field when exposed to certain chemotherapy (e.g. anthracyclines and gemcitabine). This is usually more severe than previous radiation reaction and subsides in 2 weeks.

Fatigue

Fatigue (a subjective feeling of tiredness) is a common side effect of radiotherapy and the exact cause is not known. Fatigue may increase progressively during the radiotherapy and may take weeks or months to subside after radiotherapy treatment. Measures to improve fatigue include frequent periods of rest, regular minimal aerobic exercise, and stress management. A study showed that 20–30 minutes of brisk walking 4–5 times per week improved fatigue level, symptom intensity and physical functioning.

Anorexia

Some patients experience anorexia and the exact cause is not known. A number of factors such as the primary cancer itself and its systemic treatment as well as concurrent medications can influence the degree of anorexia. Measures to improve anorexia include frequent small meals, high energy high protein diet, and sometimes appetite stimulants like megestrol acetate (400–800 mg daily) or steroids. Anorexia can cause clinically significant weight loss (loss of ≥10% prediagnosis weight loss) in which case enteral feeding is advised, particularly to those receiving radical radiotherapy.

Bone marrow suppression

Irradiation of a large area of marrow bearing bones can result in bone marrow suppression. The degree of bone marrow suppression is high if concurrent myelosuppressive chemotherapy is used. All patients at risk of bone marrow suppression need weekly blood counts and appropriate action.

Site-specific side effects

Brain

Cerebral oedema

Radiotherapy can cause cerebral oedema which manifests as headache, vomiting, seizures, neurological deficit and altered mental function. Steroids are the treatment of choice.

Alopecia

Alopecia depends on the dose and extent of radiation. Alopecia starts when the radiation dose is above 25–30 Gy and is permanent when the dose is >40 Gy. If regrowth occurs it usually starts 2–3 months after completion of radiotherapy.

Head and neck cancer

Mucositis

The initial reaction is tenderness in the mouth with associated erythema and oedema of the mucosa. Subsequently a whitish membrane is formed, which progresses to a painful ulcer with continuation of radiotherapy. Bleeding and superadded infection can occur. Concurrent chemotherapy and metallic fillings in teeth (by electron back scatter) can enhance mucosal skin reaction. Dental assessment prior to radiotherapy is important (p. 79). Measures to prevent and manage mucositis include:

- Radiotherapy planning – use of midline radiation blocks wherever appropriate and 3D planning reduce mucosal injury.
- Mouth care – frequent cleansing, tooth sponges and swabbing rather than use of a toothbrush.

- Mouth wash – sterile water, 0.9% saline or sodium bicarbonate solutions. Normal saline can be prepared by adding one teaspoon of salt to 1 litre of water and 1–2 tablespoons of sodium bicarbonate can be added if the saliva is viscous.
- Benzydamine (Difflam) is recommended for prevention of oral mucositis whereas chlorhexidine, sucralfate and antimicrobial lozenges are not.
- Pain – controlled by topical anaesthetics and analgesics and systemic analgesics.
- Diet – soft bland diet and in severe mucositis, enteral feeding.

Xerostomia

During radiotherapy, dry mouth starts within 1–2 weeks of radiotherapy which involves the region of salivary glands. Later saliva becomes thick and sticky which causes problems of retching, coughing, nausea and vomiting, difficulty in talking and disturbed sleep. Dry mouth can become chronic. Measures include:

- Mouth care – frequent cleansing.
- Improve moisture – frequent sips of fluids and saliva substitutes.
- Stimulate saliva – sucking candies, pharmacological measures (e.g. oral pilocarpine 5 mg 3–4 times daily).
- In suitable patients, intensity modulated radiotherapy (IMRT) delivery (p. 85) can avoid irradiation of at least one salivary gland and thereby reduce the degree of xerostomia.

Taste change

Radiation can change taste sensation, which may persist for years. It usually starts after doses >20 Gy and around 90% patients receiving radical radiotherapy are affected. Measures include mouth care before and after meals and modification of food and preparation. An unpleasant taste of meat is one of the common problems, which can be masked by trying additional seasoning, marinating meat in wine or sweet and sour sauce before and during cooking and serving food cold or at room temperature.

Hypopituitarism and hypothyroidism

Patients who received radiotherapy to the pituitary and thyroid regions are at risk of hormonal insufficiency. Patients need hormone replacement treatment.

Thoracic region

Cough

Cough is initially productive which becomes dry as treatment progresses. Treatment is symptomatic with adequate fluid intake, humidification of air, cessation of smoking, cough suppressants and antibiotics if there is superadded infection.

Pneumonitis

Acute pneumonitis usually occurs 1–3 months after radiotherapy and rarely earlier ('hyperacute'). It manifests initially with dry cough and later with productive cough, fever and dyspnoea. Treatment includes bed rest, steroids (prednisolone 1 mg/kg for 4–6 weeks) and antibiotics if superadded infection.

Oesophagitis

Oesophagitis develops 2–3 weeks after starting radiotherapy and the severity is high with concurrent chemotherapy, long length of oesophagus in the radiation field and increased dose per fraction. Patients develop progressive painful swallowing. Measures to improve dysphagia include liquid high calorie, high protein diet, local anaesthetics, liquid analgesics and systemic analgesics. Patients may develop superadded candidiasis and need antifungal treatment.

Radiation fibrosis

Radiation fibrosis develops 6–12 months after completion of radiotherapy and can manifest with dyspnoea. Treatment is essentially symptomatic.

Abdomen and pelvis

Vomiting

Vomiting is common with radiation involving the upper abdomen. Vomiting can occur within 6 hours of radiotherapy and may last for 3–6 hours. Patients receiving treatment to the upper abdomen, large single fractions and total body or lower hemibody irradiation are advised to have prophylactic anti-emetics with a serotonin receptor antagonist (e.g. ondansetron 8 mg, 30 minutes prior to radiotherapy). In severe vomiting continual administration of antiemetics is needed. Dietary modifications with low fat, low sugar diet and high fluid intake are also useful.

Diarrhoea

Diarrhoea can occur 2–3 weeks after starting treatment. The pattern of diarrhoea may be either increased frequency of stool or watery stools with abdominal cramps. Sulfasalazine 500 mg twice orally is suggested to reduce the incidence and severity of radiation-induced enteropathy in patients receiving pelvic radiotherapy. A low-residue, low fat (<40 g) diet and avoidance of milk products can be useful in reducing diarrhoea. Antidiarrhoeal medications such as codeine and loperamide are useful when dietary modifications are ineffective.

Proctitis

Patients with tenesmus benefit from antispasmodics and anticholinergics. Pain can be controlled by frequent sitz baths and local creams such as haemorrhoidal preparations. Patients with chronic proctitis are treated with sucralfate enema.

Cystitis

Cystitis manifests with dysuria, nocturia, urgency, hesitancy and frequency. Patients are encouraged to have an adequate fluid intake. Bladder infection should be treated. Bladder analgesics (e.g. phenazopyridine) and antispasmodics are useful in pain. Patients receiving prostatic radiotherapy can develop bladder outflow irritation which manifests with hesitancy, decreased force of flow and frequency. In these situations, alpha blockers such as terazocin (Hydrin) and tamsulosin (Flomax) result in better symptom control than NSAIDs.

Vaginal stenosis and dryness

Vaginal stenosis and dryness are late effects. Treatment is symptomatic with lubricants and vaginal dilatators.

Erectile dysfunction

Erectile dysfunction results from damage of pelvic nerves and fibrosis of pelvic vasculature. Pharmacological interventions, devices and prosthesis are useful.

Gonadal failure

Ovarian failure can induce symptoms of menopause and permanent sterility (>8 Gy fractionated dose). HRT is useful if not contraindicated. In young people needing pelvic radiotherapy, laparoscopic oophoropexy (surgically placing ovaries outside radiation field), may be protective.

Testicular irradiation (>12 Gy of fractionated RT) causes permanent sterility and hence if appropriate the testes should be shielded from radiation.

Further reading

Faithfull S, Wells M (ed). Supportive Care in Radiotherapy. Edinburgh: Churchill Livingstone, 2004.

Part III

Research in oncology

Clinical trials in cancer

25

TV Ajithkumar and HM Hatcher

Introduction

Research and development is an important aspect of cancer management. Cancer drugs have to undergo rigorous evaluation before approval for clinical use. However, technological developments, such as a new surgical or radiotherapy technique, often do not undergo such complex procedures. They are approved if they are proven not to be harmful and they meet the appropriate quality control measures. In fact, many of the new radiotherapy techniques are approved for clinical use without any robust comparative data on the clinical efficacy.

Traditionally the clinical efficacy of drugs is studied through several phases of clinical trial after initial pre clinical studies. Each of these trials is aimed at generating sufficient evidence on the safety, dosing, efficacy and feasibility of use. This process is expensive and time consuming (Figure 25.1), which often leads to very high costs of effective treatments preventing their general use and often prompting policy makers to adopt rationing strategies based on cost-effectiveness.

New methods of trial design are constantly evolving, both to address the length of time to take a drug from development into practice and to answer questions which apply to newer drugs. For example targeted treatments may incorporate an assessment of the efficiency in affecting that target or in measuring the sub-population who may benefit most from an effective but expensive treatment.

Preclinical stage

The preclinical stage involves screening of potential agents and their testing on animal models. Initial testing may be performed on cell lines or tumour explants before moving to an animal model. Preclinical studies establish that the potential agent is not lethal, safe to use and that there is some indication of activity in the medical condition studied.

Clinical trials

Phase I

Phase I studies are the first human application of a new drug or drug combination. The aim of this phase is to establish the dose and schedule of the experimental agent for efficacy testing in a phase II study based on the maximum tolerated dose (MTD) of the new agent. Phase I studies are typically single arm, open label, sequential studies that include patients with good performance status (PS 0-2) and for whom there is no standard treatment option. The MTD is determined by progressively increasing the dose in small cohorts until the dose limiting toxicity (DLT) is achieved. DLT is defined as grade 4 non-haematological toxicity or a grade 3 or more haematological toxicity graded according to the National Cancer Institute Common Terminology Criteria for Adverse Events (CTCAE) (p. 38). MTD dose is defined as the dose below the level the DLT is met or the dose level at which the DLT is seen.

© 2011, Elsevier Ltd
DOI: 10.1016/B978-0-7234-3458-0.00030-0

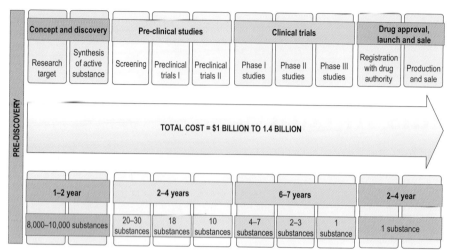

Figure 25.1
Process of drug discovery.

There are a number of components to the design of a phase I study and there are various dose escalation methods to find out the maximum tolerated dose (Box 25.1). Phase I trial design is a specialized topic and is beyond the scope of this chapter (see Further reading).

Phase II

Phase II studies are done to assess the activity, safety and feasibility of new drug. There are many options for the design of a phase II trial. A phase II study can either be completed in a single stage or as two stages. In two stage study, the first stage is to evaluate the treatment efficacy (phase IIA) and in the second stage (phase IIB) is to identify promising agents to send to phase III for additional evaluation. Phase IIA design is to test short-term tumour response, whereas phase IIB design compares two or more regimes which have demonstrated some initial efficacy.

Randomized phase II trials are increasingly being used in cancer. These studies randomize patients to new treatment or standard treatment or to a number of new treatments. Randomization is to ensure a similar patient population in each group and not to do a statistical test to compare treatment groups. These trials are not adequately powered to do this and this is the purpose of a phase III trial. Treatment outcomes are ranked according to activity, safety and feasibility to take the drug forward to phase III study.

Box 25.1: Components of phase I study design and methods of dose escalation

Design components of a phase I study
- Starting dose – usually $\frac{1}{10}$ of the animal dose
- Dose increment
- Dose escalation method
- Number of patients per dose level
- Specification of dose-limiting-toxicity (DLT)
- Target toxicity level
- Definition of maximum tolerated dose (MTD)
- Recommended dose and patient selection for phase II trial

Dose escalation methods
- Rule-based design – based on no prior assumption of the dose-toxicity curve and allows dose escalation and de-escalation of dose with diminishing fractions of preceding dose depending on the absence or presence of severe toxicity in the previous cohort of patients treated.
  - 3 + 3 design – most frequently used method. The classical assumption is toxicity increases with dose. It starts with a cohort of three patients and subsequent cohorts are treated at increasing level.
  - Accelerated titration design
  - Pharmacologically guided dose escalation
- Model based designs – are complex and use statistical models that actively seek a dose level that produces a pre-specified probability of dose toxicity using dose-toxicity curve calculated from all enrolled patients. Examples include:
  - Continual reassessment method
  - Escalation with overdose control
  - Designs that use time-to-event endpoints
  - Designs that use toxicity and efficacy as endpoints

Phase III

The aim of a phase III study (also called randomized controlled trials) is to establish the efficacy of a new treatment compared with an existing standard treatment or observation/placebo where there is no standard treatment. It also helps to establish whether the new treatment has less toxicity compared with the standard treatment. Randomization reduces bias by balancing the characteristics of study population. Design of a phase III study is complex (Box 25.2). It requires large patient numbers to ensure adequate statistical power which frequently necessitates international cooperation and is very costly. Modern trials are incorporating translational studies to try to target the new drug to the population most likely to benefit. This may affect the inclusion criteria e.g. presence of an EGFR mutation for entry into a trial for an antibody against the EGFR receptor.

Phase IV studies

Phase IV studies are post-marketing studies done to learn more about the side effects, safety, and long term risk-benefits of the drug in a wider context than in clinical trial. The various study designs are given in Box 25.3.

Ethics and good clinical practice

In order to protect patient safety and to ensure the reliability of any trial data all trials should be conducted according to good clinical practice (GCP) which has been developed according to international guidelines. Part of this process means that the trials must be peer reviewed and reviewed by an ethics committee to ensure that the trial seems appropriate, safe and adheres to these international guidelines (International Conference on Harmonization ICH). These have now been incorporated into the 2004 Medicines for Human Use (Clinical Trials) Regulations and the recent EU Directive on Good Clinical Practice, which apply to all trials within Europe. Similar practices have also been adopted in North America.

Recruiting patients into a clinical trial

A number of issues need to be considered when recruiting patients into clinical trial ranging from explaining the trial itself to giving a realistic picture of the potential risks and benefits. Consent is a complex process which does not simply refer to the signing of a form but with good clinical practice has to ensure that the patient has adequately understood what is involved and has

---

Box 25.2: Phase III study

- Identify a select group of patients and define eligibility criteria.
- Identify meaningful and reliable outcome measures (endpoints).
- Randomization process and stratification of study group.
- Statistical considerations – sample size based on expected benefit, method of data analysis etc.
- Phase III study designs:
  - Parallel-group design – patients are randomized to two or more treatment group.
  - Cross-over design – patients will receive both the new and control treatment.
  - Factorial design – includes double randomization so that the same study group is used to answer two research questions.
  - Adaptive design – starts with a number of new treatments, and the treatments found to be inactive can be dropped.
  - Discontinuation design – only patients who respond to treatment remain in the trial and then randomized to a continuation or discontinuation of treatment.

Box 25.3: Phase IV study designs

- Post-phase III 'continuation' trial – is done to identify the long-term efficacy, common dose-related adverse effects (AEs) and reasons for discontinuation.
- Phase V 'naturalistic' trial – done to analyse effectiveness and common dose-related AEs and also can assess patient reported outcomes.
- Prospective cohort design – to assess long-term effectiveness in routine practice (>2 years)
- Retrospective cohort – rapid study of a representative patient sample, often poor quality.
- Case control – to identify rare AEs.
- Large computerized databases and record linkage – to identify rare idiosyncratic AEs and to correlate AEs with laboratory value and prescribing data. This design needs >10,000 patients.

given their consent freely. It should be made clear that consent can be withdrawn at any time without affecting their future care to avoid pressurizing already vulnerable individuals into believing they have to agree to please their medical carers. Good clinical practice also states that patients should be given adequate time to reflect on the information received and be able to discuss with family, friends or their general practitioner. Key areas to be covered when discussing a trial with a patient are listed in Box 25.4.

Box 25.4: Cancer clinical trials – what to tell the patient?

- Type of study and objective – should be clear and properly explained to patients. This is important to get a right balance in the beginning in the minds of patients and their families. They should not be left with an impression that either they are simply 'guinea pigs' or the treatment is going to give them an imminent cure.

  - Phase I studies – is to decide toxicity and maximum tolerated dose and only a small percentage is expected to respond. Classically less than 5% of patients would benefit. This has improved by a few percent with targeted treatments.

  - Phase II studies – is to test the activity of a new drug for a particular type of cancer.

  - Phase III studies – standard treatment is compared with a new treatment and it may take years to show any benefit or even, harm.

- Purpose of clinical trials – it is important to tell patients that though, in many situations we have standard treatments, most of the treatments may not be the best. Hence there is a continuous attempt to improve the success of existing treatment with new clinical studies.

- All the studies discussed with patients have undergone rigorous ethical procedures before approval to ensure participants' safety and to safeguard their human rights.

- Patients have the right to decline to participate which does not compromise future care and they can withdraw from the trial at any point without affecting their future treatment.

- Need to explain the trial process – such as type of study, cannot choose the treatment in phase III study, need for frequent tests, follow-up appointments, complete a number of forms etc.

- Funding of trial – even if a trial is funded by pharmaceutical companies, the trial process is done according to national/international regulations. There is no financial incentive for the doctors or other healthcare professionals enrolling patients into the study.

Advances in clinical trials

The current process of cancer clinical trial design is costly and lengthy. Studies show that the overall cost of introduction of a drug to clinical use is approximately 1 billion dollars and that for a target molecule is 1.4 billion dollars. This process also takes an average of 12–14 years. The phase 0 trial design has been proposed as a solution (Box 25.5). This may expedite the identification of new target molecules and bring potentially active molecules into routine clinical use faster.

Other advances include development of novel trial designs or the use of alternative statistical methods. Translational studies are now integrating biological questions with clinical developments. In terms of drugs, trials are now moving on to examine the best way to combine novel agents, either with other novel agents or chemotherapy.

Box 25.5: Phase 0 trial

Phase 0 trial – are first-in-human trials with no therapeutic or diagnostic intent, in a limited number of patients (<15) using subtherapeutic doses over a limited period to establish a drug-target effect. (See Figure 25.2). These are established as means to address the pitfalls of phase I–III studies and to expedite the development of new investigational targeted agents. These methods may also be included within a classical phase I trial.

These studies help to:

- Study whether the investigational drug affects the alleged target in the desired manner.

- Provide further pharmacokinetic (PK) and pharmacodynamic (PD) data.

- Validate biomarker assays for target modulation effects.

- Select most promising molecule based further evaluations using very sensitive imaging technologies.

Under these studies, dose escalation is allowed provided it is to modulate the target, not to determine MTD. Phase 0 trials provide critical human PK and PD data which help to directly proceed to phase I/II study or a combination with an established agent, thus expediting the development of agents or combination of agents likely to have clinical activity. Using the new design, the National Cancer Institute evaluated the effect of a PARP inhibitor, ABT 888 in tumour tissue which led to a phase I study of ABT-888 with chemotherapy. The phase 0 study met its primary objective within 5 months, even before any of the planned phase I study started patient accrual (see Figure 25.2).

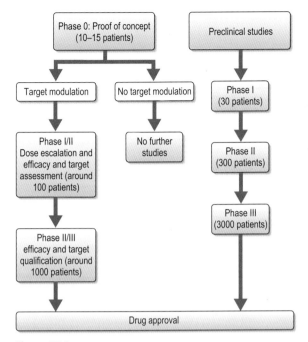

Figure 25.2
Phases of the clinical trials.

Oncology remains one of the most evidence-based specialties at the forefront of clinical trial development.

Further reading

Le Tourneau C, Lee JJ, Siu LL, Dose escalation methods in phase I cancer clinical trials. J Natl Cancer Inst 2009;101(10):708–720.

Kummar S, Doroshow JH, Tomaszewski et al. Phase 0 clinical trials: recommendations from the Task Force on Methodology for the Development of Innovative Cancer Therapies. Eur J Cancer 2009;45(5):741–746.

Eisenhauer EA, O'Dwyer PJ, Christian M, Humphrey JS. Phase I clinical trial design in cancer drug development. J Clin Oncol 2000;18:684–692.

Lee JJ, Feng L. Randomized phase II designs in cancer clinical trials: current status and future directions. J Clin Oncol 2005;23(19):4450–4457.

Green S, Bendetti J, Crowley J. Clinical Trials in Oncology. Second edition. London: Chapman and Hall, 2003.

Eisenhauer EA, Twelves C, Buyse M. Phase I cancer clinical trials. Oxford: Oxford University Press, 2006.

Understanding the strengths and weaknesses of clinical research in cancer

26

C Williams

'I hope that the cares of medical practice
have not obliterated your interest on
solving deductive problems.'

Sherlock Holmes to Watson in the
Stockbroker's Clerk*

Introduction

This chapter briefly discusses cancer clinical trials
and systematic reviews of the cancer literature,
together with the concept of critical appraisal
and evidence-based medicine (EBM). Much of
literature appraisal requires a common sense, but
systematic, approach to ascertaining answers to
key questions about potential biases in the design,
conduct and reporting of a study or review.

Appraising reports of cancer clinical trials

The difficulty in appraising clinical trials lies in
assessing the strength of the evidence. On cursory
reading the author of the report may seem to
present a strong case for the trial, but you need
to see beyond the rhetoric, the eminence of the
author or institution/trials group and the status
of the journal publishing the paper, to assess the
evidence and to see if it is strong enough to stand
on its own. Very strong evidence may be enough
to influence practice by itself, but more commonly the evidence is weaker and needs support
from further studies.

What are the important elements when assessing reports of trials?

By far the most important elements are the design
and conduct of the trial. The methods of analysis,
while still important, are generally less likely to
lead to inappropriate conclusions than inappropriate design and management of a trial. This
chapter is based on the methods recommended
by various EBM groups (Box 26.1).

Because there is such a huge volume of medical
literature published each year, it is important to
take a systematic approach to what you appraise
thoroughly (Box 26.2). The first step in appraisal
is to screen the paper to see if it is worthy of
careful reading. It may be possible to answer
these screening questions on reading the title and
abstract.

Step 1 – Screening questions

- Was there a clearly focused question? Important aspects include the population studied,
  the interventions and the outcomes used.
- Did the investigators use the right type of
  study design for the question being asked? If
  there is a clearly focused question that
  is addressed by a trial of appropriate design
  it is worth continuing on to a full appraisal
  of the results. However, do not save time
  by simply reading the abstract (Example
  Box 26.1).

Step 2 – Appraising a paper reporting a trial

There are a number of crucial questions that need
to be answered (Box 26.2):

---

*Quotes in this chapter are as those cleverly used by Jorgen
Nordenstrom in his book 'Evidence based medicine in Sherlock
Holmes' Footsteps' (Wiley Black-well, 2006).

Box 26.1: Evidence-based medicine web resources

Centre for Evidence-Based Medicine, Oxford, UK – http://www.cebm.net/?o=1013

Centre for Evidence-Based Evidence, University of Toronto, Canada – http://www.cebm.utoronto.ca/

Centre for Health Evidence – http://www.cche.net/about.asp

The Cochrane Collaboration – http://www.cochrane.org/

Users' Guides Interactive Learner Web site – http://www.usersguides.org/

Example Box 26.1: Abstracts

There is a tendency in abstracts to report only the statistically significant outcomes. Authors may ignore clinically important outcomes and may fail to report or discuss issues important to the validity of the study.

Piver MS, Barlow JJ, Vongtama V, et al. Hydroxyurea: A radiation potentiator in carcinoma of the uterine cervix: A randomized double-blind study. Am J Obstet Gynecol 1983;147:803–808.

In this trial the authors reported in the abstract and text, a highly significant benefit from the addition of hydroxyurea to radiation therapy for cervix cancer. Only when reading the table on side effects does it become evident that data on patients dying from causes other than cancer were censored. These included a significant excess of deaths from infection, bowel perforation and leukaemia in the hydroxyurea group. If these patients, whose deaths were potentially due to treatment toxicity, are included in an uncensored analysis the highly significant advantage for hydroxyurea disappears. These facts are not mentioned in the abstract or discussion.

Box 26.2: Systematic method of research appraisal

Step 1 – Screening questions
- Was there any clearly focused question?
- Did the investigators use the right type of study design?

Step 2 – Appraising the study report
1. Was there an appropriate comparison group?
   - Concurrent or historic controls?
   - Was the study randomized?
2. Was the study based on a pre-specified protocol?
   - Did the study have a narrow focus?
   - Did the study have appropriate end points?
   - Did the investigators stick to the protocol?
3. Who knew, what and when?
   - Blinding?
   - Allocation concealment?
4. Which patients were included or excluded and what happened to those lost to follow-up or who went off protocol or were left out?
   - Representative sample for the intervention studied?
   - Whether all patients randomized are included in the final analysis?
5. How much did the outcomes change and were they measured and reported appropriately?
   - Whether appropriate endpoints and validated instruments were used?
   - Were measurements appropriate and done properly?
   - Which treatment is better and how much?
   - Appropriate sample size?

1. Was there an appropriate comparison group?

'Though most of the facts were familiar to me, I had not sufficiently appreciated their relative importance, nor their connection to each other.'

Watson in Silver Blaze

The main aim is that the control group be identical to the intervention group in everything apart for the intervention itself.

Concurrent or historical controls?

When a new therapy is being tested some investigators will give the new treatment to all the patients and will then compare the outcomes with those obtained from the records of similar patients treated in the past – so-called historical controls. Any such comparison is fraught with danger as factors other than the new treatment may have change over time.

Did the authors use randomization?

The purpose of randomization is to ensure, as far as possible, that all factors (known and unknown) that may influence the treatment outcome are balanced between the treatment groups. This is done to reduce the risk of a chance bias. Randomization requires the use of a random device; this is normally a table of random numbers. Systematic allocation; i.e., alternating between treatments, odd or even birth date or hospital number is not an acceptable method, though it is sometimes referred to as pseudo-randomization. Since the researchers know which treatment each person is allocated to before they consent, selective allocation can occur, which will skew the results. Hence the process used for randomization must ensure that neither the trial subjects nor the investigator can influence the treatment arm each person ends up in ('allocation concealment').

Despite their pre-eminence, RCTs do, however, have their limitations. They are usually carried out in a narrowly defined research setting. Protocols require careful selection of patients with specific characteristics. There may be a proportion of patient eligible who chooses not to participate. Because of these factors, patients in an RCT may not be typical of patients in routine health practice.

2. Was the study based on a pre-specified protocol?

A protocol written before the trial starts is a prerequisite to good research and some journals are now recommending that the original protocol be submitted with the final paper to ensure that there was such a protocol and to identify any deviations from the original design. Any deviation from the original study design can result in skewed observation of clinical benefit.

When reading a paper bear in mind the following elements of trial design:

Was there a clearly defined research question?
A good study has limited objectives that are based on a biological hypothesis. Studies with no focus and without a clearly defined question are in danger of becoming a 'fishing expedition' with multiple comparisons.

The chances of multiple testing increases when there is numerous subgroups or endpoints or when data are reported on multiple side effects. This is particularly problematic when such comparisons are unplanned.

Did the study have appropriate end points?
Most RCTs in cancer therapy concentrate on reporting response rates (a surrogate end point of clinical benefit), disease free survival and overall survival. However, accepting that cure is out of the reach of many patients with cancer, information on symptom control and quality of life are often of major importance; they are frequently ignored in the primary research.

Optimal cut points and the problem with multiple comparisons.
'*While the individual man is an insoluble problem, in aggregate he becomes a mathematical certainty. For example you can never foretell what any one man will do, but you can say with some precision what an average number will be up to. Individuals vary, but percentages remain constant.*'
Sherlock Holmes, in The Sign of The Four

Where there is a continuous outcome measure, it is common to simplify analysis by defining one or more points that are used to characterize risk. The way that these points are selected may have a major effect on the analysis.

Subgroup analysis
Subgroup analyses are fairly common in trials; they use the data from a study to compare one endpoint across different subgroups. There are three major problems with this approach:

- The comparison is not randomized.
- The comparison is less precise as there are numbers of patients and those reaching end points is smaller.
- The power calculations for the size in a study may be invalidated by a large number of subgroups.

Where a subgroup is found to behave differently, you should consider if there is a plausible biological mechanism for this and whether other trials have found a similar finding. Where there is a statistical analysis, this should be done as a formal test of interaction. Strong empirical evidence suggests that post hoc subgroup analyses often lead to false positive results (Example Box 26.2).

3. Did the investigators stick to the protocol?

Clinical research is rarely predictable, so changes or alterations to a protocol are often needed. However, they should be clearly reported, as major deviations may reduce the reliability of the data.

Example Box 26.2: International study of infarct survival

Sleight P. Subgroup analyses in clinical trials: fun to look at – but don't believe them! Curr Control Trials Cardiovasc Med 2000;1(1):25–27.

Analysis of subgroup results in a clinical trial is surprisingly unreliable, even in a large trial. This is due to a combination of reduced statistical power, increased variance and the play of chance. Reliance on such analyses is likely to be erroneous. Plausible explanations can usually be found for effects that are, in reality, simply due to the play of chance. When clinicians believe such subgroup analyses, there is a real danger of harm to the individual patient.

In order to study the effect of examining subgroups the investigators of the ISIS trial, testing the value of aspirin and streptokinase after MI, analysed the results by astrological star sign. All of the patients had their date of birth entered as an important 'identifier'. They divided population into 12 subgroups by astrological star sign. Even in a highly positive trial such as ISIS-2, in which the overall statistical benefit for aspirin over placebo was extreme (p < 0.00001), division into only 12 subgroups threw up two (Gemini and Libra) for which aspirin had a non-significantly adverse effect (9% ± 13%).

ISIS-2 was carried out in 16 countries. For the streptokinase randomization, two countries had non-significantly negative results, and a single (different) country was non-significantly negative for aspirin.

There is no plausible explanation for such findings except for the entirely expected operation of the statistical play of chance. It is very important to realize that lack of a statistically significant effect is not evidence of lack of a real effect.

Changes in a protocol that may cause major problems includes, introducing new exclusion criteria after the trial has finished or during the course of the trial and introducing new end points. So, for instance, new exclusion criteria may improve the results by leaving only those patients who get apparent benefit. The addition of unplanned end points may turn a negative study around by concentrating the focus on positive results for the new end points, when the old endpoints were negative.

Without access to the original protocol, it may be difficult for the reader to know if there were major protocol deviations. Where a deviation is known the acid test is to ask if the change would have made sense if it had been considered when the protocol was being designed.

There is also an increase in trend towards stopping the trials too early after an interim analysis. The ethical reason for this decision is to minimize the number of patients receiving an unsafe, ineffective or inferior treatment. However, stopping trials for apparent benefit will systematically overestimate treatment effects, especially when the sample size is small. The best strategy to minimize the problems associated with early stopping is not to stop early. Alternative strategies include a low p-value as the threshold for stopping at the time of interim analysis, not to analyse before a sufficiently large number of events had accrued and continuation of enrolment and follow-up for further period.

Fraudulent conduct of clinical research

Although we all hope that such fraud is very rare, there are too many instances where there has been clear fraud (Example Box 26.3). Detecting such fraud is very difficult. Peer review may help, but in many instances journals do not have the original protocol and access to the raw data is extremely unusual. In the above example, it was an independent outside review that revealed the fraud. The review was carried out as the trial was at variance with other literature and the subject was of great importance.

4. Who knew what and when?

Blinding

While it is often not possible to blind patients and clinicians about which arm a trial patient is in, anyone who evaluates patient outcomes should be blinded to the treatment allocation. This is especially important when there is a 'surrogate' endpoint subject to individual interpretation, e.g. imaging to assess response or measurement of toxicity.

The effect of blinding on the patient

Blinding removes the placebo effect. There are three specific situations where the placebo effect is of particular concern. It is most important when doctors and patients are enthusiastic about the treatment being tested, when outcomes use patient's self-assessment (e.g. quality of life studies), and when the primary aim is symptom control. When there is an objective outcome such as survival, the placebo effect is much less important.

Example Box 26.3: On-site audit for high-dose chemotherapy

Weiss RB et al. An on-site audit of the South African Trial of high-dose chemotherapy for metastatic breast cancer and associated publications. J Clin Oncol 2001;19:2771–2777.

This article reported the results of an on-site audit to verify the results of a randomized study reported by Bezwoda et al. on high-dose chemotherapy (HDC) for treatment of metastatic breast cancer. In the original study, 90 patients were reported to have been randomized and treated. However, even after searching more than 15,000 sets of medical records only 61 of the 90 patients could be found. Of these 61, only 27 had sufficient records to verify eligibility for the trial by the published criteria. Of these 27, 18 did not meet one or more eligibility criteria. Only 25 patients appeared to have received their assigned therapy temporally associated with their enrolment date, and all but three of these 25 received HDC. The treatment details of individual patients were at great variance from the published data.

In the accompanying editorial (High-dose chemotherapy for breast cancer: 'how do you know?' J Clin Oncol 2001;19(11):2769–2770) Larry Norton wrote 'In this regard, Dr Weiss et al. ... have done a great service. They offer us unequivocal evidence that Dr Werner Bezwoda's critical study in high-dose chemotherapy for advanced breast cancer is fake and completely inadmissible information regarding the safety and efficacy of such treatment was included. This work was previously and wrongly reported as positive at ASCO's 1992 Annual Meeting, in the Journal in 1995, and in multiple subsequent publications [six] ... That the original publication, now being retracted by the Journal, has influenced major thinkers in this field and may have put patients in danger raises the stakes as we consider how we can improve the process to make sure that this never happens again.'

Blinding of investigators

Clinicians caring for the patients may also influence a trial outcome by their attitude and the way that they manage the disease overall. When unblinded studies were compared to blinded studies, the former studies tended to estimate a treatment effect that was (on average) 11% to 17% higher than in blinded studies. Blinding is of less importance where there is an objective end point such as survival.

Allocation concealment

For randomization to be effective, neither the trial subjects nor the investigators can influence the treatment each person is allocated. If either the patients or the investigators know the treatment each patient is allocated before they consent, selective allocation may occur which results in skewing of results. Similarly, if the patients know the treatment they are receiving, it can introduce bias in reporting the outcomes. Hence, it is important to conceal the randomization list from those recruiting patients. Only when an eligible patient has agreed to participate should the treatment allocation be carried out. Unblinded allocation methods show an average bias of 30–40%.

The only safe method of randomization is to carry out allocation, for a single patient at a time, by a central trials office or pharmacy.

5. Which patients were included or excluded and what happened to those lost to follow up or who went off protocol or were left out?

There is a major problem when studies, particularly RCTs, become unrepresentative of the population or setting which the treatment is potentially suitable for. Frequently, patients in trials are fitter and younger than those encountered in routine practice.

Who was lost to follow-up or dropped out during the study?

Loss of some patients in a study is inevitable. These patients may have a different prognosis than those remaining in the trial. Excluding those lost to follow-up or dropped out will often result in overestimate of treatment benefit.

All patients should be analysed in the groups they were randomized to, regardless of whether they crossed over or changed treatment, were lost to follow up or dropped out. This is known as 'intention to treat' analysis and should always be reported, even if the authors also choose to present analyses excluding selected patients (Box 26.3). Intention to treat analysis is the only way we can ensure that the original randomization has retained and thereby, the groups are comparable.

6. How much did the outcomes change and were they measured and reported appropriately?

It is important to ensure that the end points used are appropriate. There is a tendency to measure, easier and quicker, surrogate end points, rather than those that are important to the patient or

Box 26.3: Sample size slippages in randomized trials

- All randomized participants should be included in the primary analysis (an intent-to-treat analysis). Participants might ignore follow-up, leave town, or take aspartame when instructed to take aspirin.

- Exclusions before randomization do not bias the treatment comparison, but they can hurt generalizability.

- Eligibility criteria for a trial should be clear, specific, and applied before randomization. Readers should assess whether any of the criteria make the trial sample atypical or unrepresentative of the people in which they are interested.

- In reality, patients will lose follow-up. Investigators should, therefore, commit adequate resources to develop and implement procedures to maximize retention of participants.

- Researchers should provide clear, explicit information on the progress of all randomized participants through the trial by use of, for instance, a trial profile.

- Investigators can also do secondary analyses on, for instance, per-protocol or as-treated participants. Such analyses should be described as secondary and non-randomized comparisons.

- Mishandling of exclusions causes serious methodological difficulties. Unfortunately, some explanations for mishandling exclusions intuitively appeal to readers, disguising the seriousness of the issues. Creative mismanagement of exclusions can undermine trial validity.

Schulz KF and Grimes DA. Sample size slippages in randomized trials: exclusions and the lost and wayward. Lancet 2002;359:781–785.

their clinicians. Patients want information on what effect an intervention will have on their chance of survival, what the side effects will be, and whether it will change their quality of life. Use of surrogate measures, such as a fall in a tumour marker, will fail to answer these questions; even if they may provide evidence supporting potential benefit.

Were measurements appropriate and well done?

Although it is probably less of a problem in cancer studies than some other areas of medicine, be wary of end points that measure short-term outcomes. For instance, in studies concerned with management of complications of cancer or the side effects of its treatment, trials may report effectiveness of an intervention after, say, six-week therapy. Since it is easier to get a short-term

change, it is important to consider if the investigators should have been measuring long-term effectiveness. For instance, several treatments in the review 'Non-surgical interventions for late radiation proctitis in patients who have received radical radiotherapy to the pelvis,' (Denton et al., 2008), were often only given for one month and then response was assessed at one time point.

Although less of a problem in cancer studies, when compared with the general medical literature, it is sometimes difficult to obtain accurate measurements in certain types of study. If the measurement error concerns an important factor predictive of an outcome, this is of major concern. An example in the field of cancer would be the difficulty in accurately measuring dietary fat intake when studying the effect of diet on development of breast cancer.

Which is the better treatment and how much difference?

It is not sufficient to know that one treatment is better than another, it is important to quantify how much better the treatment is than the other. While a p-value may tell you which treatment is better, the confidence interval is a better measure. It not only tells you which is the better treatment, but quantifies the difference (Box 26.4). This is particularly important where any gain has to be balanced against the side effects of that treatment.

Just because a statistical test shows an intervention to be superior this does not tell you whether the difference is clinically important. This requires, in addition, an estimate of the numbers of patients seen in routine practice who might benefit from the 'better' treatment, the toxicity of the treatment, its ease of administration and cost. Assessing clinical significance requires sound judgment. The decision whether to use that treatment will also ultimately depend on the personal preferences of patients.

Were there sufficient subjects?

There has been a tendency for cancer RCTs to have too few subjects, or more accurately patients reaching the end point of the study. Investigators should provide an a priori justification of the sample size in the paper itself. If there are no power calculations, it is useful to look at the

Box 26.4: Is the result important?

In any study, the beneficial effect/risk of the experimental arm can be due to three possible reasons:

- Bias – excluded by assessing the validity of study.
- Chance variation between the treatment groups – excluded by analysing p-value and confidence interval.
- The real benefit/risk – quantified by calculating various event rates.

P-value is used to measure the probability of occurring the benefit/risk by a chance, e.g. a p-value of 0.01 means that there is a 1 in 100 (1%) probability of the result occurring by chance. Conventionally, a p value of <0.05 (<1 in 20 probability) is set as the statistically significant result.

Confidence interval (CI) is used to measure the sampling error. Since any study can only examine a sample of a population, we would expect the sample to be different from the population (sampling error). Conventionally a 95% CI is used, which specifies that there is a 95% chance that the population's true value lies between the two limits. If the 95% CI crosses the 'line of no difference' between interventions, the result is not statistically significant.

Once the bias and chance have been ruled out, the benefit/risk of intervention can be quantified using the following measures:

- Relative risk (RR) – the ratio of the risk in the experimental group divided by the risk in the control group.
- Absolute risk reduction (ARR) – the difference between the control event rate and experimental event rate. This is a more clinically relevant measure.
- Relative risk reduction (RRR) – calculated by dividing ARR with control event rate.
- Number needed to treat (NNT) – is the inverse of ARR and is the most useful measure of clinical benefit. It tells you the absolute number of patients who need to be treated to prevent one adverse outcome.

Example Box 26.4: Publication bias

Stern JM, Simes RJ. Publication bias: evidence of delayed publication in a cohort study of clinical research projects. BMJ 1997;315:640–645.

This retrospective study was undertaken to determine the extent to which publication is influenced by study outcome. Of the 218 studies analysed with tests of significance, those with positive results ($p < 0.05$) were much more likely to be published than those with negative results ($P \geq 0.10$) (hazard ratio 2.32 (95% confidence interval 1.47 to 3.66), p = 0.0003), with a significantly shorter time to publication (median 4.8 vs. 8.0 years). Studies with indefinite conclusions ($0.05 \leq P < 0.10$) tended to have an even lower publication rate and longer time to publication than studies with negative results (hazard ratio 0.39 (0.13 to 1.12), p = 0.08).

ing the results of a meta-analysis, you should ask the following questions:

- Were all the available studies included? An incomplete search of the literature can bias the findings of a meta-analysis or systematic review.
- Was it appropriate to pool the data? Heterogeneity among studies may make any pooled estimate meaningless.
- Was the quality of the trials good? The quality of a meta-analysis cannot be any better than the quality of the studies it is summarizing.

Did the reviewers find all of the trials?

One of the greatest risks of bias in a meta-analysis is omitting relevant studies. Often studies are never published; evidence suggests that such studies are likely to be negative. This is known as publication bias (Example Box 26.4). Registration of trials, before they start, is being introduced as a way of avoiding publication bias.

Duplicate publication

Studies which are positive are more likely to appear more than once in publication. This is especially problematic for multi-centre trials where an individual centres may publish results specific to their site.

The limitations of a Medline search

While a Medline search is the most convenient way to identify published research, it should not be the only source of publications for a meta-analysis. Medline searches cover only about a quarter of the medical literature.

width of the confidence intervals. If there is an inadequate sample size, the confidence intervals will be abnormally wide.

Systematic reviews and meta-analyses

Introduction

A systematic review is one carried out in accordance with a written protocol and using methodology designed to reduce the risk of bias. Meta-analysis is the quantitative pooling of data from two or more studies. When you are examin-

Foreign language publications

Some meta-analyses restrict their attention to English language publications only. This makes life easier for the reviewers, but there is evidence that researchers tend to publish reports of positive trials in English language journals. Conversely, they publish negative reports in a native language journal where the citation index is likely to be lower.

Heterogeneity

Even when the trials do not have obvious clinical heterogeneity the results may turn out to be very different. An example is RCTs testing the efficacy of adding paclitaxel to platinum therapy for the primary chemotherapy of ovarian cancer. The initial two studies, GOG 111 and OV10, showed an advantage for the addition of paclitaxel. Two subsequent trials, GOG132 and ICON3 (by far the biggest trial), have failed to show an advantage for the addition of paclitaxel. Examining the results there appears to be such an extreme heterogeneity that pooling of the data in a meta-analysis should be avoided. Despite this NICE in its appraisal did include a meta-analysis (Box 26.5).

The main areas where heterogeneity occurs include:

Heterogeneity of the treatment and control groups:
- Varying inclusion and exclusion criteria.
- Variation in general health of patients or geographical differences.
- Differences in dose or timing of a drug or co-medication.

Heterogeneity in the design of the study:
- Variation in length of follow-up.
- Variation in proportion of drop outs and how they are handled.

Heterogeneity in the management of the patients and in the outcome:
- Variation in the management of co-morbidity.
- Variation in managing side effects.

Managing heterogeneity

A degree of heterogeneity is to be expected and is acceptable. Showing that a treatment gives consistent results, with some variation, across a variety of trials, and in a large number of sub-

---

Box 26.5: NICE appraisal on addition of paclitaxel to platinum in ovarian cancer

'While design differences between the four trials, in terms of severity of disease of included patients, differences in treatment and control drugs and doses, length of follow-up, and the extent of cross-over (before and after disease progression), may hamper statistical pooling of results, meta-analyses have been undertaken ... These take account of statistical heterogeneity as far as possible, and their results appear consistent, reporting that the findings for progression-free survival (hazard ratios = 0.84, 95% CI = 0.70 to 1.02 [MRC] and 0.87, 95% CI 0.72 to 1.05 [BMS]) and overall survival (hazard ratios = 0.82, 95% CI 0.66 to 1.01 [MRC] and 0.82, 95% CI 0.68 to 1.00 [BMS]) across the trials do not show statistically significant differences between paclitaxel/platinum and the alternatives.'

'The four trials showed consistently that treatment with paclitaxel in combination with platinum leads to more side effects ...'

'The Committee took account of this range of trial evidence as well as other factors that would differentiate between the two regimens including the side-effect profiles of the treatments ... On this basis the Committee considered that paclitaxel/platinum combination treatment should no longer be recommended exclusively as standard therapy for women receiving first-line chemotherapy for ovarian cancer. [The original recommendation was made when ICON3 had not been published.] ... both platinum therapy alone and a combination of paclitaxel and a platinum compound were appropriate first-line treatments for women with ovarian cancer.'

This guidance allows clinicians to exercise their prejudice, either to believe the two positive trials or the two negative trials, containing many more patients. The meta-analysis, although showing no statistical benefit for the addition of paclitaxel, has not added to the guidance since its conclusion has been ignored. The statistical heterogeneity was so great that it would have been better to have discussed the two pairs of trials in narrative fashion, rather than to have produced a meta-analysis of the four trials.

---

jects, increases confidence in that treatment. Where there is excessive heterogeneity pooling of data should be avoided. The results can be explored in various ways.

Subgroup analysis

When there is substantial heterogeneity, you can look and compare subgroups of the studies. As the case in Box 26.5, of the use of paclitaxel chemotherapy in ovarian cancer, suggests rather than pooling all the data, the review could have pooled the data from the two groups of positive and negative trials and then discussed the reasons for the different outcomes.

Meta-regression
You can try to adjust for heterogeneity in a meta-analysis. This works similarly to the adjustment for covariates in a regression model.

Sensitivity analysis
Another approach to heterogeneity is to examine the sensitivity of the results by looking at selected groups of studies. This may mean only including those trials selected to be of good quality factor or some other element likely to reduce bias.

Was the quality of the trials good?
Meta-analysis cannot correct or compensate for poorly designed or conducted studies. It is for this reason that poor quality trials should be excluded or a sensitivity analysis carried out based on trial quality.

Reporting of trials is often poor so that it is impossible to assess the quality of the study. There is evidence that poorly reported trials are more likely to be of poor quality and incomplete reporting is associated with poor quality.

Taking the easy option – a narrative review

> 'The temptation to form premature theories upon insufficient data is the bane of our profession.'
>> Sherlock Holmes in the Tragedy of Birlstone

A classical narrative review frequently suffers from a lack of systematic ways of avoiding bias. There is also a worrying tendency to choose papers that support the reviewer's own point of view. This is fine in an opinion piece designed to make people think, but is very dangerous if the reviewer purports to give a balanced assessment of the literature.

Traditional narrative reviews generally do not use meta-analysis, but will often undertake an exercise often referred to as vote counting. In such a process, there is a sum of the number of positive and negative studies; the overall interpretation depending on whether or not the number of positive studies exceeds the negative group or vice versa. However, there is a major flaw with this approach as it ignores the possibility that some studies are negative because they are simply too small.

How to avoid bias from exclusion of publications
The major bibliographic databases, registries for clinical trials, and the grey literature should all be searched. In addition the bibliographies of all articles found should be checked to see if there are relevant trial reports.

Intentional exclusion of studies
In any meta-analysis, you have to draw a line somewhere. Studies that fail to meet your criteria will not be included in the results. Where the cut-off point is based on judgment, such as trial quality, this can sometimes cause serious controversy. A Cochrane Review of mammographic screening for breast cancer found seven eligible studies, but only two were deemed to be of sufficient quality to include in the review; meta-analysis of the two studies found no benefit from screening. If all seven studies were included the outcome was positive. This Cochrane review provoked a furious response and intense debate over the rights and wrongs of excluding most of the available trials (Example Box 26.5).

Objectivity in a systematic review

> 'It is capital mistake to theorize before one has data. One begins to twist the facts to fit theories, instead of theories to fit facts.'
>> Sherlock Holmes in Scandal in Bohemia

A systematic review or meta-analysis should have a written protocol, though most published meta-analyses do not state if a protocol was used. This protocol should state: the inclusion/exclusion criteria for studies, how quality will be assessed, a detailed search strategy and the statistical methods used to combine results. The protocol is there to reduce bias, increase transparency and to make it possible to see how the review was done. As well as including information on included studies, a systematic review should report on which studies were excluded and on what grounds.

Example Box 26.5: Screening for breast cancer with mammography

Olsen O and Gøtzsche PC. Screening for breast cancer with mammography. Cochrane Database Syst Rev 2001;(4):CD001877.

MAIN RESULTS: Seven completed and eligible trials involving half a million women were identified. The two best trials provided medium-quality data and, when combined, yield a relative risk for overall mortality of 1.00 (95% CI 0.96–1.05) after 13 years. However, the trials are underpowered for all-cause mortality, and confidence intervals include a possible worthwhile effect as well as a possible detrimental effect. If data from all eligible trials (excluding flawed studies) are considered then the relative risk for overall mortality after 13 years is 1.01 (95% CI 0.99–1.03). The best trials failed to show a significant reduction in breast cancer mortality with a relative risk of 0.97 (95% CI 0.82–1.14). If data from all eligible trials (excluding flawed studies) are considered then the relative risk for breast cancer mortality after 13 years is 0.80 (95% CI 0.71–0.89). However, breast cancer mortality is considered to be an unreliable outcome and biased in favour of screening. Flaws are due to differential exclusion of women with breast cancer from analysis and differential misclassification of cause of death.

Evidence-based medicine (EBM)

Evidence-based medicine (EBM) brings together best research evidence with clinical expertise and patient expectations. Best research evidence means clinically relevant research (basic sciences), clinical research into the accuracy of diagnostic tests (includes clinical examination), the power of prognostic and predictive markers, and the efficacy and safety of all types of interventions. Clinical expertise includes the ability to use our clinical skills and past experience to recognize a patient's individual diagnosis and general health, the potential risks and benefits of interventions, and to integrate this with their personal expectations.

Why do we need EBM?

Clinicians are hungry for edible sized bites of reliable information:

- Traditional sources are often out-of-date, frequently wrong, overly didactic and too unfocused.

- Clinicians need valid information about patient management up to five times per in-patient and twice for every three out-patients.
- While our diagnostic skills and clinical judgment increase with experience, our up-to-date knowledge declines.
- There is too little time to see patients or to look for information and to keep up-to-date.

EBM has helped to find ways to support clinicians through:

- The creation of systematic reviews, with succinct summaries, by groups such as the Cochrane Collaboration.
- The creation of evidence-based journals that publish summaries of the small proportion of clinical papers that are valid and useful to us in seconds.

Further reading

Moher D, Schulz KF and Altman DG. The CONSORT statement: revised recommendations for improving the quality of reports of parallel-group randomised trials. Lancet 2001;357(9263):1191–1194.

Denton AS, Clarke N and Maher J. Non-surgical interventions for late radiation proctitis in patients who have received radical radiotherapy to the pelvis. Cochrane Database of Systematic Reviews 2008; Issue 4.

Straus SE and Sackett DL. Using research findings in clinical practice. BMJ 1998;317(7154):339–342.

Montori VM and Guyatt GH. Intention-to-treat principle. CMAJ 2001;165(10):1339–1341.

Straus SE and Sackett DL. Applying evidence to the individual patient. Ann Oncol 1999;10(1):29–32.

Straus SE and McAlister FA. Evidence-based medicine: a commentary on common criticisms. CMAJ 2000;163(7):837–841.

Jackson R, Ameratunga S, Broad J et al. The GATE frame: critical appraisal with pictures. Evid Based Med 2006;11(2):35–38.

Sackett DL and Straus SE. Finding and applying evidence during clinical rounds: the 'evidence cart'. JAMA 1998;280(15):1336–1338.

Williams CJ. The pitfalls of narrative reviews in clinical medicine. Ann Oncol 1998;9:601–605.

Appendix:
A glossary of common targets with examples

HM Hatcher

There is now a better understanding of the molecular mechanisms involved in the development of cancer. In addition to specific genetic changes seen in individual cancers, some cellular pathways are common to many types of cancer and have been the focus of targeted therapies. This glossary highlights two of these processes and gives examples of where and how new drugs work in specific malignancies.

It should also be noted that the toxicities of these targeted agents are different from those of traditional chemotherapy (Table A.1).

Epidermal growth factor receptor (EGFR)

The EGFR is a cell surface growth factor receptor which is activated by the binding of an EGFR ligand. This activation causes the formation of a dimer (Figure A.1), leading to phosphorylation of the intracellular kinases and a cascade of signal transduction proteins which regulate DNA synthesis and cell proliferation (Figure A.2).

EGFR is part of the ErbB family of receptors which also includes HER-2 (also known as ErbB2).

In many types of cancer there are mutations within part of the EGFR which make it a potentially useful target for novel treatments. Increased HER-2 expression is also seen in breast cancer. There are several areas within this signalling process which can be targeted, such as the receptor binding site, the tyrosine kinases or any of the downstream signalling proteins.

Figure A.3 shows the location of some of the drugs developed to date. Cetuximab is a monoclonal EGFR antibody which has demonstrated

Table A.1 Toxicities of common targeted agents

Drug	Action	Common toxicity
Cetuximab	EGFR antibody	Rash, diarrhoea
Erlotinib, gefitinib	EGFR TKIs	Rash
Bevacizumab	VEGF antibody	Hypertension, bleeding, clots (arterial + venous)
Transtuzumab	HER-2 antibody	Anaphylaxis, cardiac failure
Sunitinib	TKI multi target	Skin changes, stomatitis
Imatinib	TKI (SCF/c-KIT)	Peripheral oedema, rash, diarrhoea

activity, both with chemotherapy or as a single agent, in metastatic colorectal cancer (p. 169). Used in combination with irinotecan and 5-FU it showed a benefit in progression free survival over chemotherapy without cetuximab. Erlotinib and gefitinib are selective tyrosine kinase inhibitors (TKIs) (p. 102) which have shown improvements in clinical symptoms and response rates in metastatic lung cancer. Their use in the adjuvant setting combined with chemotherapy has only been shown to be of benefit in a small subset of patients (lifelong non-smokers, adenocarcinoma, females and those of Asian origin). Further analysis has shown that the greatest benefits are seen

DOI: 10.1016/B978-0-7234-3458-0.00032-4

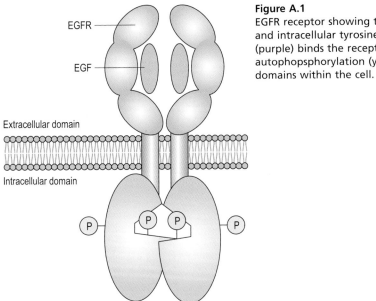

Figure A.1
EGFR receptor showing the extracellular binding domain (pink) and intracellular tyrosine kinases (blue). When the EGF (ligand) (purple) binds the receptor it causes heterodimerization and autophopsphorylation (yellow P symbols) of the tyrosine kinase domains within the cell.

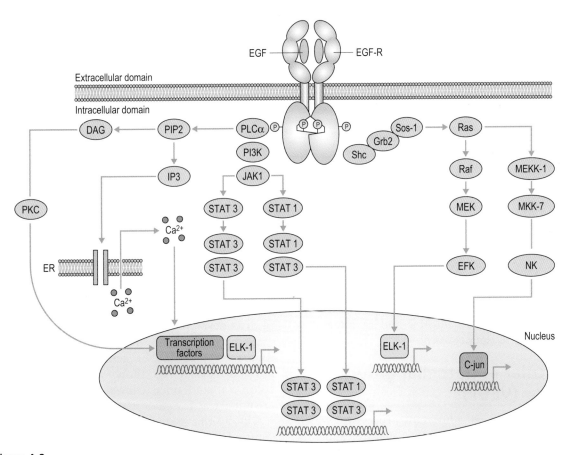

Figure A.2
The complex signalling pathways following activation of EGFR.

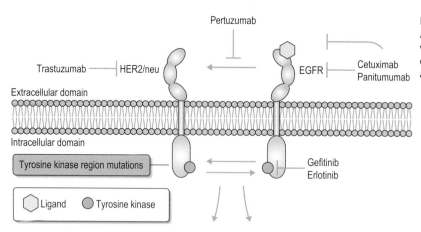

Figure A.3
Areas of the EGFR or HER-2 for which targeted drugs have been developed and examples of drugs acting at these sites.

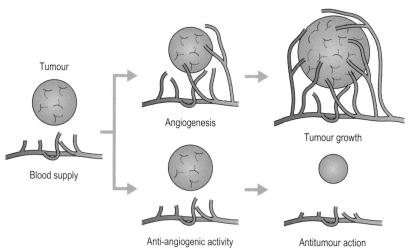

Figure A.4
The effect of angiogenesis on tumour growth (above) and the effect of inhibiting angiogenesis (below).

with those who have specific EGFR mutations. Transtuzumab (Herceptin™) is an antibody against HER-2 and has shown significant activity in breast cancer. In the adjuvant setting, combined with chemotherapy, it has shown significant improvements in progression free survival. (p. 128). Lapatinib is a small molecule which has activity against both HER-2 and EGFR and is also active in breast cancer.

Vascular endothelial growth factor (VEGF)

Angiogenesis is an important process by which tumours gain increased vasculature allowing them to grow and spread. A major contributory factor to angiogenesis is increased expression of VEGF. VEGF is another growth factor receptor which, like EGFR, leads to an intracellular cascade of proteins which regulate cell growth. Increased VEGF expression is also observed in many cancers (e.g. ovarian and renal). Interfering with this process by reducing VEGF expression or its subsequent signalling has been another major target of drug developers (Figures A.4 and A.5).

As with EGFR, antibodies can be developed to the receptor and bevacizumab is a VEGFR antibody which has shown activity in breast, colorectal and renal cancer and investigations are underway for other malignancies. TKIs which work on this pathway include sorafenib and sunitinib both of which have shown significant improvements in survival in metastatic renal cancer (Figure A.6).

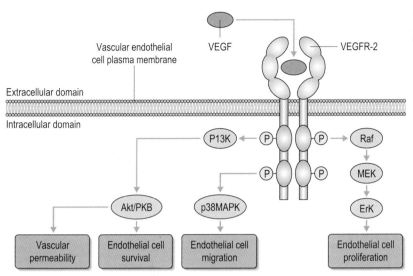

Figure A.5
Potential downstream effects of VEGF.

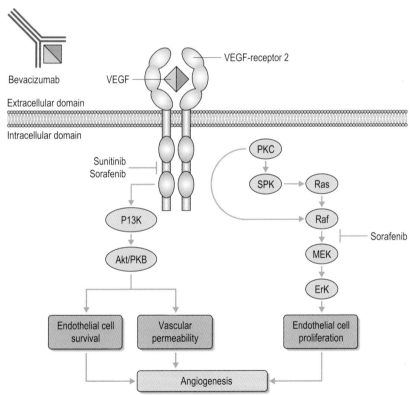

Figure A.6
Sites of action of various drugs which work in the VEGF/ angiogenesis pathway.

Other molecules

Sorafenib and sunitinib are also examples of TKIs which can target more than one receptor pathway. For example, sunitinib also has activity against the c-KIT and PDGF (platelet derived growth factor) receptors.

Other new target developments include targeting small intracellular proteins further down the signalling cascades described above, e.g. mTOR

373

inhibitors and PI3K inhibitors which are under investigation. The mTOR inhibitor Terosilimus has already shown activity in metastatic renal cancer.

Antisense agents are those which recognize abnormal proteins or products of transcription, bind to them and inactivate them. An example is the bcl-2 antisense Oblimersen sodium which in early trials has shown activity in pre-clinical and pilot studies of lung cancer and melanoma.

Future areas involve targeting many parts of the signalling pathway at the same time to see if this leads to synergistic activity and is safe.

Index

375